HEALTH AND WELLNESS

ISSN 1549-0971

HEALTH AND WELLNESS

Barbara Wexler

INFORMATION PLUS® REFERENCE SERIES
Formerly Published by Information Plus, Wylie, Texas

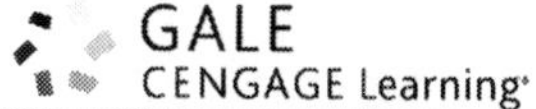

Farmington Hills, Mich • San Francisco • New York • Waterville, Maine
Meriden, Conn • Mason, Ohio • Chicago

GALE
CENGAGE Learning®

Health and Wellness

Barbara Wexler

Kepos Media, Inc.: Steven Long and Janice Jorgensen, Series Editors

Project Editors: Laura Avery, Tracie Moy

Rights Acquisition and Management: Ashley M. Maynard, Carissa Poweleit

Composition: Evi Abou-El-Seoud, Mary Beth Trimper

Manufacturing: Rita Wimberley

For product information and technology assistance, contact us at
Gale Customer Support, 1-800-877-4253.
For permission to use material from this text or product,
submit all requests online at **www.cengage.com/permissions.**
Further permissions questions can be e-mailed to
permissionrequest@cengage.com

Cover photograph: © v. schlichting/Shutterstock.com.

Gale
27500 Drake Rd.
Farmington Hills, MI 48331-3535

ISBN-13: 978-0-7876-5103-9 (set)
ISBN-13: 978-1-57302-700-7

ISSN 1549-0971

This title is also available as an e-book.
ISBN-13: 978-1-57302-710-6 (set)
Contact your Gale sales representative for ordering information.

Printed in the United States of America
1 2 3 4 5 20 19 18 17 16

TABLE OF CONTENTS

PREFACE

Health and Wellness is part of the *Information Plus Reference Series.* The purpose of each volume of the series is to present the latest facts on a topic of pressing concern in modern American life. These topics include the most controversial and studied social issues of the 21st century: abortion, capital punishment, care for older adults, crime, the environment, immigration, race and ethnicity, social welfare, women, world poverty, youth, and many more. Although this series is written especially for high school and undergraduate students, it is an excellent resource for anyone in need of factual information on current affairs.

By presenting the facts, it is the intention of Gale, Cengage Learning, to provide its readers with everything they need to reach an informed opinion on current issues. To that end, there is a particular emphasis in this series on the presentation of scientific studies, surveys, and statistics. These data are generally presented in the form of tables, charts, and other graphics placed within the text of each book. Every graphic is directly referred to and carefully explained in the text. The source of each graphic is presented within the graphic itself. The data used in these graphics are drawn from the most reputable and reliable sources, such as from the various branches of the U.S. government and from private organizations and associations. Every effort has been made to secure the most recent information available. Readers should bear in mind that many major studies take years to conduct and that additional years often pass before the data from these studies are made available to the public. Therefore, in many cases the most recent information available in 2016 is dated from 2013 or 2014. Older statistics are sometimes presented as well, if they are landmark studies or of particular interest and no more-recent information exists.

Although statistics are a major focus of the *Information Plus Reference Series*, they are by no means its only content. Each book also presents the widely held positions and important ideas that shape how the book's subject is discussed in the United States. These positions are explained in detail and, where possible, in the words of their proponents. Some of the other material to be found in these books includes historical background, descriptions of major events related to the subject, relevant laws and court cases, and examples of how these issues play out in American life. Some books also feature primary documents or have pro and con debate sections that provide the words and opinions of prominent Americans on both sides of a controversial topic. All material is presented in an evenhanded and unbiased manner; readers will never be encouraged to accept one view of an issue over another.

HOW TO USE THIS BOOK

"Health" describes the condition of being free from disease. "Wellness," however, is an important complement to health that represents a person's overarching efforts to live happily and successfully—emotionally, intellectually, occupationally, physically, socially, and spiritually. This book examines health and wellness among Americans, including the ways in which illness is currently prevented, identified, and treated. Many common types of chronic, degenerative, genetic, and infectious diseases are described, as are the concepts of mental health and illness. Both traditional and selected complementary and integrative medicine approaches are described.

Health and Wellness consists of nine chapters and three appendixes. Each chapter is devoted to a particular aspect of health and wellness in the United States. For a summary of the information that is covered in each chapter, please see the synopses that are provided in the Table of Contents. Chapters generally begin with an overview of the basic facts and background information on the chapter's topic, then proceed to examine subtopics of particular interest. For example, Chapter 2: Prevention of Disease explains that preventing disease involves a wide range of interrelated programs, actions, and activities. The chapter describes the organizations and groups responsible for local and global disease prevention. Next, it distinguishes between primary, secondary, and tertiary prevention programs and provides examples of each. It concludes with a description of U.S. prevention research and goals and a discussion of the roles that work, social activities, and personal relationships play in preventing disease. Readers can find their way through a chapter by looking for the section and subsection headings, which are clearly set off from the text. They can also refer to the book's extensive Index if they already know what they are looking for.

Statistical Information

The tables and figures featured throughout *Health and Wellness* will be of particular use to readers in learning about this issue. These tables and figures represent an extensive collection of the most recent and important statistics on health and wellness, as well as related issues—for example, graphics cover the prevalence of overweight and obesity, how Americans assess their own health, leading causes of death in the United States, recommended immunizations, and the symptoms of depression. Gale, Cengage Learning, believes that making this information available to readers is the most important way to fulfill the goal of this book: to help readers understand the issues and controversies surrounding health and wellness in the United States and reach their own conclusions.

Each table or figure has a unique identifier appearing above it, for ease of identification and reference. Titles for the tables and figures explain their purpose. At the end of each table or figure, the original source of the data is provided.

To help readers understand these often complicated statistics, all tables and figures are explained in the text. References in the text direct readers to the relevant statistics. Furthermore, the contents of all tables and figures are fully indexed. Please see the opening section of the Index at the back of this volume for a description of how to find tables and figures within it.

Appendixes

Besides the main body text and images, *Health and Wellness* has three appendixes. The first is the Important Names and Addresses directory. Here, readers will find contact information for a number of government and private organizations that can provide further information on aspects of health and wellness. The second appendix is the Resources section, which can also assist readers in conducting their own research. In this section, the author and editors of *Health and Wellness* describe some of the sources that were most useful during the compilation of this book. The final appendix is the detailed Index. It has been greatly expanded from previous editions and should make it even easier to find specific topics in this book.

COMMENTS AND SUGGESTIONS

The editors of the *Information Plus Reference Series* welcome your feedback on *Health and Wellness*. Please direct all correspondence to:

Editors
Information Plus Reference Series
27500 Drake Rd.
Farmington Hills, MI 48331-3535

CHAPTER 1
DEFINING HEALTH AND WELLNESS

Most Americans can benefit from making small shifts in their daily eating habits to improve their health over the long run. Small shifts in food choices—over the course of a week, a day, or even a meal—can make a difference in working toward a healthy eating pattern that works for you. Remember physical activity! Regular physical activity is one of the most important things individuals can do to improve their health. According to the Department of Health and Human Services' Physical Activity Guidelines for Americans, adults need at least 150 minutes of moderate intensity physical activity each week and should perform muscle-strengthening exercises on two or more days each week. Children ages 6 to 17 years need at least 60 minutes of physical activity per day, including aerobic, muscle-strengthening, and bone-strengthening activities.

—Office of Disease Prevention and Health Promotion, Office of the Assistant Secretary for Health, Office of the Secretary, U.S. Department of Health and Human Services, in "Top 10 Things You Need to Know about the 2015–2020 Dietary Guidelines for Americans" (March 14, 2016)

Many definitions of health exist. Most definitions consider health as an outcome—the result of actions to produce it, such as good nutrition, immunization to prevent disease, or medical treatment to cure disease. The *American Heritage Dictionary* (2016, https://www.ahdictionary.com/word/search.html?q=health&submit.x=65&submit.y=28) defines health as fixed and measurable: "The overall condition of an organism at a given time." It also defines health as "soundness, especially of body or mind; freedom from disease or abnormality." However, health may also be viewed as the active process used by individuals and communities to adapt to ever-changing environments.

In 1948 the constitution of the World Health Organization (WHO; October 2006, http://www.who.int/governance/eb/who_constitution_en.pdf) defined health as "a state of complete physical, mental and social well-being and not merely the absence of disease or infirmity." This still widely used definition is broader and more positive than simply defining health as the absence of illness or disability.

Expanding on the WHO definition of health and the commonly understood idea of well-being, the concept of wellness has been defined by the National Wellness Institute in "About Wellness" (2016, http://www.nationalwellness.org/?page=AboutWellness) as "a conscious, self-directed and evolving process of achieving full potential [and] is multidimensional and holistic, encompassing lifestyle, mental and spiritual well-being, and the environment." Wellness encompasses how people feel about various aspects of their life. Six interrelated aspects of human life are commonly known to make up wellness:

- Emotional wellness refers to awareness, sensitivity, and acceptance of feelings and the ability to successfully express and manage one's feelings. Emotional wellness enables people to cope with stress, maintain satisfying relationships with family and friends, and assume responsibility for their actions.
- Intellectual wellness emphasizes knowledge, learning, creativity, problem solving, and lifelong interest in learning and new ideas.
- Occupational wellness relates to preparing for and pursuing work that is meaningful, satisfying, and consistent with one's interests, aptitudes, and personal beliefs.
- Physical wellness is more than simply freedom from disease. The physical dimension of wellness concentrates on the prevention of illness and encourages exercise, healthy diet, and knowledgeable, appropriate use of the health care system. Physical wellness requires individuals to take personal responsibility for actions and choices that affect their health. Examples of healthy choices include wearing a seat belt in automobiles, wearing a helmet when bicycling, and avoiding tobacco and illegal drugs.

- Social wellness is acting in harmony with nature, family, and others in the community. The pursuit of social wellness may involve actions to protect or preserve the environment or contribute to the health and well-being of the community by performing volunteer work.
- Spiritual wellness involves finding meaning in life and acting purposefully in a manner that is consistent with one's deeply held values and beliefs.

The concept of wellness is broader and includes more facets of human life than the traditional definition of health, and the two differ in an important way. When defined as the absence of disease, health may be measured and assessed objectively. For example, a physical examination and the results of laboratory testing enable a physician to determine that a patient is free of disease and thereby healthy.

In comparison, wellness is a more subjective quality and is more difficult to measure. The determination of wellness relies on self-assessment and self-report. Furthermore, it is not necessarily essential that individuals satisfy the traditional definition of good health to rate themselves high in terms of wellness. For instance, many people with chronic (ongoing or long-term) conditions—such as diabetes, heart disease, or asthma—or disabilities report high levels of satisfaction with each of the six dimensions of wellness. Similarly, people in apparently good health may not necessarily give themselves high scores in all six aspects of wellness.

MEASURES OF QUALITY OF LIFE

Quality of life encompasses multiple subjective measures of many interrelated aspects of life. Along with health, quality of life takes into consideration one's work life, housing, schooling, neighborhood, and community as well as spiritual life, values, and interpersonal relationships. There are many measures of quality of life. For example, the United Nations explains in "The Human Development Index" (2016, http://hdr.undp.org/en/statistics/hdi/) that it has used the Human Development Index (HDI) since 1993 to compare countries in terms of life expectancy, poverty, literacy, education, and other indicators. The WHO (Five) Well-Being Index (1998, http://www.cure4you.dk/354/WHO-5_English.pdf) is a short, self-administered questionnaire that poses five questions about the frequency of positive mood (good spirits and relaxation), vitality (being active and waking fresh and rested), and general interests.

Other measures include the:

- Physical Quality of Life Index, which is used to rank countries and summarizes infant mortality, life expectancy at age one, and basic literacy on a 0 to 100 scale.
- Happy Planet Index, which compares countries based on a combined score of environmental impact and well-being to measure the environmental efficiency with which people live long and happy lives.
- Self-Perceived Quality of Life, which provides a measurement of health-related and nonhealth-related aspects of well-being, such as emotions and physical and mental health indices.
- Popsicle Index, which is the percentage of people in a community who believe that a child can leave his or her home, go to the nearest store to buy a Popsicle, and return home alone safely; it is a measure of feelings of safety and security.

HEALTH-RELATED QUALITY OF LIFE

In "Health-Related Quality of Life" (March 17, 2011, http://www.cdc.gov/hrqol/concept.htm/), the Centers for Disease Control and Prevention (CDC) defines health-related quality of life (HRQoL) as "those aspects of overall quality of life that can be clearly shown to affect health—either physical or mental." For individuals, assessment of HRQoL includes measures of health risks and medical conditions; functional status; the presence and extent of social support such as family, friends, and community; and socioeconomic status. HRQoL cannot be assessed directly using a single measure; instead, it is measured using a set of indicators. Figure 1.1 shows the predictors and indicators that contribute to the HRQoL measure that the CDC uses in its Behavioral Risk Factor Surveillance System (http://www.cdc.gov/brfss/).

At the population or community level, HRQoL considers resources such as the availability of medical care, conditions such as sanitation and safe food and water supplies, policies such as the provision of nutritious school lunches, and practices such as smoking, physical activity, and use of preventive services that influence a population's health. Tracking and analyzing HRQoL enables the development of public health policy and the allocation of resources to determine the burden of preventable disease, injuries, and disabilities and identifies health needs. Since its inception in 1993, HRQoL has been used by the CDC (March 17, 2011, http://www.cdc.gov/hrqol/applications/index.htm) to identify vulnerable populations and population disparities and to inform the design of interventions to help individuals and communities with less than optimal perceived health.

HRQoL serves as a key measure of the health of the nation. Healthy People 2020 (http://www.healthypeople.gov/2020/default.aspx), the 10-year agenda for improving the nation's health, names quality of life improvement as a key public health goal. Healthy People 2020 evaluates HRQoL using the following measures:

FIGURE 1.1

Predictors and indicators of health-related quality of life

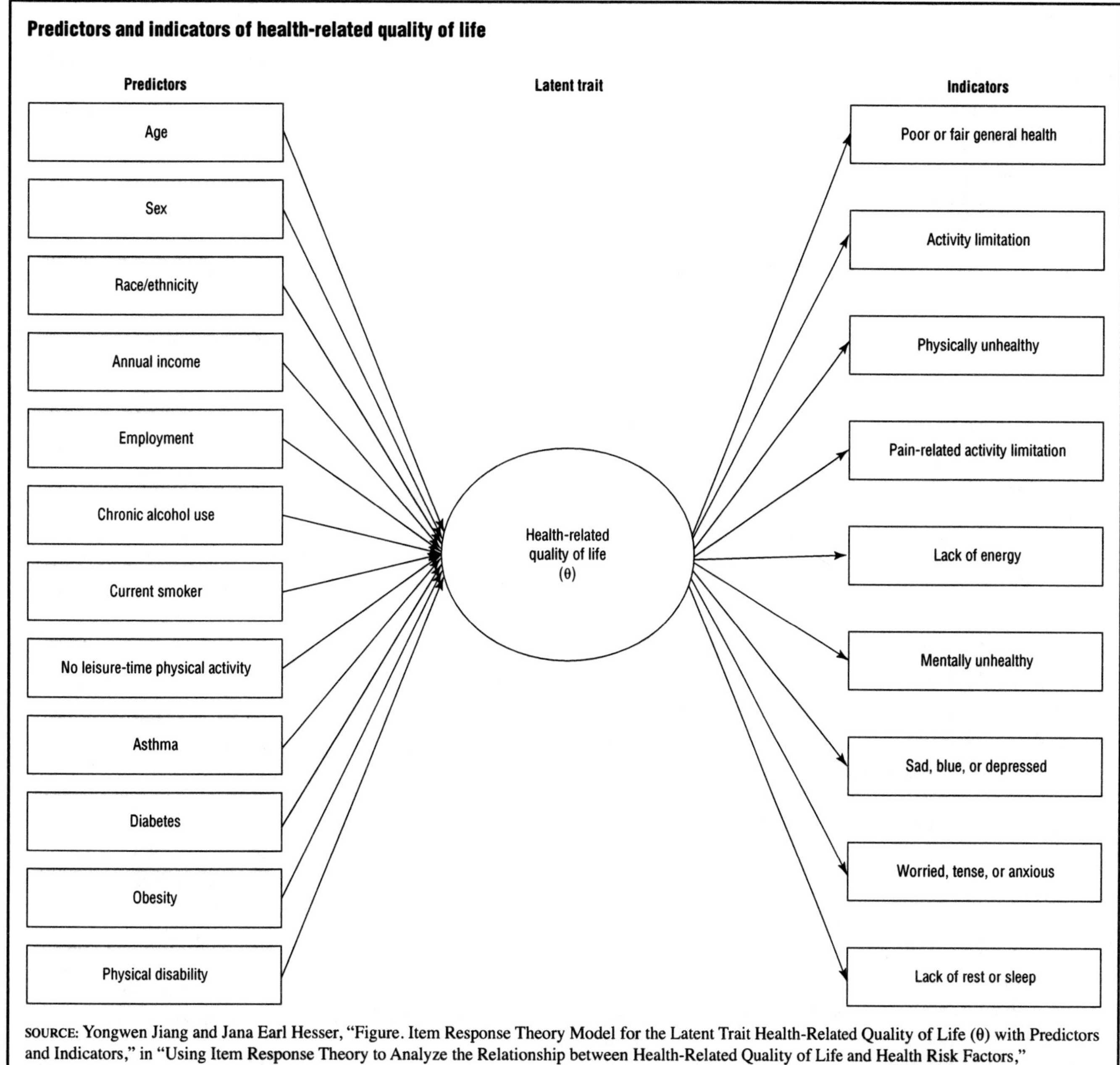

SOURCE: Yongwen Jiang and Jana Earl Hesser, "Figure. Item Response Theory Model for the Latent Trait Health-Related Quality of Life (θ) with Predictors and Indicators," in "Using Item Response Theory to Analyze the Relationship between Health-Related Quality of Life and Health Risk Factors," *Preventing Chronic Disease*, vol. 6, no. 1, January 2009, http://www.cdc.gov/Pcd/issues/2009/jan/07_0272.htm (accessed December 15, 2015)

- The Global Health Measure evaluates physical, mental, and social HRQoL by querying people about self-rated health, physical HRQoL, mental HRQoL, fatigue, pain, emotional distress, and social activities.
- The Well-Being Measures consider how people feel in terms of their health and satisfaction with life, fulfillment of their ambitions and potential, and the quality of their relationships. These measures also assess positive emotions and emotional resilience (how well people endure and manage stress).
- The Participation Measures look at individuals' assessments of the impact of their health on their social participation in education, employment, civic, social, and leisure activities. Participation Measures show that individuals with functional limitations such as vision loss, walking problems, or intellectual disability are able to live long, productive lives.

The CDC explains that many measures, such as the Medical Outcomes Study Short Forms, the Sickness Impact Profile, and the Quality of Well-Being Scale, have been used to assess HRQoL and functional status, but because most are time- and labor-intensive to administer, they are not appropriate for population-wide surveillance. HRQoL is increasingly important in view of Americans' increasing life expectancy because it can be used to help improve older adults' lives as they age.

Healthy Days Help to Assess HRQoL

Another measure of HRQoL used by the CDC is Healthy Days (March 15, 2011, http://www.cdc.gov/hrqol/hrqol14_measure.htm), which assesses an individual's perceived sense of physical and mental health and well-being using responses to the following four questions:

- Would you say that in general your health is excellent, very good, good, fair, or poor?
- Now thinking about your physical health, which includes physical illness and injury, for how many days during the past 30 days was your physical health not good?
- Now thinking about your mental health, which includes stress, depression, and problems with emotions, for how many days during the past 30 days was your mental health not good?
- During the past 30 days, for about how many days did poor physical or mental health keep you from doing your usual activities, such as self-care, work, or recreation?

THE HEALTH OF THE UNITED STATES

A primary indicator of the well-being of a nation is the health of its people. Many factors can affect a person's health: heredity, race or ethnicity, gender, income, education, geography, exposure to violent crime, exposure to environmental agents, exposure to infectious diseases, and access to and availability of health care.

Whereas physicians and other health practitioners observe the influences of these factors as they care for individual patients, epidemiologists (public health researchers who study the occurrence of disease) examine the distribution and rates of diseases and injuries in the population. Practitioners and epidemiologists each identify problems and analyze data to achieve their objectives, but they do it differently. For instance, practitioners use history and physical examination to determine a patient's health, whereas epidemiologists use surveillance and description. Practitioners deliver appropriate treatment to individual patients, whereas epidemiologists recommend actions to prevent the spread of disease or otherwise improve the health of a community or population.

Epidemiologists assess health by determining the incidence and prevalence rates of disease and disability in a given community. Incidence is a measure of the rate at which people without a disease develop the disease during a specific period, and it describes the continuing occurrence of disease over time. For example, a researcher might report that men in a given community aged 65 years and older have a 2% incidence of heart disease. Prevalence describes a group or population at a specific point in time. For example, the prevalence of high blood pressure found during screening at a health fair on a specific day might be 22%.

Other measures of the health of a population, such as natality (birth) and mortality (death) rates, are known as vital health statistics. This chapter provides an overview of vital health statistics and the health status of Americans.

BIRTH RATES AND FERTILITY RATES

The birth rate is the number of live births per 1,000 women. The fertility rate is the number of live births per 1,000 women between 15 and 44 years of age, generally considered equivalent to a woman's prime childbearing years.

In "Births: Preliminary Data for 2014" (*National Vital Statistics Reports*, vol. 64, no. 6, June 17, 2015), Brady E. Hamilton et al. of the CDC report that there were nearly 4 million births in the United States in 2014, up 1% since 2013. The general fertility rate also increased 1% in 2014, to 62.9 births per 1,000 women aged 15 to 44 years. Figure 1.2 shows changes in the number of births and the fertility rate between 1920 and 2014.

Birth rates have continued to decline for teenagers aged 15 to 19 years. In 2014 the number of live births per 1,000 teens aged 15 to 19 years was 24.2, down 9% from 2013. (See Figure 1.3.) Hamilton et al. report that the rate for this age group declined more than 7% annually since 2007, and dropped 61% since 1991, when it was 61.8.

By contrast, the birth rates for women aged 20 to 29 years has declined only slightly. (See Figure 1.3.) The birth rate for women aged 30 to 34 years increased 3%, from 98 births per 1,000 women in 2013 to 100.8 in 2014. There was a comparable increase (2%) among women aged 40 to 44 years. However, the rate for women over the age of 45 years was unchanged from 2011.

Hamilton et al. report that the fertility rate in 2014 remained below the replacement level—replacement is the rate at which a given generation can exactly replace itself, which is estimated to be approximately 2,100 births per 1,000 women. The rate has not been above replacement since 2007.

Prenatal Care, Prematurity, and Low Birth Weight

Early prenatal care, which is pregnancy-related care started during the first trimester (one to three months), can detect, prevent, and often correct many health problems early in pregnancy. Regular prenatal visits give the mother-to-be information and support for eating properly, exercising regularly, taking prenatal vitamins, and avoiding harmful substances such as alcohol, drugs, and tobacco. The benefits of these preventive measures can literally make a lifetime of difference for a newborn.

FIGURE 1.2

Number of births and fertility rates, 1920–2014

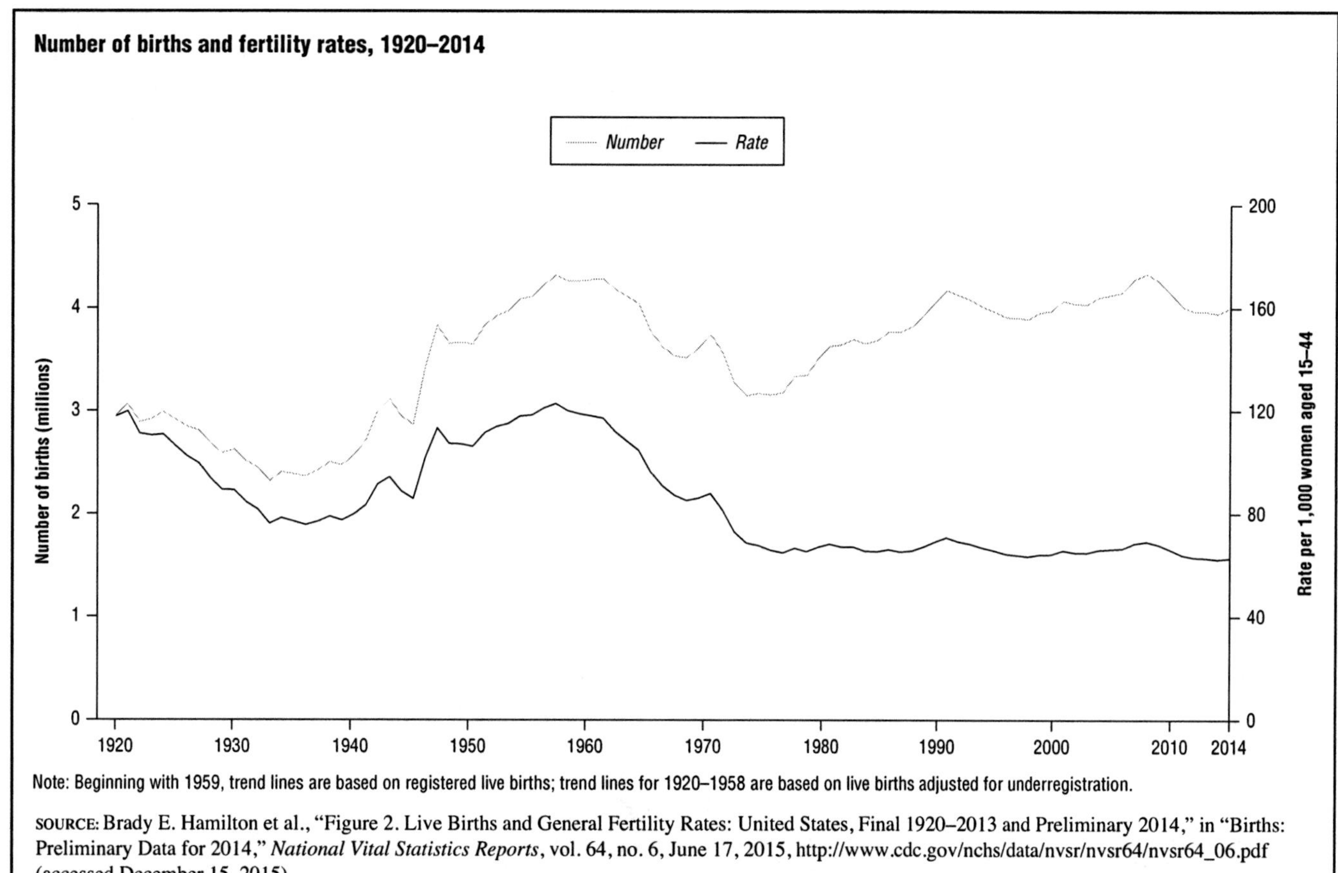

Note: Beginning with 1959, trend lines are based on registered live births; trend lines for 1920–1958 are based on live births adjusted for underregistration.

SOURCE: Brady E. Hamilton et al., "Figure 2. Live Births and General Fertility Rates: United States, Final 1920–2013 and Preliminary 2014," in "Births: Preliminary Data for 2014," *National Vital Statistics Reports*, vol. 64, no. 6, June 17, 2015, http://www.cdc.gov/nchs/data/nvsr/nvsr64/nvsr64_06.pdf (accessed December 15, 2015)

Diagnostic medical procedures, such as ultrasound scans and amniocentesis, can be performed to detect possible birth defects and other prenatal problems. Ultrasound uses high-frequency sound waves to compose a picture of the fetus and is used to detect and assess fetal development and malformations. During amniocentesis, a physician inserts a needle through the abdominal wall into the uterus to obtain a small sample of the amniotic fluid surrounding the fetus. When tested in a laboratory, this fluid can reveal chromosomal abnormalities, metabolic disorders, and physical abnormalities.

Pregnant women older than age 35 are generally advised to undergo amniocentesis and other diagnostic testing, because they are at greater risk than younger women of giving birth to babies with chromosomal abnormalities such as Down syndrome. Instead of the normal 46 chromosomes, newborns with Down syndrome have an extra copy of chromosome 21, giving them a total of 47 chromosomes. These children have varying degrees of mental retardation, and, according to the National Down Syndrome Society, in "Down Syndrome Facts" (2016, http://www.ndss.org/Down-Syndrome/Down-Syndrome-Facts/), are at increased risk for congenital heart defects, Alzheimer's disease, respiratory and hearing problems, leukemia, and thyroid conditions. In the United States, an estimated one in every 691 babies is born with Down syndrome.

Ideally, every woman should receive prenatal care, and according to the National Center for Health Statistics (NCHS), the United States is capable of delivering prenatal care to nearly all pregnant women during the first trimester of pregnancy. However, not all mothers-to-be seek or receive early or adequate prenatal care. The Adequacy of Prenatal Care Utilization Index explains that adequate/adequate plus prenatal care is defined as pregnancy-related care beginning during the first four months of pregnancy with the appropriate number of visits for gestational age. In 2007, 70.8% of pregnant women received early and adequate prenatal care. Healthy People 2020 (https://www.healthypeople.gov/2020/topics-objectives/topic/maternal-infant-and-child-health/objectives) aims for a 10% improvement, which would mean more than three-quarters (77.6%) of pregnant women would receive appropriate prenatal care.

The percentage of expectant mothers receiving prenatal care beginning during the first trimester varies by race, ethnicity, age, and educational attainment. According to the U.S. Department of Health and Human Services, in *Healthy Child USA 2014* (March 2015, http://mchb.hrsa.gov/chusa14/dl/chusa14.pdf), in 2012, 79% of non-Hispanic white women, 78% of Asian American

FIGURE 1.3

Birth rates by age of mother, 1990–2014

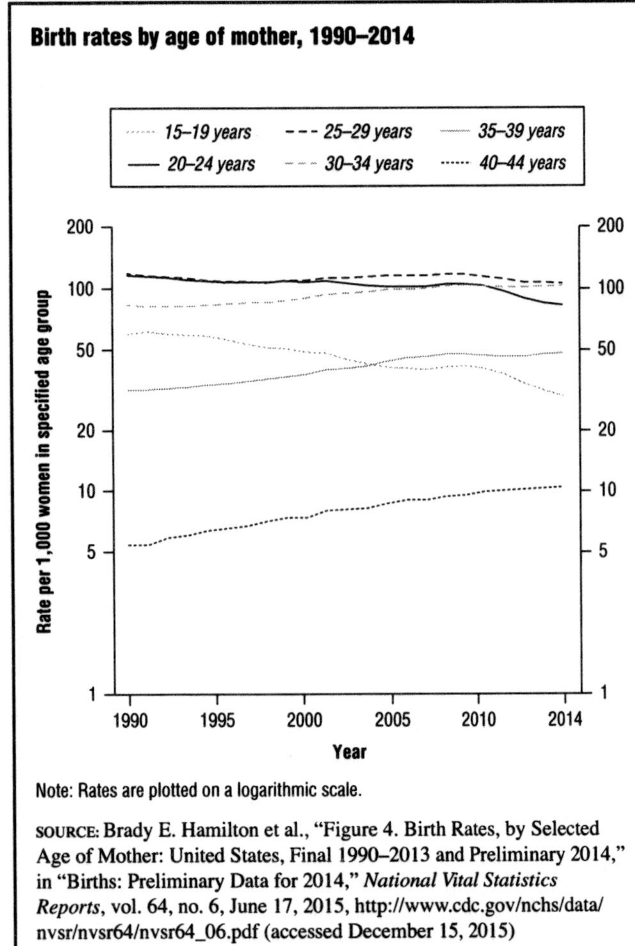

Note: Rates are plotted on a logarithmic scale.

SOURCE: Brady E. Hamilton et al., "Figure 4. Birth Rates, by Selected Age of Mother: United States, Final 1990–2013 and Preliminary 2014," in "Births: Preliminary Data for 2014," *National Vital Statistics Reports*, vol. 64, no. 6, June 17, 2015, http://www.cdc.gov/nchs/data/nvsr/nvsr64/nvsr64_06.pdf (accessed December 15, 2015)

women, 69% of Hispanic women, 70.7% of non-Hispanic multiple race women, 63.6% of non-Hispanic African American women, 59.4% of Native American/Alaskan Native women, and 54.7% of Native Hawaiian/other Pacific Islander women received prenatal care during the first trimester of pregnancy. Fewer women with less than a high school education (58.5%) received first trimester prenatal care than did those with a bachelor's degree or higher (86.1%).

In "Barriers and Facilitators Related to Use of Prenatal Care by Inner-City Women: Perceptions of Health Care Providers" (*BMC Pregnancy & Childbirth*, vol. 15, no. 2, January 16, 2015), Maureen I. Heaman et al. cite a number of barriers that may prevent expectant mothers from receiving prenatal care, such as a shortage of health care providers who offer prenatal care, providers' lack of time to devote to it, fear of tests and examinations, lack of transportation or child care, distrust of the health care system, lengthy office waits, lack of understanding of the importance of prenatal care, and cultural and personal factors.

Early prenatal care can prevent or reduce the risk of low birth weight (LBW). Infants who weigh less than 5 pounds, 8 ounces (2,500 g) at birth are considered to be of LBW. Those born weighing less than 3 pounds, 4 ounces (1,500 g) are called very low birth weight (VLBW). LBW may result from premature birth (infants born before 37 weeks of pregnancy are considered premature), poor maternal nutrition, teen pregnancy, drug and alcohol use, smoking, or sexually transmitted infections.

Infants who are premature or have an LBW are at greater risk of death and disability than infants of normal weight. About 80% of women at risk for delivering an LBW infant can be identified during the first prenatal visit, and interventions can be made to try to prevent problems. Between 1990 and 2013 the proportion of newborn babies weighing less than 5 pounds, 8 ounces increased from 7% to 8%. (See Table 1.1.)

As with access to prenatal care, the percentage of LBW live births varies by geography, race, and ethnicity. Among non-Hispanic African Americans, 13.2% of live births in 2011–13 were LBW, compared with 8.3% of Asian or Pacific Islander births, 7.6% of Native American or Alaskan Native births, 7% of non-Hispanic white births, and 7% of Hispanic births. (See Table 1.2.) In 2011–13 more than 14% of live births to non-Hispanic African American mothers in Alabama, Arkansas, Louisiana, Mississippi, Oklahoma, and South Carolina were LBW. During the same period less than 10% of live births to non-Hispanic African American mothers in Alaska, Idaho, Maine, North Dakota, Oregon, South Dakota, Vermont, and Washington were LBW. A similar trend was seen for non-Hispanic white mothers: more than 8% of live births to non-Hispanic white mothers in Colorado, Kentucky, Louisiana, Mississippi, New Mexico, West Virginia, and Wyoming were LBW, but less than 6% of live births to non-Hispanic white mothers in Alaska, California, Hawaii, Minnesota, Oregon, South Dakota, and Washington were LBW.

The usual length of pregnancy is 40 weeks from the first day of the woman's last menstrual period. Infants born prematurely do not have fully formed organ systems. If, however, the premature infant is born with a birth weight that is comparable to a full-term baby and has organ systems that are only slightly undeveloped, the chances of survival are great. Premature infants of VLBW are susceptible to many risks and are less likely to survive than full-term infants. If they survive, they may suffer from mental retardation, developmental disabilities, and other abnormalities of the nervous system.

A severe medical condition called hyaline membrane disease (or respiratory distress syndrome) commonly affects premature infants. It is caused by the inability of immature lungs to function properly. Occurring immediately after birth, the disease may cause infant death within hours. Intensive care of affected infants includes the use of a mechanical ventilator to facilitate breathing. Also, premature infants' immature gastrointestinal systems preclude them from taking in nourishment properly. Unable to suck and swallow, they must be fed through a nasogastric

TABLE 1.1

Low-birthweight live births, by selected characteristics, selected years 1970–2013

[Data are based on birth certificates]

Birthweight, maternal race, and Hispanic origin	1970	1980	1985	1990	1995	2000	2005	2010	2012	2013
Low birthweight (less than 2,500 grams)					Percent of live births[a]					
All races	7.93	6.84	6.75	6.97	7.32	7.57	8.19	8.15	7.99	8.02
White	6.85	5.72	5.65	5.70	6.22	6.55	7.16	7.08	6.96	7.00
Black or African American	13.90	12.69	12.65	13.25	13.13	12.99	13.59	13.21	12.84	12.76
American Indian or Alaska Native	7.97	6.44	5.86	6.11	6.61	6.76	7.36	7.61	7.61	7.48
Asian or Pacific Islander[b]	—	6.68	6.16	6.45	6.90	7.31	7.98	8.49	8.21	8.34
Hispanic or Latina[c]	—	6.12	6.16	6.06	6.29	6.41	6.88	6.97	6.97	7.09
Mexican	—	5.62	5.77	5.55	5.81	6.01	6.49	6.49	6.48	6.62
Puerto Rican	—	8.95	8.69	8.99	9.41	9.30	9.92	9.55	9.40	9.38
Cuban	—	5.62	6.02	5.67	6.50	6.49	7.64	7.30	7.43	7.35
Central and South American	—	5.76	5.68	5.84	6.20	6.34	6.78	6.55	6.64	6.85
Other and unknown Hispanic or Latina	—	6.96	6.83	6.87	7.55	7.84	8.27	8.38	8.00	7.99
Not Hispanic or Latina:[c]										
White	—	5.69	5.61	5.61	6.20	6.60	7.29	7.14	6.97	6.98
Black or African American	—	12.71	12.62	13.32	13.21	13.13	14.02	13.53	13.18	13.08
Very low birthweight (less than 1,500 grams)										
All races	1.17	1.15	1.21	1.27	1.35	1.43	1.49	1.45	1.42	1.41
White	0.95	0.90	0.94	0.95	1.06	1.14	1.20	1.17	1.15	1.14
Black or African American	2.40	2.48	2.71	2.92	2.97	3.07	3.15	2.90	2.85	2.82
American Indian or Alaska Native	0.98	0.92	1.01	1.01	1.10	1.16	1.17	1.28	1.33	1.32
Asian or Pacific Islander[b]	—	0.92	0.85	0.87	0.91	1.05	1.14	1.17	1.13	1.18
Hispanic or Latina[c]	—	0.98	1.01	1.03	1.11	1.14	1.20	1.20	1.22	1.21
Mexican	—	0.92	0.97	0.92	1.01	1.03	1.12	1.09	1.13	1.13
Puerto Rican	—	1.29	1.30	1.62	1.79	1.93	1.87	1.82	1.77	1.65
Cuban	—	1.02	1.18	1.20	1.19	1.21	1.50	1.42	1.55	1.27
Central and South American	—	0.99	1.01	1.05	1.13	1.20	1.19	1.09	1.13	1.15
Other and unknown Hispanic or Latina	—	1.01	0.96	1.09	1.28	1.42	1.36	1.46	1.38	1.37
Not Hispanic or Latina:[c]										
White	—	0.87	0.91	0.93	1.04	1.14	1.21	1.16	1.13	1.11
Black or African American	—	2.47	2.67	2.93	2.98	3.10	3.27	2.98	2.94	2.90

—Data not available.

[a]Excludes live births with unknown birthweight. Percentage based on live births with known birthweight.

[b]Estimates are not available for Asian or Pacific Islander subgroups because not all states have adopted the 2003 revision of the U.S. Standard Certificate of Live Birth.

[c]Prior to 1993, data from states that did not report Hispanic origin on the birth certificate were excluded. Data for non-Hispanic white and non-Hispanic black women for years prior to 1989 are not nationally representative and are provided solely for comparison with Hispanic data.

Notes: The race groups, white, black, American Indian or Alaska Native, and Asian or Pacific Islander, include persons of Hispanic and non-Hispanic origin. Persons of Hispanic origin may be of any race. Starting with 2003 data, some states reported multiple-race data. The multiple-race data for these states were bridged to the single-race categories of the 1977 Office of Management and Budget standards, for comparability with other states. Interpretation of trend data for Hispanic births should take into consideration expansion of reporting areas. Data for additional years are available.

SOURCE: "Table 6. Low Birthweight Live Births, by Detailed Race and Hispanic Origin of Mother: United States, Selected Years 1970–2013," in *Health, United States, 2014: With Special Feature on Adults Aged 55–64*, Centers for Disease Control and Prevention, National Center for Health Statistics, 2015, http://www.cdc.gov/nchs/data/hus/hus14.pdf (accessed December 15, 2015)

feeding tube (nutrient-rich formula enters through a tube inserted into the stomach via the nose).

LBW and VLBW are major predictors of infant morbidity (illness or disease) and mortality. For LBW infants, the risk of dying during the first year of life is more than five times that of normal-weight infants; the risk for VLBW infants is nearly 100 times higher. The risk of delivering an LBW infant is greatest among the youngest and oldest mothers; however, many of the LBW births among older mothers are attributable to their higher rates of multiple births.

Birth Weight Influences the Risk of Infant Death and Future Disease

Although the precise mechanisms of the relationship between birth weight and the development of disease in adulthood have not yet been completely described, there is ample evidence that lower- and higher-than-average birth weight are associated with health in later life. LBW infants are more likely than normal-weight infants to develop disease as they age and male LBW infants—who gain weight rapidly before their first birthday—are disproportionately affected and seem to be at the highest risk for future health problems. Researchers conjecture that LBW infants have fewer muscle cells at birth and that rapid weight gain during the first year of life may lead to different ratios of fat to muscle and above-average body mass. LBW infants who later develop above-average body mass are at higher risk of developing diseases such as type 2 diabetes, hypertension (high blood pressure), and cardiovascular disease (heart disease and stroke) than normal-weight infants who do not gain weight rapidly during their first year of life.

TABLE 1.2

Low-birthweight births by race, ethnicity, state, and territory, selected years 2000–13

[Data are based on birth certificates]

	All races			Not Hispanic or Latina					
				White			Black or African American		
State and territory	2000–2002	2003–2005	2011–2013	2000–2002	2003–2005	2011–2013	2000–2002	2003–2005	2011–2013
	Percent of live births weighing less than 2,500 grams[a]								
United States[b]	**7.69**	**8.07**	**8.04**	**6.75**	**7.18**	**7.01**	**13.19**	**13.77**	**13.20**
Alabama	9.75	10.35	9.98	7.77	8.46	7.95	14.10	15.02	14.85
Alaska	5.71	6.02	5.81	4.84	5.34	5.14	10.70	11.74	9.01
Arizona	6.91	7.05	6.95	6.78	7.01	6.56	13.16	12.38	12.00
Arkansas	8.64	9.04	8.84	7.48	7.83	7.62	13.81	14.86	14.45
California	6.29	6.71	6.76	5.86	6.30	5.97	11.66	12.46	11.50
Colorado	8.60	9.04	8.77	8.24	8.81	8.32	14.59	15.20	13.62
Connecticut	7.52	7.74	7.80	6.48	6.60	6.56	12.28	12.88	12.09
Delaware	9.29	9.31	8.32	7.80	7.62	6.77	14.08	14.32	12.41
District of Columbia	11.85	11.06	9.83	6.35	6.28	6.06	14.60	13.96	12.60
Florida	8.18	8.59	8.59	6.98	7.38	7.21	12.58	13.28	12.91
Georgia	8.79	9.27	9.36	6.92	7.44	7.29	12.98	13.81	13.33
Hawaii	7.98	8.23	8.19	6.17	6.42	5.99	11.01	11.44	11.22
Idaho	6.41	6.65	6.47	6.29	6.60	6.35	*	*7.03	*6.71
Illinois	8.04	8.40	8.19	6.74	7.22	6.89	14.04	14.70	13.57
Indiana	7.54	8.10	7.97	6.95	7.54	7.35	12.89	13.46	12.86
Iowa	6.39	6.92	6.58	6.19	6.72	6.36	11.77	12.22	11.22
Kansas	6.96	7.28	7.12	6.66	6.97	6.63	12.37	13.42	12.78
Kentucky	8.38	8.86	8.82	7.84	8.50	8.42	13.84	13.52	13.55
Louisiana	10.40	11.02	10.88	7.56	8.12	8.19	14.44	15.33	15.33
Maine	6.12	6.58	6.82	6.13	6.57	6.73	*9.47	8.47	8.91
Maryland	8.88	9.17	8.71	6.79	7.19	6.69	13.00	13.13	12.34
Massachusetts	7.26	7.77	7.63	6.56	7.15	6.95	11.54	11.82	10.42
Michigan	7.94	8.28	8.34	6.55	7.00	6.96	14.24	14.43	13.67
Minnesota	6.23	6.43	6.47	5.80	5.93	5.84	10.54	10.71	10.03
Mississippi	10.82	11.62	11.67	7.97	8.67	8.51	14.48	15.60	16.06
Missouri	7.74	8.12	7.89	6.79	7.18	6.85	13.27	13.90	13.67
Montana	6.65	7.02	7.31	6.60	6.81	7.03	*	*15.58	*10.50
Nebraska	6.88	6.97	6.58	6.52	6.76	6.07	13.07	12.16	12.25
Nevada	7.44	8.11	8.08	7.19	7.78	7.46	13.40	13.98	12.97
New Hampshire	6.40	6.65	7.06	6.24	6.59	7.00	10.58	10.85	10.62
New Jersey	7.89	8.19	8.32	6.59	7.11	7.26	13.20	13.48	12.44
New Mexico	7.99	8.38	8.82	7.89	8.33	8.44	13.88	15.01	13.31
New York	7.76	8.11	8.00	6.48	6.82	6.71	12.02	12.78	12.35
North Carolina	8.90	9.07	8.87	7.49	7.73	7.37	13.83	14.33	13.59
North Dakota	6.28	6.49	6.42	6.13	6.37	6.23	*9.02	*9.43	9.00
Ohio	8.07	8.51	8.57	7.08	7.53	7.47	13.45	13.83	13.59
Oklahoma	7.75	7.92	8.17	7.35	7.63	7.79	13.57	13.62	14.06
Oregon	5.65	6.09	6.19	5.44	6.02	5.91	10.32	11.16	9.43
Pennsylvania	7.93	8.20	8.09	6.78	7.06	6.95	13.79	13.67	12.92
Rhode Island	7.47	8.12	7.46	6.75	7.39	6.68	12.32	11.22	11.53
South Carolina	9.74	10.15	9.70	7.40	7.82	7.59	14.29	15.19	14.49
South Dakota	6.58	6.71	6.24	6.37	6.62	5.80	*11.51	*7.27	9.47
Tennessee	9.20	9.35	9.11	7.95	8.26	7.98	14.23	14.51	13.98
Texas	7.54	8.07	8.35	6.81	7.43	7.44	12.82	13.91	13.48
Utah	6.48	6.68	6.92	6.28	6.45	6.63	13.09	12.05	11.38
Vermont	6.15	6.57	6.51	6.12	6.55	6.43	*	*	*8.25
Virginia	7.90	8.23	8.04	6.54	7.01	6.68	12.56	12.83	12.56
Washington	5.75	6.13	6.23	5.43	5.63	5.66	10.34	10.63	9.65
West Virginia	8.60	9.16	9.40	8.39	9.03	9.28	13.81	13.15	13.46
Wisconsin	6.58	6.93	7.12	5.83	6.18	6.31	13.25	13.59	13.46
Wyoming	8.35	8.71	8.43	8.12	8.74	8.31	*13.29	*	*12.05
American Samoa[c]	3.51	3.75	4.32	—	—	*	—	—	. . .
Guam[c]	7.88	8.81	8.77	*4.13	*4.01	3.24	*	*	*
Northern Marianas[c]	8.05	7.55	7.12	—	—	*	—	—	. . .
Puerto Rico[c]	11.14	11.92	11.58	—	—	11.44	—	—	12.66
Virgin Islands[c]	10.21	11.14	9.43	*8.37	*5.90	10.08	9.89	12.51	9.99

LBW is an important predictor of infant health risks and a leading cause of infant deaths. Brady E. Hamilton et al. report in "Annual Summary of Vital Statistics: 2010–2011" (*Pediatrics*, vol. 131, no. 3, March 1, 2013) that in 2011, 17.2% of infant deaths were attributable to disorders related to "short gestation and low birth weight." The researchers observe that the percentage of infants born with LBW rose more than 20% from the mid-1980s through 2006, but has declined by 2% from 2006 through 2011.

In "Low Birth Weight and Increased Cardiovascular Risk: Fetal Programming" (*International Journal of Cardiology*, vol. 144, no. 1, September 24, 2010), Mustafa Mucahit

TABLE 1.2

Low-birthweight births by race, ethnicity, state, and territory, selected years 2000–13 [CONTINUED]

[Data are based on birth certificates]

State and territory	Hispanic or Latina[d] 2000–2002	Hispanic or Latina[d] 2003–2005	Hispanic or Latina[d] 2011–2013	American Indian or Alaska Native[e] 2000–2002	American Indian or Alaska Native[e] 2003–2005	American Indian or Alaska Native[e] 2011–2013	Asian or Pacific Islander[e] 2000–2002	Asian or Pacific Islander[e] 2003–2005	Asian or Pacific Islander[e] 2011–2013
	Percent of live births weighing less than 2,500 grams[a]								
United States[b]	**6.48**	**6.79**	**7.03**	**7.11**	**7.39**	**7.55**	**7.54**	**7.89**	**8.30**
Alabama	6.95	6.92	6.41	9.68	10.53	11.17	7.38	8.02	8.62
Alaska	6.07	5.31	6.41	5.81	5.86	6.12	7.33	6.57	7.30
Arizona	6.56	6.69	6.64	6.85	7.11	7.03	7.95	7.92	7.81
Arkansas	5.79	6.54	6.38	8.11	8.86	7.93	7.73	6.74	9.71
California	5.66	6.10	6.23	6.21	6.49	6.35	7.15	7.42	7.84
Colorado	8.33	8.53	8.53	9.05	9.45	9.39	10.17	10.26	10.70
Connecticut	8.25	8.49	8.24	10.06	7.45	9.43	8.07	7.83	8.61
Delaware	6.81	7.03	6.34	*	*	*	9.89	9.33	7.53
District of Columbia	8.04	7.46	8.00	*	*	*	*7.00	8.97	7.31
Florida	6.61	6.98	7.23	7.11	7.38	7.47	8.35	8.73	8.56
Georgia	5.77	5.96	6.52	9.29	9.00	9.21	8.18	8.35	8.48
Hawaii	8.00	8.34	8.88	*4.99	*	*	8.45	8.84	8.91
Idaho	6.95	6.67	6.82	6.15	8.31	7.30	7.38	6.67	7.60
Illinois	6.31	6.60	6.93	8.60	9.46	10.49	8.49	8.28	8.97
Indiana	6.09	6.33	6.65	*7.74	*10.00	*10.30	7.41	7.87	7.80
Iowa	6.01	6.12	5.49	7.23	9.15	6.80	7.13	7.71	7.36
Kansas	5.93	6.09	6.43	6.20	7.09	8.80	6.69	7.34	8.25
Kentucky	7.73	6.85	6.89	*7.17	*8.54	*10.61	7.75	7.56	7.65
Louisiana	6.56	7.62	7.32	9.06	10.11	8.26	7.89	8.46	8.92
Maine	*6.03	*4.74	*8.01	*	*	*	*5.46	8.69	8.50
Maryland	6.73	7.18	6.99	9.74	10.87	8.09	7.42	7.93	8.31
Massachusetts	8.37	8.41	8.24	*7.11	*7.62	*8.14	7.57	7.63	8.13
Michigan	6.26	6.46	7.12	7.26	6.98	7.67	7.46	8.33	9.09
Minnesota	6.02	5.70	6.21	7.10	6.87	8.26	7.28	7.43	7.52
Mississippi	6.61	6.42	6.23	7.30	6.24	*5.86	6.83	8.06	8.76
Missouri	6.18	6.33	6.53	8.67	7.63	7.88	7.34	7.61	7.07
Montana	7.44	8.63	7.54	7.14	7.80	8.48	*5.95	*8.70	*9.93
Nebraska	6.30	6.20	6.60	7.27	6.78	5.93	8.05	7.61	6.42
Nevada	6.34	6.74	6.87	6.80	7.58	7.78	7.56	10.35	9.94
New Hampshire	4.84	6.55	7.26	*	*	*	5.95	7.75	7.36
New Jersey	7.15	7.27	7.42	11.09	9.83	10.54	7.57	8.10	9.16
New Mexico	8.13	8.45	8.98	6.88	7.32	7.88	7.67	8.60	10.91
New York	7.38	7.59	7.63	7.81	7.31	7.06	7.33	7.89	8.07
North Carolina	6.13	6.27	6.77	10.30	11.01	10.44	8.20	7.77	8.23
North Dakota	*8.10	*5.84	6.07	6.62	6.78	7.20	*	*8.39	*5.44
Ohio	7.20	7.13	7.82	8.86	10.22	9.90	7.86	8.27	8.26
Oklahoma	6.41	6.46	6.64	6.48	6.69	7.14	7.87	6.82	8.22
Oregon	5.54	5.43	6.14	7.23	7.34	7.43	6.78	7.00	7.69
Pennsylvania	8.97	9.00	8.48	9.15	10.95	9.38	7.48	7.99	8.42
Rhode Island	7.20	8.61	7.58	*10.32	13.66	*9.91	9.31	10.11	8.69
South Carolina	6.87	6.66	6.17	10.22	10.75	9.13	8.02	8.13	8.16
South Dakota	6.89	5.94	7.69	6.84	7.04	7.13	*11.39	*9.50	9.07
Tennessee	6.28	6.04	6.56	*7.11	*6.63	7.54	8.60	7.76	8.28
Texas	6.88	7.23	7.66	6.67	7.33	7.35	7.78	8.33	9.52
Utah	7.20	7.26	7.40	6.37	7.46	7.89	7.23	8.20	8.87
Vermont	*	*	*	*	*	*	*	*8.08	*8.42
Virginia	6.07	6.28	6.43	*10.73	*9.20	8.66	7.50	7.71	8.41
Washington	5.31	5.93	6.24	7.08	7.31	7.37	6.37	6.90	7.38
West Virginia	*	*6.06	*6.80	*	*	*	*9.16	*9.51	*6.54
Wisconsin	6.13	6.34	6.62	6.12	6.04	6.50	6.97	7.50	7.74
Wyoming	8.81	8.43	8.48	9.55	8.39	8.95	*12.04	*	*6.78
American Samoa[c]	—	—	—	—	—	—	3.46	3.75	4.30
Guam[c]	*	*	*	*	. . .	*	7.78	9.33	9.13
Northern Marianas[c]	—	—	. . .	—	—	—	8.12	7.65	7.17
Puerto Rico[c]	—	—	11.59	—	—	—	—	—	—
Virgin Islands[c]	10.84	8.29	9.40	*12.50	. . .	—	*	*	*

Balci, Sadik Acikel, and Ramazan Akdemir posit that LBW infants may have hyper-responsive immune systems that predispose them to inflammatory conditions such as certain forms of heart disease, diabetes, arthritis, and asthma.

Evidence also indicates that LBW is related to a risk of developing asthma. Min Mu et al. review 18 studies with data from more than 90,000 children in "Birth Weight and Subsequent Risk of Asthma: A Systematic Review and Meta-analysis" (*Heart Lung and Circulation*, vol. 23, no. 6, June 2014) and determine that LBW but not high birth weight is associated with increased risk of asthma in childhood and adulthood.

In "Birth Weight and Subsequent Risk of Cancer" (*Cancer Epidemiology*, vol. 38, no. 5, October 2014), Cassandra N. Spracklen et al. report that high birth weight is associated with increased risk of developing

TABLE 1.2

Low-birthweight births by race, ethnicity, state, and territory, selected years 2000–13 [CONTINUED]

[Data are based on birth certificates]

*Percentages preceded by an asterisk are based on fewer than 50 births. Percentages not shown are based on fewer than 20 births.
—Data not available.
. . . Quantity zero.
[a]Excludes live births with unknown birthweight.
[b]Excludes data for American Samoa, Guam, Northern Marianas, Puerto Rico, and Virgin Islands.
[c]Comparable data were not available for all time periods and racial and ethnicity groups. Therefore, only selected low birthweight percentages are presented for the territories.
[d]Persons of Hispanic origin may be of any race.
[e]Includes persons of Hispanic and non-Hispanic origin.
Notes: Starting with 2003 data, some states and territories reported multiple-race data. The multiple-race data for these areas were bridged to the single-race categories of the 1977 Office of Management and Budget standards, for comparability with other areas. Data for the territories are shown by race and ethnicity only if race-specific data are available for all years in the 3-year period.

SOURCE: "Table 7. Low Birthweight Live Births, by Race and Hispanic Origin of Mother, State and Territory: United States and U.S. Dependent Areas, 2000–2002, 2003–2005, and 2011–2013," in *Health, United States, 2014: With Special Feature on Adults Aged 55–64*, Centers for Disease Control and Prevention, National Center for Health Statistics, 2015, http://www.cdc.gov/nchs/data/hus/hus14.pdf (accessed December 15, 2015)

selected cancers, including breast cancer, gynecological cancers (which include uterine, vaginal, cervical, and vulvar cancer), endometrial (the lining of the uterus) cancer, as well as lung cancer and colon cancer. An exception to this trend of increasing cancer risk with increasing birth weight was observed for leukemia. Women born weighing 6 pounds (2.7 kg) or less had a significantly higher risk of developing leukemia.

The only action able to alter the birth weight of an infant is to modify weight gain by the mother during pregnancy. In 2016 health professionals concurred that for normal-weight women the ideal weight gain during pregnancy ranges from 25 to 35 pounds (11.3 to 15.9 kg) of fat and lean mass. Furthermore, a newborn's birth weight and a mother's postpregnancy weight are influenced not only by how much weight is gained during pregnancy but also by the source of the excess weight. In the landmark study "Composition of Gestational Weight Gain Impacts Maternal Fat Retention and Infant Birth Weight" (*American Journal of Obstetrics and Gynecology*, vol. 189, no. 5, November 2003), Nancy F. Butte et al. of the Children's Nutrition Research Center in Houston, Texas, conducted body scans of 63 women before, during, and after their pregnancies and recorded changes in the women's weight from water, protein, fat, and potassium—a marker for changes in muscle tissue, which is one component of lean mass. The researchers find that only increases in lean mass, not fat mass, appeared to influence infant size. Independent of how much fat was gained by women during pregnancy, only lean body mass increased the birth weight of the infant, with women who gained more lean body mass giving birth to larger infants.

Women with a higher prepregnancy weight and those who gain large amounts of weight during pregnancy are more likely to give birth to heavier infants. In "Maternal Pre-pregnant Body Mass Index, Maternal Weight Change and Offspring Birthweight" (*Acta Obstetricia et Gynecologica Scandinavica*, vol. 91, no. 2, February 2012), Unni Mette Stamnes Koepp et al. analyze the association between prepregnancy weight and the infant's birth weight and determine that prepregnancy weight is an important predictor of birth weight. The researchers conclude that overweight and obese women should be encouraged to attain a healthy weight before becoming pregnant and should aim for moderate weight gain during pregnancy.

Kathleen M. Rasmussen et al. report in *Weight Gain during Pregnancy: Reexamining the Guidelines* (May 28, 2009, http://iom.edu/Reports/2009/Weight-Gain-During-Pregnancy-Reexamining-the-Guidelines.aspx) that in 2009 the Institute of Medicine and the National Research Council issued updated recommendations for pregnancy weight gain. (See Table 1.3.) The updated guidelines caution that obese expectant mothers (with a body mass index [a measure of body fat based on weight and height] of 30 or higher) should limit weight gain to between 11 and 20 pounds (5 and 9.1 kg). This recommendation replaces the 1990 guideline, which advised obese expectant mothers to gain no less than 15 pounds (6.8 kg). The updated guidelines are based on the findings that the offspring of overweight or obese women face increased risk for preterm birth or being larger than normal at delivery, with extra fat. Large babies may suffer stuck shoulders and broken collar bones during birth and are at greater risk of becoming overweight, obese, and diabetic in adulthood.

Birth Defects

In "Data & Statistics" (February 29, 2016, http://www.cdc.gov/ncbddd/birthdefects/data.html), the CDC states that birth defects affect one out of 33 babies and that birth defects account for more than 20% of all infant deaths. A birth defect may be a structural defect, a deficiency of function, or a disease that an infant has at birth (congenital). Some common birth defects are genetic—inherited abnormalities such as Tay-Sachs disease (a fatal

TABLE 1.3

Updated recommendations for weight gain during pregnancy by prepregnancy body mass index, 2009

Prepregnancy BMI	BMI (kg/m²)	Total weight gain (lbs)	Rates of weight gain 2nd and 3rd trimester (lbs/week)
Underweight	<18.5	28–40	1 (1–1.3)
Normal weight	18.5–24.9	25–35	1 (0.8–1)
Overweight	25.0–29.9	15–25	0.6 (0.5–0.7)
Obese (includes all classes)	≥30.0	11–20	0.5 (0.4–0.6)

Notes: To calculate BMI go to www.nhlbisupport.com/bmi. Calculations assume a 0.5 = 2 kg (1.1–4.4 lbs) weight gain in the first trimester (based on Siega-Riz et al., 1994; Abrams et al., 1995; Carmichael et al., 1997)
BMI = Body mass index.

SOURCE: Kathleen M. Rasmussen et al., "Table 1. New Recommendations for Total and Rate of Weight Gain during Pregnancy, by Prepregnancy BMI," in *Weight Gain during Pregnancy: Reexamining the Guidelines*, Institute of Medicine of the National Academies, May 28, 2009, http://www.iom.edu/~/media/Files/Report%20Files/2009/Weight-Gain-During-Pregnancy-Reexamining-the-Guidelines/Resource%20Page%20-%20Weight%20Gain%20During%20Pregnancy.ashx (accessed December 12, 2013). Copyright © 2009 by the National Academy of Sciences. All rights reserved.

disease that generally affects children of east European Jewish ancestry) or chromosomal irregularities such as Down syndrome. Other birth defects result from environmental factors—infections during pregnancy, such as rubella (German measles), or drugs used by the pregnant woman. Although the specific causes of some birth defects are unknown, many result from a combination of genetic and environmental factors.

Prenatal testing can detect and diagnose many birth defects. Blood tests and ultrasound, which creates images of the fetus, are used to detect problems such as chromosomal or heart defects. High-resolution ultrasound may be used to produce more detailed images. Chorionic villus sampling involves an examination of a tiny bit of the placenta (an organ that lines the uterus during pregnancy, joining the mother and fetus and enabling transfer of oxygen and nutrients from the mother to the fetus and the release of carbon dioxide and waste products from the fetus) to check for chromosomal or genetic disorders. Amniocentesis tests the fluid that surrounds the baby in the uterus for specific proteins, which may indicate a birth defect such as Down syndrome and genetic problems such as cystic fibrosis (a condition in which a defective gene causes the body to produce abnormally thick mucus that builds up in the lungs and pancreas, the organ that helps break down and absorb food) or Tay-Sachs disease.

NEURAL TUBE DEFECTS. Neural tube defects (NTDs) are abnormalities of the brain and spinal cord resulting from the failure of the neural tube to develop properly during early pregnancy. The neural tube is the embryonic nerve tissue that eventually develops into the brain and the spinal cord. The two most common NTDs are anencephaly and spina bifida.

ANENCEPHALY. According to the U.S. National Library of Medicine's Genetics Home Reference, in "Anencephaly" (March 7, 2016, http://www.nlm.nih.gov/medlineplus/ency/article/001580.htm), anencephaly (the absence of a major part of the brain, skull, and scalp) occurs in about one out of 10,000 births. The exact number is unknown because many of these pregnancies end in miscarriage. Infants with anencephaly either die before birth (in utero or stillborn) or shortly thereafter.

SPINA BIFIDA. Spina bifida, which literally means "divided spine," is caused by the failure of the vertebrae (backbone) to completely cover the spinal cord early in fetal development, leaving the spinal cord exposed. Depending on the amount of nerve tissue exposed, spina bifida defects range from minor developmental disabilities to paralysis. The March of Dimes reports in "Spina Bifida" (May 2014, http://www.marchofdimes.com/professionals/14332_1224.asp) that spina bifida occurs in about 1,500 to 2,000 infants per year.

PREVENTION. Daily consumption of 400 micrograms of the B vitamin folic acid by women before and during the first trimester of pregnancy greatly reduces the risk of spina bifida and other birth defects. Because half of all pregnancies in the United States are unplanned or incorrectly timed and because NTDs occur during the first month of pregnancy—before most women know they are pregnant—the U.S. Public Health Service began recommending in 1992 that all women of childbearing age consume 400 micrograms of folic acid daily. Since January 1998 all enriched cereal grain products must be fortified with folic acid. According to the March of Dimes, in "Perinatal Data Snapshots" (October 2015, https://www.marchofdimes.com/peristats/pdflib/999/pds_99_4.pdf), the occurrence of NTDs can be reduced by up to 70% if women consume the recommended amount of folic acid before conception and throughout the first weeks of pregnancy.

According to the CDC, in "Key Findings: Folic Acid Fortification Continues to Prevent Neural Tube Defect" (January 15, 2015, http://www.cdc.gov/ncbddd/folicacid/features/folicacid-prevents-ntds.html), the prevalence of spina bifida has decreased 35% since 1998, when mandatory fortification of grain products began. This decline is an indicator of the successful efforts to prevent birth defects by increasing folic acid consumption and folate levels among women of childbearing age.

INFANT MORTALITY

Since 1958 infant mortality has declined or remained unchanged, except for a slight increase in 2002. In 2012 there were 6 deaths per 1,000 live births, 356 fewer than in 2011. (See Figure 1.4.)

Advances in neonatology (the medical subspecialty that is concerned with the care of newborns, especially

FIGURE 1.4

Infant, neonatal, and postneonatal mortality rates, 1940–2012

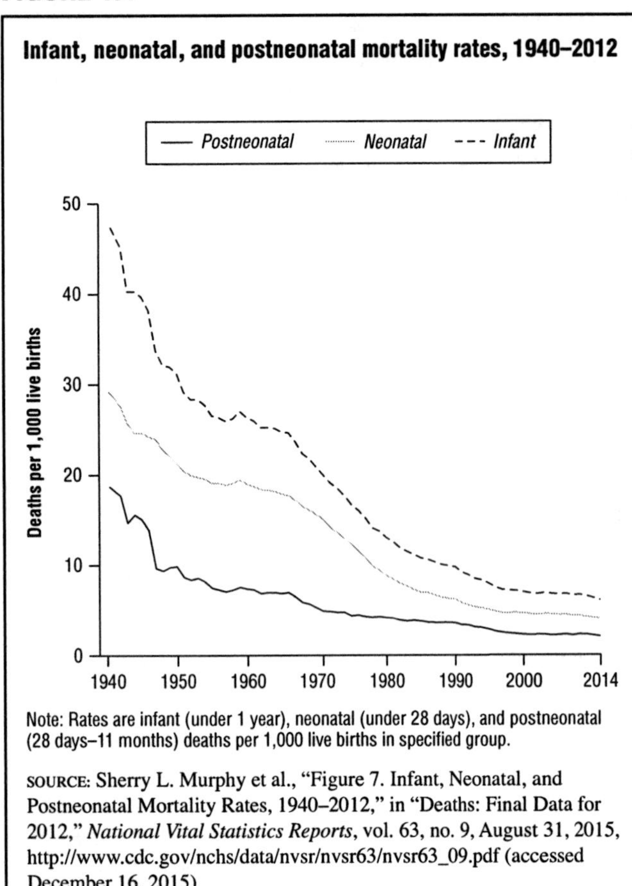

Note: Rates are infant (under 1 year), neonatal (under 28 days), and postneonatal (28 days–11 months) deaths per 1,000 live births in specified group.

SOURCE: Sherry L. Murphy et al., "Figure 7. Infant, Neonatal, and Postneonatal Mortality Rates, 1940–2012," in "Deaths: Final Data for 2012," *National Vital Statistics Reports*, vol. 63, no. 9, August 31, 2015, http://www.cdc.gov/nchs/data/nvsr/nvsr63/nvsr63_09.pdf (accessed December 16, 2015)

FIGURE 1.5

Life expectancy at birth and aged 65, by sex, 2013 and 2014

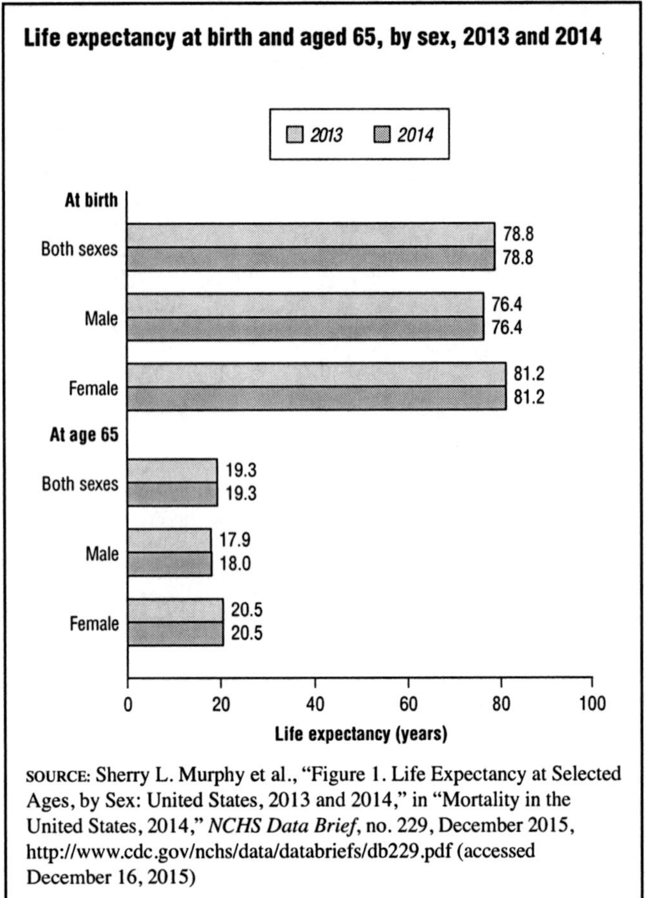

SOURCE: Sherry L. Murphy et al., "Figure 1. Life Expectancy at Selected Ages, by Sex: United States, 2013 and 2014," in "Mortality in the United States, 2014," *NCHS Data Brief*, no. 229, December 2015, http://www.cdc.gov/nchs/data/databriefs/db229.pdf (accessed December 16, 2015)

those at risk) have contributed to the huge decline in infant death rates. Infants born prematurely or with LBWs, who were once likely to die, can survive life-threatening conditions due to the development of neonatal intensive care units. Improved access to health care has also contributed to the decline, as have public health initiatives such as education about how to prevent sudden infant death syndrome—specifically, the Back to Sleep campaign, which teaches caregivers to place sleeping infants on their back.

According to the NCHS, in *Health, United States, 2014* (2015, http://www.cdc.gov/nchs/data/hus/hus14.pdf), in 2011 (the most current year for which data were available) the United States had a higher infant mortality rate than 26 other countries and at least twice the rate of infant deaths as the Czech Republic, Finland, Iceland, Ireland, Italy, Japan, Norway, South Korea, and Sweden.

LIFE EXPECTANCY

Along with infant mortality, life expectancy rates are an important measure of the health of the population. Life expectancy at birth is strongly influenced by infant and child mortality. Life expectancy in adulthood reflects death rates at or beyond specified ages and is independent of the effect of mortality at younger ages.

Sherry L. Murphy et al. of the CDC report in "Mortality in the United States, 2014" (December 2015, http://www.cdc.gov/nchs/data/databriefs/db229.pdf) that overall life expectancy in the United States was 78.8 years in 2014, unchanged from 2013. Figure 1.5 shows life expectancy at birth and at age 65 by sex in 2013 and 2014.

Figure 1.6 shows the upward trend between 1980 and 2013 in U.S. life expectancy for males and females at birth. In *Health, United States, 2014*, the NCHS indicates that life expectancy increased throughout the latter part of the 20th century, from 70 years in 1980 to 76.4 years in 2013 for males and from 77.4 years in 1980 to 81.2 years in 2013 for females. Although racial disparities in life expectancy at birth were still evident, the gap had narrowed since 1990.

Similarly, life expectancy at age 65 also increased during the 20th century. Unlike life expectancy at birth, which rose early in the 20th century, much of the rise in life expectancy at age 65 occurred after 1950, in response to improved access to health care, advances in medicine, healthier current lifestyles, and better health throughout the life span. (See Table 1.4.) Nonetheless, the United States does not boast the longest life expectancy. According to the NCHS, in 2012 life expectancy at birth for males

FIGURE 1.6

Life expectancy at birth, by selected characteristics, 1980–2013

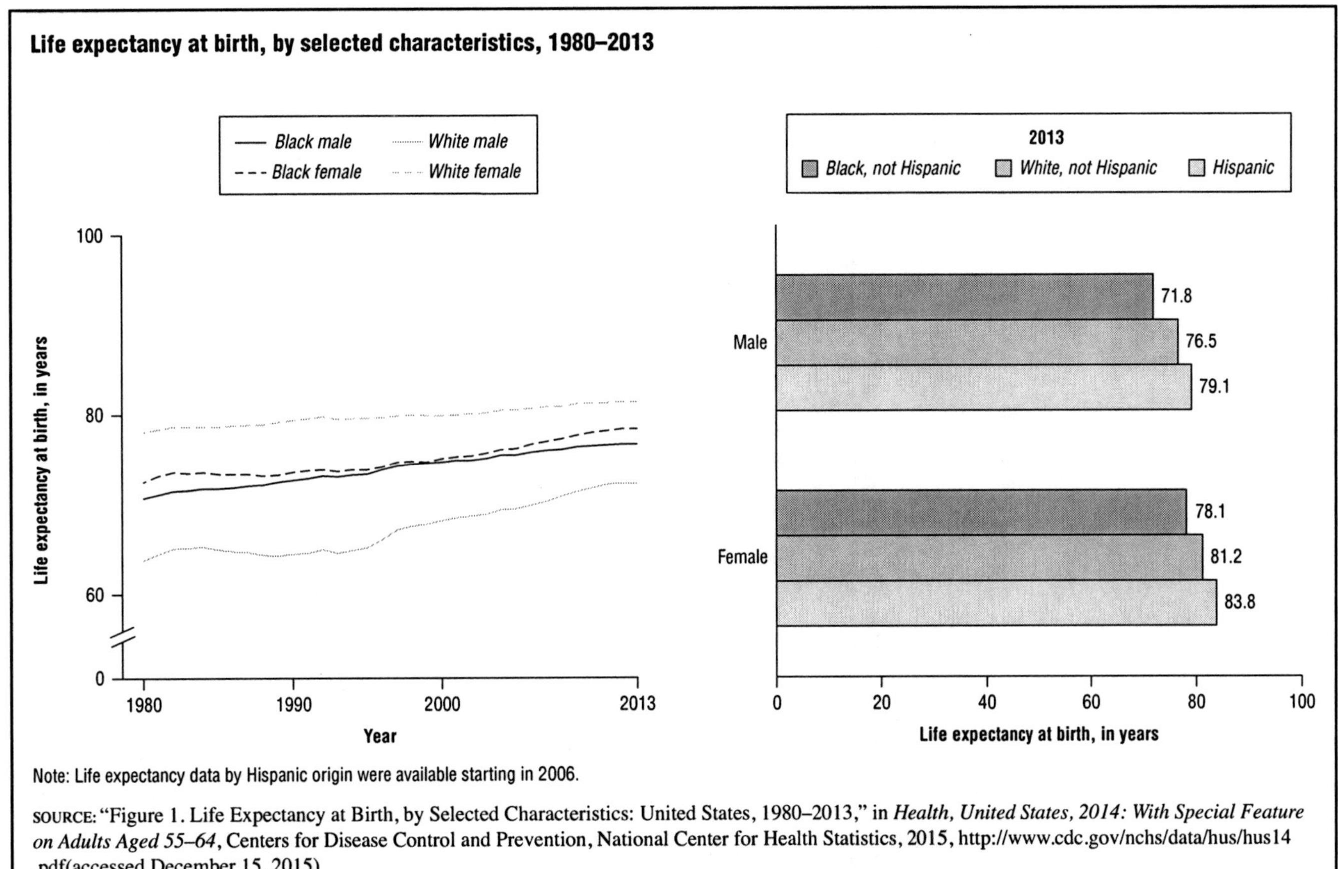

Note: Life expectancy data by Hispanic origin were available starting in 2006.

SOURCE: "Figure 1. Life Expectancy at Birth, by Selected Characteristics: United States, 1980–2013," in *Health, United States, 2014: With Special Feature on Adults Aged 55–64*, Centers for Disease Control and Prevention, National Center for Health Statistics, 2015, http://www.cdc.gov/nchs/data/hus/hus14.pdf(accessed December 15, 2015)

was longer in Australia, Austria, Belgium, Canada, Denmark, Finland, France, Germany, Greece, Iceland, Ireland, Israel, Italy, Japan, Luxembourg, the Netherlands, New Zealand, Norway, Portugal, Slovenia, South Korea, Spain, Sweden, Switzerland, and the United Kingdom.

Specific segments of the U.S. population have even lower life expectancy. For example, African American men continue to trail in terms of life expectancy. Several factors contribute to this group's significantly lower life expectancy. Besides issues of access to health care, some observers suggest that African American men must deal with greater social, economic, and psychological stress than other men, leaving them more susceptible to various diseases. Among African American males in 2013, the NCHS indicates that the observed number of deaths resulting from homicides, the human immunodeficiency virus (HIV; the virus that produces the acquired immunodeficiency syndrome), and cardiovascular disease was much higher than would be expected based on their proportion of the overall population.

Over time, the causes of death and threats to longevity have changed. As deaths from infectious diseases declined, mortality from chronic diseases, such as heart disease, cancer, and diabetes, increased. Table 1.5 displays the 10 leading causes of death in the United States in 1980 and 2013. Being overweight or obese is considered to be a contributing factor to at least four of the 10 leading causes of death in 2013: diseases of the heart, malignant neoplasms (cancer), cerebrovascular diseases (diseases affecting the supply of blood to the brain), and diabetes mellitus. Obesity may also be implicated in another leading cause of death: nephritis, nephrotic syndrome, and nephrosis (kidney disease or chronic renal failure). Table 1.5 also reveals the rise of diabetes as a cause of death. In 1980 it was the seventh-leading cause of death, claiming 34,851 lives. In 2013 it was still the seventh-leading cause of death; however, it claimed more lives: 75,578. Epidemiologists and medical researchers believe the increasing prevalence of diabetes in the U.S. population and the resultant rise in deaths that are attributable to diabetes are direct consequences of the obesity epidemic in the United States.

Recent research suggests that the steady increase in life expectancy the United States has experienced over the past two centuries is likely to end in the coming years and that life expectancy may actually decline. In "Optimizing Health in Aging Societies" (*Public Policy & Aging Report*, vol. 25, no. 2, May 2015), Laura L. Carstensen et al. observe that since the 1960s all-cause mortality rates have decreased steadily in most developed countries and life expectancy has increased. The researchers note that

TABLE 1.4

Life expectancy at birth and aged 65 and 75, by sex, race, and Hispanic origin, selected years 1900–2013

[Data are based on death certificates]

Specified age and year	All races			White			Black or African American[a]		
	Both sexes	Male	Female	Both sexes	Male	Female	Both sexes	Male	Female
At birth	Life expectancy, in years								
1900[b,c]	47.3	46.3	48.3	47.6	46.6	48.7	33.0	32.5	33.5
1950[c]	68.2	65.6	71.1	69.1	66.5	72.2	60.8	59.1	62.9
1960[c]	69.7	66.6	73.1	70.6	67.4	74.1	63.6	61.1	66.3
1970	70.8	67.1	74.7	71.7	68.0	75.6	64.1	60.0	68.3
1980	73.7	70.0	77.4	74.4	70.7	78.1	68.1	63.8	72.5
1990	75.4	71.8	78.8	76.1	72.7	79.4	69.1	64.5	73.6
1995	75.8	72.5	78.9	76.5	73.4	79.6	69.6	65.2	73.9
2000	76.8	74.1	79.3	77.3	74.7	79.9	71.8	68.2	75.1
2001	77.0	74.3	79.5	77.5	74.9	80.0	72.0	68.5	75.3
2002	77.0	74.4	79.6	77.5	74.9	80.1	72.2	68.7	75.4
2005	77.6	75.0	80.1	78.0	75.5	80.5	73.0	69.5	76.2
2006	77.8	75.2	80.3	78.3	75.8	80.7	73.4	69.9	76.7
2007	78.1	75.5	80.6	78.5	76.0	80.9	73.8	70.3	77.0
2008	78.2	75.6	80.6	78.5	76.1	80.9	74.3	70.9	77.3
2009	78.5	76.0	80.9	78.8	76.4	81.2	74.7	71.4	77.7
2010	78.7	76.2	81.0	78.9	76.5	81.3	75.1	71.8	78.0
2011	78.7	76.3	81.1	79.0	76.6	81.3	75.3	72.2	78.2
2012	78.8	76.4	81.2	79.1	76.7	81.4	75.5	72.3	78.4
2013	78.8	76.4	81.2	79.1	76.7	81.4	75.5	72.3	78.4
At 65 years									
1950[c]	13.9	12.8	15.0	14.1	12.8	15.1	13.9	12.9	14.9
1960[c]	14.3	12.8	15.8	14.4	12.9	15.9	13.9	12.7	15.1
1970	15.2	13.1	17.0	15.2	13.1	17.1	14.2	12.5	15.7
1980	16.4	14.1	18.3	16.5	14.2	18.4	15.1	13.0	16.8
1990	17.2	15.1	18.9	17.3	15.2	19.1	15.4	13.2	17.2
1995	17.4	15.6	18.9	17.6	15.7	19.1	15.6	13.6	17.1
2000	17.6	16.0	19.0	17.7	16.1	19.1	16.1	14.1	17.5
2001	17.9	16.2	19.2	18.0	16.3	19.3	16.2	14.2	17.7
2002	17.9	16.3	19.2	18.0	16.4	19.3	16.3	14.4	17.8
2005	18.4	16.9	19.6	18.5	17.0	19.7	16.9	15.0	18.3
2006	18.7	17.2	19.9	18.7	17.3	19.9	17.2	15.2	18.6
2007	18.8	17.4	20.0	18.9	17.4	20.1	17.3	15.4	18.8
2008	18.8	17.4	20.0	18.9	17.5	20.0	17.5	15.5	18.9
2009	19.1	17.7	20.3	19.2	17.7	20.3	17.8	15.9	19.2
2010	19.1	17.7	20.3	19.2	17.8	20.3	17.8	15.9	19.3
2011	19.2	17.8	20.3	19.2	17.8	20.4	18.0	16.2	19.4
2012	19.3	17.9	20.5	19.3	18.0	20.4	18.1	16.2	19.5
2013	19.3	17.9	20.5	19.3	18.0	20.5	18.1	16.3	19.5
At 75 years									
1980	10.4	8.8	11.5	10.4	8.8	11.5	9.7	8.3	10.7
1990	10.9	9.4	12.0	11.0	9.4	12.0	10.2	8.6	11.2
1995	11.0	9.7	11.9	11.1	9.7	12.0	10.2	8.8	11.1
2000	11.0	9.8	11.8	11.0	9.8	11.9	10.4	9.0	11.3
2001	11.2	9.9	12.0	11.2	10.0	12.1	10.5	9.0	11.5
2002	11.2	10.0	12.0	11.2	10.0	12.1	10.5	9.1	11.5
2005	11.5	10.4	12.3	11.5	10.4	12.3	10.9	9.4	11.2
2006	11.7	10.6	12.5	11.1	10.6	12.5	11.1	9.1	12.0
2007	11.9	10.7	12.6	11.9	10.8	12.6	11.2	9.8	12.1
2008	11.8	10.7	12.6	11.8	10.7	12.6	11.3	9.8	12.2
2009	12.1	11.0	12.9	12.1	10.4	12.9	11.6	10.2	12.5
2010	12.1	11.0	12.9	12.1	11.0	12.8	11.6	10.2	12.5
2011	12.1	11.1	12.9	12.1	11.0	12.8	11.7	10.4	12.5
2012	12.2	11.2	12.9	12.1	11.1	12.9	11.8	10.4	12.7
2013	12.2	11.2	12.9	12.1	11.1	12.9	11.8	10.4	12.7

improvements in health have been extended into old age and that in 2012 the U.S. population included more people 60 years and older than under the age of 15 years. Nonetheless, Carstensen et al. caution that "many experts today believe that in a single generation, obesity may erase all of the health gains made in the last 50 years."

MORTALITY

Years of Potential Life Lost

Years of potential life lost (YPLL) is a term used by medical and public health professionals to describe the number of years deceased people might have lived if they had not died prematurely (before their life expectancy). In 2013 most

TABLE 1.4

Life expectancy at birth and aged 65 and 75, by sex, race, and Hispanic origin, selected years 1900–2013 [CONTINUED]

[Data are based on death certificates]

Specified age and year	White, not Hispanic			Black, not Hispanic			Hispanic[d]		
	Both sexes	Male	Female	Both sexes	Male	Female	Both sexes	Male	Female
	Life expectancy, in years								
At birth									
2006	78.2	75.7	80.6	73.1	69.5	76.4	80.3	77.5	82.9
2007	78.4	75.9	80.8	73.5	69.9	76.7	80.7	77.8	83.2
2008	78.4	76.0	80.7	73.9	70.5	77.0	80.8	78.0	83.3
2009	78.7	76.3	81.1	74.3	70.9	77.4	81.1	78.4	83.5
2010	78.8	76.4	81.1	74.7	71.4	77.7	81.2	78.5	83.8
2011	78.8	76.4	81.1	74.9	71.7	77.8	81.4	78.8	83.7
2012	78.9	76.6	81.2	75.1	71.8	78.1	81.6	79.1	83.9
2013	78.9	76.5	81.2	75.1	71.8	78.1	81.6	79.1	83.8
At 65 years									
2006	18.7	17.2	19.9	17.1	15.1	18.5	20.2	18.5	21.5
2007	18.8	17.4	20.0	17.2	15.3	18.7	20.5	18.7	21.7
2008	18.8	17.4	20.0	17.4	15.4	18.8	20.4	18.7	21.6
2009	19.1	17.7	19.5	17.7	15.8	19.1	20.7	19.0	21.9
2010	19.1	17.7	20.3	17.7	15.8	19.1	20.6	18.8	22.0
2011	19.1	17.8	20.3	17.9	16.1	19.2	20.7	19.1	21.8
2012	19.3	17.9	20.4	18.0	16.1	19.4	21.0	19.5	22.1
2013	19.3	17.9	20.4	18.0	16.1	19.4	20.9	19.3	22.0
At 75 years									
2006	11.7	10.6	12.5	11.1	9.6	12.0	13.0	11.7	13.7
2007	11.8	10.7	12.6	11.2	9.7	12.1	13.1	11.8	13.8
2008	11.8	10.7	12.6	11.3	9.8	12.2	13.0	11.7	13.8
2009	12.0	11.0	12.9	11.6	10.1	12.4	13.3	12.0	13.8
2010	12.0	11.0	12.8	11.6	10.1	12.5	13.2	11.7	14.1
2011	12.0	11.0	12.8	11.7	10.4	12.5	13.2	12.0	13.9
2012	12.1	11.1	12.9	11.7	10.4	12.6	13.5	12.3	14.2
2013	12.1	11.1	12.9	11.7	10.4	12.6	13.4	12.3	14.1

[a]Data shown for 1900–1960 are for the nonwhite population.
[b]Death registration area only. The death registration area increased from 10 states and the District of Columbia (D.C.) in 1900 to the coterminous United States in 1933.
[c]Includes deaths of persons who were not residents of the 50 states and D.C.
[d]Hispanic origin was added to the U.S. standard death certificate in 1989 and was adopted by every state in 1997. To estimate life expectancy, age-specific death rates were corrected to address racial and ethnic misclassification, which underestimates deaths in the Hispanic population. Life expectancies for the Hispanic population are adjusted for underreporting on the death certificate of Hispanic ethnicity, but are not adjusted to account for the potential effects of return migration. To address the effects of age misstatement at the oldest ages, the probability of death for Hispanic persons older than 80 years is estimated as a function of non-Hispanic white mortality with the use of the Brass relational logit model.
Notes: Populations for computing life expectancy for 1991–1999 are 1990-based postcensal estimates of the U.S. resident population. Starting with *Health, United States, 2012*, populations for computing life expectancy for 2001–2009 were based on intercensal population estimates of the U.S. resident population. Populations for computing life expectancy for 2010 were based on 2010 census counts. Life expectancy for 2011 and beyond was computed using 2010-based postcensal estimates. In 2000, the life table methodology was revised. The revised methodology is similar to that developed for the 1999–2001 decennial life tables. In 2008, the life table methodology was further refined. Starting with 2003 data, some states allowed the reporting of more than one race on the death certificate. The multiple-race data for these states were bridged to the single-race categories of the 1977 Office of Management and Budget standards, for comparability with other states. The race groups, white and black include persons of Hispanic and non-Hispanic origin. Persons of Hispanic origin may be of any race.

SOURCE: "Table 16. Life Expectancy at Birth, at Age 65, and at Age 75, by Sex, Race and Hispanic Origin: United States, Selected Years 1900–2013," in *Health, United States, 2014: With Special Feature on Adults Aged 55–64*, Centers for Disease Control and Prevention, National Center for Health Statistics, 2015, http://www.cdc.gov/nchs/data/hus/hus14.pdf (accessed December 15, 2015)

YPLL resulted from heart disease, malignant neoplasms, or unintentional injuries (accidents). (See Table 1.6.)

The increase in life expectancy during the 20th and 21st centuries has meant a decrease in the YPLL rate. In 1980 a total of 10,448.4 years per 100,000 population were lost to people younger than the age of 75 years; by 2013 this number had declined to 6,593.1 total years lost. (See Table 1.6.) Although heart disease remains the number-one killer in the United States (see Table 1.5), it has been responsible for a smaller proportion of YPLL since 1980 (2,238.7 in 1980 and 952.3 in 2013). Similarly, the years lost to cerebrovascular diseases (e.g., strokes), liver diseases, influenza and pneumonia, and motor vehicle accidents have also declined since 1980. However, YPLL rates for diabetes increased over this same period, dropping slightly between 2000 and 2010, and chronic lower respiratory diseases followed a similar pattern. The years lost to HIV infection steadily decreased between 1990 and 2013.

Except for suicide, the YPLL due to all causes was significantly higher for African Americans than it was for whites. In 2013 for all causes, African Americans lost 9,528.5 years per 100,000 population, compared with 6,338.2 years for whites. (See Table 1.6.) African Americans lost considerably more years of life to heart disease, cerebrovascular diseases, cancers, HIV, and homicide than did whites.

RACIAL AND SEX DIFFERENCES. In *Health, United States, 2014*, the NCHS notes that significant racial and ethnic variations exist in the 10 leading causes of death. In 2013 chronic liver disease and cirrhosis were not listed as

TABLE 1.5

Leading causes of death and numbers of deaths by sex, race, and Hispanic origin, 1980 and 2013

[Data are based on death certificates]

Sex, race, Hispanic origin, and rank order	1980		2013*	
	Cause of death	Deaths	Cause of death	Deaths
All persons				
Rank	All causes	1,989,841	All causes	2,596,993
1	Diseases of heart	761,085	Diseases of heart	611,105
2	Malignant neoplasms	416,509	Malignant neoplasms	584,881
3	Cerebrovascular diseases	170,225	Chronic lower respiratory diseases	149,205
4	Unintentional injuries	105,718	Unintentional injuries	130,557
5	Chronic obstructive pulmonary diseases	56,050	Cerebrovascular diseases	128,978
6	Pneumonia and influenza	54,619	Alzheimer's disease	84,767
7	Diabetes mellitus	34,851	Diabetes mellitus*	75,578
8	Chronic liver disease and cirrhosis	30,583	Influenza and pneumonia	56,979
9	Atherosclerosis	29,449	Nephritis, nephrotic syndrome and nephrosis*	47,112
10	Suicide	26,869	Suicide	41,149
Male				
Rank	All causes	1,075,078	All causes	1,306,034
1	Diseases of heart	405,661	Diseases of heart	321,347
2	Malignant neoplasms	225,948	Malignant neoplasms	307,559
3	Unintentional injuries	74,180	Unintentional injuries	81,916
4	Cerebrovascular diseases	69,973	Chronic lower respiratory diseases	70,317
5	Chronic obstructive pulmonary diseases	38,625	Cerebrovascular diseases	53,691
6	Pneumonia and influenza	27,574	Diabetes mellitus*	39,841
7	Suicide	20,505	Suicide	32,055
8	Chronic liver disease and cirrhosis	19,768	Influenza and pneumonia	26,804
9	Homicide	18,779	Alzheimer's disease	25,836
10	Diabetes mellitus	14,325	Chronic liver disease and cirrhosis	23,709
Female				
Rank	All causes	914,763	All causes	1,290,959
1	Diseases of heart	355,424	Diseases of heart	289,758
2	Malignant neoplasms	190,561	Malignant neoplasms	277,322
3	Cerebrovascular diseases	100,252	Chronic lower respiratory diseases	78,888
4	Unintentional injuries	31,538	Cerebrovascular diseases	75,287
5	Pneumonia and influenza	27,045	Alzheimer's disease	58,931
6	Diabetes mellitus	20,526	Unintentional injuries	48,641
7	Atherosclerosis	17,848	Diabetes mellitus*	35,737
8	Chronic obstructive pulmonary diseases	17,425	Influenza and pneumonia	30,175
9	Chronic liver disease and cirrhosis	10,815	Nephritis, nephrotic syndrome and nephrosis*	23,619
10	Certain conditions originating in the perinatal period	9,815	Septicemia	20,162
White				
Rank	All causes	1,738,607	All causes	2,217,103
1	Diseases of heart	683,347	Diseases of heart	522,645
2	Malignant neoplasms	368,162	Malignant neoplasms	498,116
3	Cerebrovascular diseases	148,734	Chronic lower respiratory diseases	136,682
4	Unintentional injuries	90,122	Unintentional injuries	112,803
5	Chronic obstructive pulmonary diseases	52,375	Cerebrovascular diseases	107,909
6	Pneumonia and influenza	48,369	Alzheimer's disease	77,387
7	Diabetes mellitus	28,868	Diabetes mellitus*	58,925
8	Atherosclerosis	27,069	Influenza and pneumonia	49,013
9	Chronic liver disease and cirrhosis	25,240	Nephritis, nephrotic syndrome and nephrosis	37,270
10	Suicide	24,829	Suicide	37,154
Black or African American				
Rank	All causes	233,135	All causes	302,969
1	Diseases of heart	72,956	Diseases of heart	72,010
2	Malignant neoplasms	45,037	Malignant neoplasms	67,953
3	Cerebrovascular diseases	20,135	Cerebrovascular diseases	16,269
4	Unintentional injuries	13,480	Unintentional injuries	13,413
5	Homicide	10,172	Diabetes mellitus*	13,385
6	Certain conditions originating in the perinatal period	6,961	Chronic lower respiratory diseases	9,918
7	Pneumonia and influenza	5,648	Nephritis, nephrotic syndrome and nephrosis*	8,393
8	Diabetes mellitus	5,544	Homicide	8,059
9	Chronic liver disease and cirrhosis	4,790	Septicemia	6,250
10	Nephritis, nephrotic syndrome and nephrosis	3,416	Alzheimer's disease	5,714

leading causes of death for all Americans; they were, however, listed as leading causes of death among Native Americans or Alaskan Natives and Hispanics. (See Table 1.5.) Homicide was a leading cause of death for African American, Hispanic, and Native American or Alaskan Native men; however, it was not among the top-10 causes of death for white and Asian or Pacific Islander men. Essential hypertension and hypertensive renal disease was a leading cause of

TABLE 1.5

Leading causes of death and numbers of deaths by sex, race, and Hispanic origin, 1980 and 2013 [CONTINUED]

[Data are based on death certificates]

Sex, race, Hispanic origin, and rank order	1980		2013*	
	Cause of death	Deaths	Cause of death	Deaths
American Indian or Alaska Native				
Rank	All causes	6,923	All causes	17,052
1	Diseases of heart	1,494	Diseases of heart	3,139
2	Unintentional injuries	1,290	Malignant neoplasms	3,109
3	Malignant neoplasms	770	Unintentional injuries	1,833
4	Chronic liver disease and cirrhosis	410	Diabetes mellitus*	959
5	Cerebrovascular diseases	322	Chronic liver disease and cirrhosis	944
6	Pneumonia and influenza	257	Chronic lower respiratory diseases	757
7	Homicide	217	Cerebrovascular diseases	595
8	Diabetes mellitus	210	Suicide	521
9	Certain conditions originating in the perinatal period	199	Influenza and pneumonia	375
10	Suicide	181	Nephritis, nephrotic syndrome and nephrosis*	302
Asian or Pacific Islander				
Rank	All causes	11,071	All causes	59,869
1	Diseases of heart	3,265	Malignant neoplasms	15,703
2	Malignant neoplasms	2,522	Diseases of heart	13,311
3	Cerebrovascular diseases	1,028	Cerebrovascular diseases	4,205
4	Unintentional injuries	810	Unintentional injuries	2,508
5	Pneumonia and influenza	342	Diabetes mellitus[1]	2,309
6	Suicide	249	Influenza and pneumonia	2,024
7	Certain conditions originating in the perinatal period	246	Chronic lower respiratory diseases	1,848
8	Diabetes mellitus	227	Alzheimer's disease	1,428
9	Homicide	211	Nephritis, nephrotic syndrome and nephrosis*	1,147
10	Chronic obstructive pulmonary diseases	207	Suicide	1,121
Hispanic or Latino				
Rank	—	—	All causes	163,241
1	—	—	Malignant neoplasms	35,147
2	—	—	Diseases of heart	33,243
3	—	—	Unintentional injuries	12,015
4	—	—	Cerebrovascular diseases	8,127
5	—	—	Diabetes mellitus*	7,632
6	—	—	Chronic liver disease and cirrhosis	5,141
7	—	—	Chronic lower respiratory diseases	4,827
8	—	—	Alzheimer's disease	4,127
9	—	—	Influenza and pneumonia	3,592
10	—	—	Nephritis, nephrotic syndrome and nephrosis*	3,083
White male				
Rank	All causes	933,878	All causes	1,110,956
1	Diseases of heart	364,679	Diseases of heart	275,101
2	Malignant neoplasms	198,188	Malignant neoplasms	263,167
3	Unintentional injuries	62,963	Unintentional injuries	70,161
4	Cerebrovascular diseases	60,095	Chronic lower respiratory diseases	63,757
5	Chronic obstructive pulmonary diseases	35,977	Cerebrovascular diseases	44,203
6	Pneumonia and influenza	23,810	Diabetes mellitus*	31,745
7	Suicide	18,901	Suicide	28,943
8	Chronic liver disease and cirrhosis	16,407	Alzheimer's disease	23,648
9	Diabetes mellitus	12,125	Influenza and pneumonia	22,907
10	Atherosclerosis	10,543	Chronic liver disease and cirrhosis	20,884
Black or African American male				
Rank	All causes	130,138	All causes	154,767
1	Diseases of heart	37,877	Diseases of heart	37,096
2	Malignant neoplasms	25,861	Malignant neoplasms	34,671
3	Unintentional injuries	9,701	Unintentional injuries	9,017
4	Cerebrovascular diseases	9,194	Cerebrovascular diseases	7,338
5	Homicide	8,274	Homicide	6,937
6	Certain conditions originating in the perinatal period	3,869	Diabetes mellitus*	6,378
7	Pneumonia and influenza	3,386	Chronic lower respiratory diseases	5,073
8	Chronic liver disease and cirrhosis	3,020	Nephritis, nephrotic syndrome and nephrosis*	3,976
9	Chronic obstructive pulmonary diseases	2,429	Septicemia	2,882
10	Diabetes mellitus	2,010	Influenza and pneumonia	2,696

death for African American and Asian or Pacific Islander women, but it was not a leading cause of death for white, Native American or Alaskan Native, or Hispanic women.

AGE DIFFERENCES. The 10 leading causes of death vary by age. In 2013 accidents (unintentional injuries) were the leading cause of death for children one to four

TABLE 1.5

Leading causes of death and numbers of deaths by sex, race, and Hispanic origin, 1980 and 2013 [CONTINUED]

[Data are based on death certificates]

Sex, race, Hispanic origin, and rank order	1980 Cause of death	1980 Deaths	2013* Cause of death	2013* Deaths
American Indian or Alaska Native male				
Rank	All causes	4,193	All causes	9,331
1	Unintentional injuries	946	Diseases of heart	1,843
2	Diseases of heart	917	Malignant neoplasms	1,650
3	Malignant neoplasms	408	Unintentional injuries	1,177
4	Chronic liver disease and cirrhosis	239	Chronic liver disease and cirrhosis	511
5	Cerebrovascular diseases	163	Diabetes mellitus*	490
6	Homicide	162	Suicide	401
7	Pneumonia and influenza	148	Chronic lower respiratory diseases	370
8	Suicide	147	Cerebrovascular diseases	253
9	Certain conditions originating in the perinatal period	107	Influenza and pneumonia	190
10	Diabetes mellitus	86	Homicide	187
Asian or Pacific Islander male				
Rank	All causes	6,809	All causes	30,980
1	Diseases of heart	2,174	Malignant neoplasms	8,071
2	Malignant neoplasms	1,485	Diseases of heart	7,307
3	Unintentional injuries	556	Cerebrovascular diseases	1,897
4	Cerebrovascular diseases	521	Unintentional injuries	1,561
5	Pneumonia and influenza	227	Diabetes mellitus*	1,228
6	Suicide	159	Chronic lower respiratory diseases	1,117
7	Chronic obstructive pulmonary diseases	158	Influenza and pneumonia	1,011
8	Homicide	151	Suicide	820
9	Certain conditions originating in the perinatal period	128	Nephritis, nephrotic syndrome and nephrosis*	574
10	Diabetes mellitus	103	Alzheimer's disease	447
Hispanic or Latino male				
Rank	—	—	All causes	88,880
1	—	—	Diseases of heart	18,377
2	—	—	Malignant neoplasms	18,371
3	—	—	Unintentional injuries	8,760
4	—	—	Diabetes mellitus*	3,934
5	—	—	Cerebrovascular diseases	3,841
6	—	—	Chronic liver disease and cirrhosis	3,552
7	—	—	Chronic lower respiratory diseases	2,536
8	—	—	Suicide	2,279
9	—	—	Homicide	2,132
10	—	—	Influenza and pneumonia	1,816
White female				
Rank	All causes	804,729	All causes	1,106,147
1	Diseases of heart	318,668	Diseases of heart	247,544
2	Malignant neoplasms	169,974	Malignant neoplasms	234,949
3	Cerebrovascular diseases	88,639	Chronic lower respiratory diseases	72,925
4	Unintentional injuries	27,159	Cerebrovascular diseases	63,706
5	Pneumonia and influenza	24,559	Alzheimer's disease	53,739
6	Diabetes mellitus	16,743	Unintentional injuries	42,642
7	Atherosclerosis	16,526	Diabetes mellitus*	27,180
8	Chronic obstructive pulmonary diseases	16,398	Influenza and pneumonia	26,106
9	Chronic liver disease and cirrhosis	8,833	Nephritis, nephrotic syndrome and nephrosis*	18,470
10	Certain conditions originating in the perinatal period	6,512	Septicemia	16,287
Black or African American female				
Rank	All causes	102,997	All causes	148,202
1	Diseases of heart	35,079	Diseases of heart	34,914
2	Malignant neoplasms	19,176	Malignant neoplasms	33,282
3	Cerebrovascular diseases	10,941	Cerebrovascular diseases	8,931
4	Unintentional injuries	3,779	Diabetes mellitus*	7,007
5	Diabetes mellitus	3,534	Chronic lower respiratory diseases	4,845
6	Certain conditions originating in the perinatal period	3,092	Nephritis, nephrotic syndrome and nephrosis*	4,417
7	Pneumonia and influenza	2,262	Unintentional injuries	4,396
8	Homicide	1,898	Alzheimer's disease	4,050
9	Chronic liver disease and cirrhosis	1,770	Septicemia	3,368
10	Nephritis, nephrotic syndrome and nephrosis	1,722	Essential hypertension and hypertensive renal disease	2,959

TABLE 1.5

Leading causes of death and numbers of deaths by sex, race, and Hispanic origin, 1980 and 2013 [CONTINUED]

[Data are based on death certificates]

Sex, race, Hispanic origin, and rank order	1980 Cause of death	1980 Deaths	2013* Cause of death	2013* Deaths
American Indian or Alaska Native female				
Rank	All causes	2,730	All causes	7,721
1	Diseases of heart	577	Malignant neoplasms	1,459
2	Malignant neoplasms	362	Diseases of heart	1,296
3	Unintentional injuries	344	Unintentional injuries	656
4	Chronic liver disease and cirrhosis	171	Diabetes mellitus*	469
5	Cerebrovascular diseases	159	Chronic liver disease and cirrhosis	433
6	Diabetes mellitus	124	Chronic lower respiratory diseases	387
7	Pneumonia and influenza	109	Cerebrovascular diseases	342
8	Certain conditions originating in the perinatal period	92	Influenza and pneumonia	185
9	Nephritis, nephrotic syndrome and nephrosis	56	Alzheimer's disease	161
10	Homicide	55	Nephritis, nephrotic syndrome and nephrosis*	159
Asian or Pacific Islander female				
Rank	All causes	4,262	All causes	28,889
1	Diseases of heart	1,091	Malignant neoplasms	7,632
2	Malignant neoplasms	1,037	Diseases of heart	6,004
3	Cerebrovascular diseases	507	Cerebrovascular diseases	2,308
4	Unintentional injuries	254	Diabetes mellitus*	1,081
5	Diabetes mellitus	124	Influenza and pneumonia	1,013
6	Certain conditions originating in the perinatal period	118	Alzheimer's disease	981
7	Pneumonia and influenza	115	Unintentional injuries	947
8	Congenital anomalies	104	Chronic lower respiratory diseases	731
9	Suicide	90	Nephritis, nephrotic syndrome and nephrosis*	573
10	Homicide	60	Essential hypertension and hypertensive renal disease	550
Hispanic or Latino female				
Rank	—	—	All causes	74,361
1	—	—	Malignant neoplasms	16,776
2	—	—	Diseases of heart	14,866
3	—	—	Cerebrovascular diseases	4,286
4	—	—	Diabetes mellitus*	3,698
5	—	—	Unintentional injuries	3,255
6	—	—	Alzheimer's disease	2,829
7	—	—	Chronic lower respiratory diseases	2,291
8	—	—	Influenza and pneumonia	1,776
9	—	—	Chronic liver disease and cirrhosis	1,589
10	—	—	Nephritis, nephrotic syndrome and nephrosis*	1,500

—Data not available. Complete coverage of all states for the Hispanic origin variable began in 1997.
*Starting with 2011 data, the rules for selecting Renal failure as the underlying cause of death were changed, affecting the number of deaths in the Nephritis, nephrotic syndrome and nephrosis and Diabetes categories. These changes directly affect deaths with mention of Renal failure and other associated conditions, such as Diabetes mellitus with renal complications. The result is a decrease in the number of deaths for Nephritis, nephrotic syndrome and nephrosis and an increase in the number of deaths for Diabetes mellitus. Therefore, trend data for these two causes of death should be interpreted with caution.
Notes: Starting with 2003 data, some states allowed the reporting of more than one race on the death certificate. The multiple-race data for these states were bridged to the single-race categories of the 1977 Office of Management and Budget standards, for comparability with other states. The race groups, white, black, Asian or Pacific Islander, and American Indian or Alaska Native, include persons of Hispanic and non-Hispanic origin. Persons of Hispanic origin may be of any race.

SOURCE: "Table 20. Leading Causes of Death and Numbers of Deaths, by Sex, Race, and Hispanic Origin: United States, 1980 and 2013," in *Health, United States, 2014: With Special Feature on Adults Aged 55–64*, Centers for Disease Control and Prevention, National Center for Health Statistics, 2015, http://www.cdc.gov/nchs/data/hus/hus14.pdf (accessed December 15, 2015)

years of age, followed by congenital malformations, deformations, and chromosomal abnormalities, homicide, and malignant neoplasms. (See Table 1.7.) Among children five to 14 years old, accidents were a leading cause of death, followed by cancer, suicide, and congenital malformations, deformations, and chromosomal abnormalities.

Accidents were the leading cause of death in 2013 for young people aged 15 to 24 years. (See Table 1.7.) Suicide was the second-leading cause of death, followed by homicide. Cancer was the fourth-leading cause of death among this age group.

Among adults aged 25 to 44 years in 2010, accidents were the most frequent cause of death, and cancer was second. (See Table 1.7.) Heart disease and suicide were the third- and fourth-leading causes of death, respectively, followed by homicide, chronic liver disease and cirrhosis, and diabetes.

TABLE 1.6

Years of potential life lost before aged 75 for selected causes of death, by sex, race, and Hispanic origin, selected years 1980–2013

[Data are based on death certificates]

Sex, race, Hispanic origin, and cause of death	Crude	Age-adjusted[a]					
	2013	1980	1990	2000	2010	2012	2013
All persons	Years lost before age 75 per 100,000 population under age 75						
All causes	7,002.7	10,448.4	9,085.5	7,578.1	6,642.9	6,588.0	6,593.1
Diseases of heart	1,070.9	2,238.7	1,617.7	1,253.0	972.4	951.9	952.3
Ischemic heart disease	630.4	1,729.3	1,153.6	841.8	577.3	558.4	546.1
Cerebrovascular diseases	177.2	357.5	259.6	223.3	169.3	161.6	158.1
Malignant neoplasms	1,527.1	2,108.8	2,003.8	1,674.1	1,395.8	1,356.2	1,328.6
Trachea, bronchus, and lung	362.1	548.5	561.4	443.1	331.3	309.9	298.2
Colorectal	139.2	190.0	164.7	141.9	125.0	123.0	123.5
Prostate[b]	57.6	84.9	96.8	63.6	52.2	48.1	47.5
Breast[c]	278.5	463.2	451.6	332.6	262.4	256.0	250.0
Chronic lower respiratory diseases	211.1	169.1	187.4	188.1	172.4	171.6	176.6
Influenza and pneumonia	88.8	160.2	141.5	87.1	71.4	67.4	82.3
Chronic liver disease and cirrhosis	192.0	300.3	196.9	164.1	163.9	173.3	176.9
Diabetes mellitus[f]	189.3	134.4	155.9	178.4	158.2	164.3	168.3
Alzheimer's disease	14.0	†	†	10.9	11.7	11.0	11.1
Human immunodeficiency virus (HIV) disease	57.7	...	383.8	174.6	76.6	61.8	58.1
Unintentional injuries	1,027.8	1,543.5	1,162.1	1,026.5	1,025.2	1,046.1	1,051.2
Motor vehicle-related injuries	378.6	912.9	716.4	574.3	400.6	402.4	386.6
Poisoning	417.1	68.0	81.2	163.6	379.7	408.8	430.9
Nephritis, nephrotic syndrome and nephrosis[d]	74.4	—	50.4	70.7	73.1	65.2	65.7
Suicide[e]	394.4	392.0	393.1	334.5	385.2	402.1	401.6
Homicide[e]	222.1	425.5	417.4	266.5	239.0	240.9	229.8
Male							
All causes	8,678.3	13,777.2	11,973.5	9,572.2	8,329.5	8,249.1	8,249.5
Diseases of heart	1,473.5	3,352.1	2,356.0	1,766.0	1,370.8	1,336.6	1,338.2
Ischemic heart disease	917.1	2,715.1	1,766.3	1,255.4	864.8	831.8	816.2
Cerebrovascular diseases	200.3	396.7	286.6	244.6	190.7	183.7	182.1
Malignant neoplasms	1,609.9	2,360.8	2,214.6	1,810.8	1,500.8	1,450.9	1,415.9
Trachea, bronchus, and lung	408.5	821.1	764.8	554.9	390.5	361.1	345.1
Colorectal	162.4	214.9	194.3	167.3	148.0	144.4	146.8
Prostate	57.6	84.9	96.8	63.6	52.2	48.1	47.5
Chronic lower respiratory diseases	215.0	235.1	224.8	206.0	182.8	179.7	185.2
Influenza and pneumonia	100.5	202.5	180.0	102.8	82.6	77.5	94.1
Chronic liver disease and cirrhosis	260.0	415.0	283.9	236.9	226.9	237.2	242.1
Diabetes mellitus[d]	229.4	140.4	170.4	203.8	194.8	203.5	208.6
Alzheimer's disease	12.1	†	†	10.6	10.7	10.2	10.2
Human immunodeficiency virus (HIV) disease	83.8	...	686.2	258.9	109.5	87.0	84.3
Unintentional injuries	1,441.8	2,342.7	1,715.1	1,475.6	1,432.1	1,459.7	1,463.5
Motor vehicle-related injuries	546.7	1,359.7	1,018.4	796.4	569.2	574.3	552.2
Poisoning	557.4	96.4	123.6	242.1	503.8	541.5	573.1
Nephritis, nephrotic syndrome and nephrosis[d]	83.3	—	58.9	81.1	82.3	75.3	75.3
Suicide[e]	612.0	605.6	634.8	539.1	607.0	625.9	619.8
Homicide[e]	359.7	675.0	658.0	410.5	380.3	383.6	365.9
Female							
All causes	5,337.8	7,350.3	6,333.1	5,644.6	4,994.0	4,959.6	4,967.9
Diseases of heart	670.8	1,246.0	948.5	774.6	593.6	585.4	584.5
Ischemic heart disease	345.4	852.1	600.3	457.6	305.2	299.3	290.0
Cerebrovascular diseases	154.2	324.0	235.9	203.9	149.1	140.7	135.4
Malignant neoplasms	1,444.9	1,896.8	1,826.6	1,555.3	1,301.0	1,271.0	1,250.3
Trachea, bronchus, and lung	315.9	310.4	382.2	342.1	276.9	262.8	255.1
Colorectal	116.2	168.7	138.7	118.7	103.4	102.8	101.5
Breast	278.5	463.2	451.6	332.6	262.4	256.0	250.0
Chronic lower respiratory diseases	207.2	114.0	155.9	172.3	162.8	164.1	168.7
Influenza and pneumonia	77.1	122.0	106.2	72.3	60.7	57.8	70.9
Chronic liver disease and cirrhosis	124.3	194.5	115.1	94.5	103.5	111.9	114.4
Diabetes mellitus[d]	149.5	128.5	142.3	154.4	123.5	127.0	129.8
Alzheimer's disease	15.8	†	†	11.1	12.6	11.8	12.0
Human immunodeficiency virus (HIV) disease	31.8	...	87.8	92.0	44.4	37.2	32.5
Unintentional injuries	616.4	755.3	607.4	573.2	616.4	629.6	635.7
Motor vehicle-related injuries	211.5	470.4	411.6	348.5	230.5	228.7	219.0
Poisoning	277.7	40.2	39.1	85.0	255.1	275.1	287.7
Nephritis, nephrotic syndrome and nephrosis[d]	65.5	—	42.4	60.8	64.6	55.6	56.6
Suicide[e]	178.3	184.2	153.3	129.1	163.7	177.6	182.5
Homicide[e]	85.4	181.3	174.3	118.9	94.9	94.9	90.4

Among adults 45 to 64 years old, cancer and heart disease were ranked the first- and second-leading causes of death, respectively. (See Table 1.7.) Among those aged 65 years and older, these two categories were reversed.

TABLE 1.6

Years of potential life lost before aged 75 for selected causes of death, by sex, race, and Hispanic origin, selected years 1980–2013 [CONTINUED]

[Data are based on death certificates]

Sex, race, Hispanic origin, and cause of death	Crude	Age-adjusted[a]					
	2013	1980	1990	2000	2010	2012	2013
White[f]	Years lost before age 75 per 100,000 population under age 75						
All causes	6,864.3	9,554.1	8,159.5	6,949.5	6,342.8	6,321.6	6,338.2
Diseases of heart	1,032.2	2,100.8	1,490.3	1,149.4	900.9	882.5	881.8
Ischemic heart disease	640.1	1,682.7	1,113.4	805.3	563.7	544.8	532.0
Cerebrovascular diseases	157.7	300.7	213.1	187.1	142.7	138.7	135.1
Malignant neoplasms	1,572.4	2,035.9	1,929.3	1,627.8	1,375.8	1,340.7	1,317.7
Trachea, bronchus, and lung	383.0	529.9	544.2	436.3	332.8	311.4	300.4
Colorectal	138.5	186.8	157.8	134.1	118.4	117.9	118.6
Prostate[b]	53.9	74.8	86.6	54.3	45.3	42.1	41.9
Breast[c]	272.0	460.2	441.7	315.6	245.0	239.3	236.0
Chronic lower respiratory diseases	228.7	165.4	182.3	185.3	176.1	175.3	180.1
Influenza and pneumonia	86.7	130.8	116.9	77.7	66.7	63.2	78.4
Chronic liver disease and cirrhosis	210.6	257.3	175.8	162.7	173.5	185.9	189.3
Diabetes mellitus[d]	174.3	115.7	133.7	155.6	139.0	145.4	149.2
Alzheimer's disease	15.8	†	†	11.4	12.4	11.7	11.8
Human immunodeficiency virus (HIV) disease	31.6	...	309.0	94.7	39.9	32.8	31.5
Unintentional injuries	1,089.1	1,520.4	1,139.7	1,031.8	1,098.6	1,119.7	1,125.2
Motor vehicle-related injuries	387.4	939.9	726.7	586.1	419.0	420.1	401.2
Poisoning	472.2	64.9	74.4	167.2	435.4	467.6	493.0
Nephritis, nephrotic syndrome and nephrosis[d]	62.1	—	37.0	52.5	57.4	51.1	52.7
Suicide[e]	440.3	414.5	417.7	362.0	430.8	450.8	451.2
Homicide[e]	120.6	271.7	234.9	156.6	138.7	135.9	127.7
Black or African American[f]							
All causes	9,508.1	17,873.4	16,593.0	12,897.1	9,832.5	9,555.7	9,528.5
Diseases of heart	1,597.4	3,619.9	2,891.8	2,275.2	1,691.1	1,645.0	1,647.0
Ischemic heart disease	757.2	2,305.1	1,676.1	1,300.1	818.8	792.0	776.7
Cerebrovascular diseases	309.9	883.2	656.4	507.0	358.1	326.5	319.2
Malignant neoplasms	1,645.8	2,946.1	2,894.8	2,294.7	1,796.7	1,724.1	1,666.7
Trachea, bronchus, and lung	363.6	776.0	811.3	593.0	405.6	377.5	362.4
Colorectal	169.2	232.3	241.8	222.4	188.6	177.0	174.2
Prostate[b]	100.7	200.3	223.5	171.0	127.3	113.6	109.9
Breast[c]	384.2	524.2	592.9	500.0	420.8	406.2	389.8
Chronic lower respiratory diseases	198.2	203.7	240.6	232.7	187.7	192.8	200.1
Influenza and pneumonia	121.4	384.9	330.8	161.2	109.8	106.2	122.9
Chronic liver disease and cirrhosis	120.5	644.0	371.8	185.6	120.2	116.2	122.4
Diabetes mellitus[d]	314.4	305.3	361.5	383.4	316.4	316.6	323.8
Alzheimer's disease	8.9	†	†	8.3	10.0	9.3	9.8
Human immunodeficiency virus (HIV) disease	224.4	...	1,014.7	763.3	329.5	259.0	238.4
Unintentional injuries	955.2	1,751.5	1,392.7	1,152.8	896.7	925.8	953.0
Motor vehicle-related injuries	408.4	750.2	699.5	580.8	393.4	404.0	402.6
Poisoning	253.2	99.4	144.3	196.6	218.9	242.1	265.6
Nephritis, nephrotic syndrome and nephrosis[d]	161.1	—	160.9	216.9	193.2	172.4	165.7
Suicide[e]	208.7	238.0	261.4	208.7	196.4	210.4	207.0
Homicide[e]	847.5	1,580.8	1,612.9	941.6	821.2	842.9	813.5
American Indian or Alaska Native[f]							
All causes	6,359.5	13,390.9	9,506.2	7,758.2	6,771.3	6,842.6	6,698.8
Diseases of heart	708.1	1,819.9	1,391.0	1,030.1	820.6	797.4	807.4
Ischemic heart disease	419.3	1,208.2	901.8	709.3	487.6	486.4	484.4
Cerebrovascular diseases	107.6	269.3	223.3	198.1	129.7	121.5	124.1
Malignant neoplasms	755.5	1,101.3	1,141.1	995.7	929.5	856.9	852.4
Trachea, bronchus, and lung	141.6	181.1	268.1	227.8	211.0	188.5	166.0
Colorectal	91.4	78.8	82.4	93.8	95.8	90.0	103.3
Prostate[b]	26.3	66.7	42.0	44.5	36.8	36.7	32.6
Breast[c]	97.7	205.5	213.4	174.1	145.0	120.0	108.5
Chronic lower respiratory diseases	116.0	89.3	129.0	151.8	154.5	133.2	135.6
Influenza and pneumonia	99.6	307.9	206.3	124.0	99.3	80.8	109.0
Chronic liver disease and cirrhosis	497.9	1,190.3	535.1	519.4	510.8	553.3	562.2
Diabetes mellitus[d]	248.2	305.5	292.3	305.6	267.6	286.4	281.7
Alzheimer's disease	4.5	†	†	*	8.8	6.2	5.7
Human immunodeficiency virus (HIV) disease	30.2	...	70.1	68.4	46.1	32.1	33.8
Unintentional injuries	1,389.5	3,541.0	2,183.9	1,700.1	1,377.7	1,505.2	1,388.2
Motor vehicle-related injuries	603.5	2,102.4	1,301.5	1,032.2	570.6	637.0	575.7
Poisoning	464.0	92.9	119.5	180.1	449.6	514.1	487.3
Nephritis, nephrotic syndrome and nephrosis[d]	65.3	—	88.5	102.0	81.7	67.5	73.7
Suicide[e]	480.9	515.0	495.9	403.1	437.9	437.6	463.0
Homicide[e]	234.9	628.9	434.2	278.5	256.4	244.5	227.8

TABLE 1.6

Years of potential life lost before aged 75 for selected causes of death, by sex, race, and Hispanic origin, selected years 1980–2013 [CONTINUED]

[Data are based on death certificates]

. . .Category not applicable.
—Data not available.
†Data for Alzheimer's disease are only presented for data years 1999 and beyond.
*Rates based on fewer than 20 deaths are considered unreliable and are not shown.
[a]Age-adjusted rates are calculated using the year 2000 standard population. Prior to 2001, age-adjusted rates were calculated using standard million proportions based on rounded population numbers. Starting with 2001 data, unrounded population numbers are used to calculate age-adjusted rates.
[b]Rate for male population only.
[c]Rate for female population only.
[d]Starting with 2011 data, the rules for selecting Renal failure as the underlying cause of death were changed, affecting the number of deaths in the Nephritis, nephrotic syndrome and nephrosis and Diabetes categories. These changes directly affect deaths with mention of Renal failure and other associated conditions, such as Diabetes mellitus with renal complications. The result is a decrease in the number of deaths for Nephritis, nephrotic syndrome and nephrosis and an increase in the number of deaths for Diabetes mellitus. Therefore, trend data for these two causes of death should be interpreted with caution.
[e]Figures for 2001 include September 11-related deaths for which death certificates were filed as of October 24, 2002.
[f]The race groups, white, black, Asian or Pacific Islander, and American Indian or Alaska Native, include persons of Hispanic and non-Hispanic origin. Persons of Hispanic origin may be of any race. Death rates for Hispanic, American Indian or Alaska Native, and Asian or Pacific Islander persons should be interpreted with caution because of inconsistencies in reporting Hispanic origin or race on the death certificate (death rate numerators) compared with population figures (death rate denominators). The net effect of misclassification is an underestimation of deaths and death rates for races other than white and black.
Notes: Starting with *Health, United States, 2003,* rates for 1991–1999 were revised using intercensal population estimates based on the 1990 and 2000 censuses. For 2000, population estimates are bridged-race April 1 census counts. Starting with *Health, United States, 2012,* rates for 2001–2009 were revised using intercensal population estimates based on the 2000 and 2010 censuses. For 2010, population estimates are bridged-race April 1 census counts. Rates for 2011 and beyond were computed using 2010-based postcensal estimates. Starting with 2003 data, some states allowed the reporting of more than one race on the death certificate. The multiple-race data for these states were bridged to the single-race categories of the 1977 Office of Management and Budget standards, for comparability with other states.

SOURCE: Adapted from "Table 19. Years of Potential Life Lost before Age 75 for Selected Causes of Death, by Sex, Race, and Hispanic Origin: United States, Selected Years 1980–2013," in *Health, United States, 2014: With Special Feature on Adults Aged 55–64*, Centers for Disease Control and Prevention, National Center for Health Statistics, 2015, http://www.cdc.gov/nchs/data/hus/hus14.pdf (accessed December 15, 2015)

SELF-ASSESSED HEALTH STATUS

The NCHS regularly asks respondents to the National Health Interview Survey to evaluate their health status. Figure 1.7 shows that between 1997 and June 2015 the percentage of people who considered their health to be excellent or very good was relatively unchanged, ranging from a high of 69.1% in 1998 but hovering around 66% for most years. Between January and June 2015, 66.2% of respondents assessed their health as excellent or very good.

Overall, men were slightly more likely to rate their health as excellent. (See Figure 1.8.) For both men and women, however, the percentage who considered their health as excellent or very good decreased with advancing age—85% for those under the age of 18 years, 64% for those aged 18 to 64 years, and 45% for those aged 65 years and older. (See Figure 1.9.) Compared with the 70.8% of non-Hispanic white survey respondents who assessed their health as excellent or very good, fewer non-Hispanic African American (59.2%) and Hispanic (59.3%) survey respondents rated their health status as excellent or very good. (See Figure 1.10.)

TABLE 1.7

Leading causes of death and numbers of deaths by age, 1980 and 2013

[Data are based on death certificates]

	1980		2013*	
Age and rank order	**Cause of death**	**Deaths**	**Cause of death**	**Deaths**
Under 1 year				
Rank	All causes	45,526	All causes	23,440
1	Congenital anomalies	9,220	Congenital malformations, deformations and chromosomal abnormalities	4,758
2	Sudden infant death syndrome	5,510	Disorders related to short gestation and low birthweight, not elsewhere classified	4,202
3	Respiratory distress syndrome	4,989	Newborn affected by maternal complications of pregnancy	1,595
4	Disorders relating to short gestation and unspecified low birthweight	3,648	Sudden infant death syndrome	1,563
5	Newborn affected by maternal complications of pregnancy	1,572	Unintentional injuries	1,156
6	Intrauterine hypoxia and birth asphyxia	1,497	Newborn affected by complications of placenta, cord and membranes	953
7	Unintentional injuries	1,166	Bacterial sepsis of newborn	578
8	Birth trauma	1,058	Respiratory distress of newborn	522
9	Pneumonia and influenza	1,012	Diseases of circulatory system	458
10	Newborn affected by complications of placenta, cord, and membranes	985	Neonatal hemorrhage	389
1–4 years				
Rank	All causes	8,187	All causes	4,068
1	Unintentional injuries	3,313	Unintentional injuries	1,316
2	Congenital anomalies	1,026	Congenital malformations, deformations and chromosomal abnormalities	476
3	Malignant neoplasms	573	Homicide	337
4	Diseases of heart	338	Malignant neoplasms	328
5	Homicide	319	Diseases of heart	169
6	Pneumonia and influenza	267	Influenza and pneumonia	102
7	Meningitis	223	Chronic lower respiratory diseases	64
8	Meningococcal infection	110	Septicemia	53
9	Certain conditions originating in the perinatal period	84	In situ neoplasms, benign neoplasms and neoplasms of uncertain or unknown behavior	47
10	Septicemia	71	Certain conditions originating in the perinatal period	45
5–14 years				
Rank	All causes	10,689	All causes	5,340
1	Unintentional injuries	5,224	Unintentional injuries	1,521
2	Malignant neoplasms	1,497	Malignant neoplasms	895
3	Congenital anomalies	561	Suicide	395
4	Homicide	415	Congenital malformations, deformations and chromosomal abnormalities	340
5	Diseases of heart	330	Homicide	277
6	Pneumonia and influenza	194	Diseases of heart	173
7	Suicide	142	Chronic lower respiratory diseases	155
8	Benign neoplasms	104	Influenza and pneumonia	128
9	Cerebrovascular diseases	95	Cerebrovascular diseases	89
10	Chronic obstructive pulmonary diseases	85	In situ neoplasms, benign neoplasms and neoplasms of uncertain or unknown behavior	65
15–24 years				
Rank	All causes	49,027	All causes	28,486
1	Unintentional injuries	26,206	Unintentional injuries	11,619
2	Homicide	6,537	Suicide	4,878
3	Suicide	5,239	Homicide	4,329
4	Malignant neoplasms	2,683	Malignant neoplasms	1,496
5	Diseases of heart	1,223	Diseases of heart	941
6	Congenital anomalies	600	Congenital malformations, deformations and chromosomal abnormalities	362
7	Cerebrovascular diseases	418	Influenza and pneumonia	197
8	Pneumonia and influenza	348	Diabetes mellitus*	193
9	Chronic obstructive pulmonary diseases	141	Pregnancy, childbirth, and the puerperium	178
10	Anemias	133	Chronic lower respiratory diseases	155

TABLE 1.7

Leading causes of death and numbers of deaths by age, 1980 and 2013 [CONTINUED]

[Data are based on death certificates]

	1980		2013*	
Age and rank order	**Cause of death**	**Deaths**	**Cause of death**	**Deaths**
25–44 years				
Rank	All causes	108,658	All causes	115,036
1	Unintentional injuries	26,722	Unintentional injuries	31,563
2	Malignant neoplasms	17,551	Malignant neoplasms	15,022
3	Diseases of heart	14,513	Diseases of heart	13,599
4	Homicide	10,983	Suicide	12,899
5	Suicide	9,855	Homicide	6,817
6	Chronic liver disease and cirrhosis	4,782	Chronic liver disease and cirrhosis	3,167
7	Cerebrovascular diseases	3,154	Diabetes mellitus*	2,636
8	Diabetes mellitus	1,472	Cerebrovascular diseases	2,195
9	Pneumonia and influenza	1,467	Human immunodeficiency virus (HIV) disease	1,877
10	Congenital anomalies	817	Influenza and pneumonia	1,330
45–64 years				
Rank	All causes	425,338	All causes	515,851
1	Diseases of heart	148,322	Malignant neoplasms	159,509
2	Malignant neoplasms	135,675	Diseases of heart	107,735
3	Cerebrovascular diseases	19,909	Unintentional injuries	37,414
4	Unintentional injuries	18,140	Chronic liver disease and cirrhosis	20,736
5	Chronic liver disease and cirrhosis	16,089	Chronic lower respiratory diseases	20,561
6	Chronic obstructive pulmonary diseases	11,514	Diabetes mellitus*	18,960
7	Diabetes mellitus	7,977	Cerebrovascular diseases	16,789
8	Suicide	7,079	Suicide	15,756
9	Pneumonia and influenza	5,804	Septicemia	7,790
10	Homicide	4,019	Influenza and pneumonia	7,012
65 years and over				
Rank	All causes	1,341,848	All causes	1,904,640
1	Diseases of heart	595,406	Diseases of heart	488,156
2	Malignant neoplasms	258,389	Malignant neoplasms	407,558
3	Cerebrovascular diseases	146,417	Chronic lower respiratory diseases	127,194
4	Pneumonia and influenza	45,512	Cerebrovascular diseases	109,602
5	Chronic obstructive pulmonary diseases	43,587	Alzheimer's disease	83,786
6	Atherosclerosis	28,081	Diabetes mellitus*	53,751
7	Diabetes mellitus	25,216	Influenza and pneumonia	48,031
8	Unintentional injuries	24,844	Unintentional injuries	45,942
9	Nephritis, nephrotic syndrome, and nephrosis	12,968	Nephritis, nephrotic syndrome and nephrosis*	39,080
10	Chronic liver disease and cirrhosis	9,519	Septicemia	28,815

*Starting with 2011 data, the rules for selecting renal failure as the underlying cause of death were changed, affecting the number of deaths in the nephritis, nephrotic syndrome and nephrosis and diabetes categories. These changes directly affect deaths with mention of renal failure and other associated conditions, such as diabetes mellitus with renal complications. The result is a decrease in the number of deaths for nephritis, nephrotic syndrome and nephrosis and an increase in the number of deaths for diabetes mellitus. Therefore, trend data for these two causes of death should be interpreted with caution.

SOURCE: "Table 21. Leading Causes of Death and Numbers of Deaths, by Age: United States, 1980 and 2013," in *Health, United States, 2014: With Special Feature on Adults Aged 55–64*, Centers for Disease Control and Prevention, National Center for Health Statistics, 2015, http://www.cdc.gov/nchs/data/hus/hus14.pdf (accessed December 15, 2015)

FIGURE 1.7

Percentage of persons of all ages who said their health was excellent or very good, 1997–June 2015

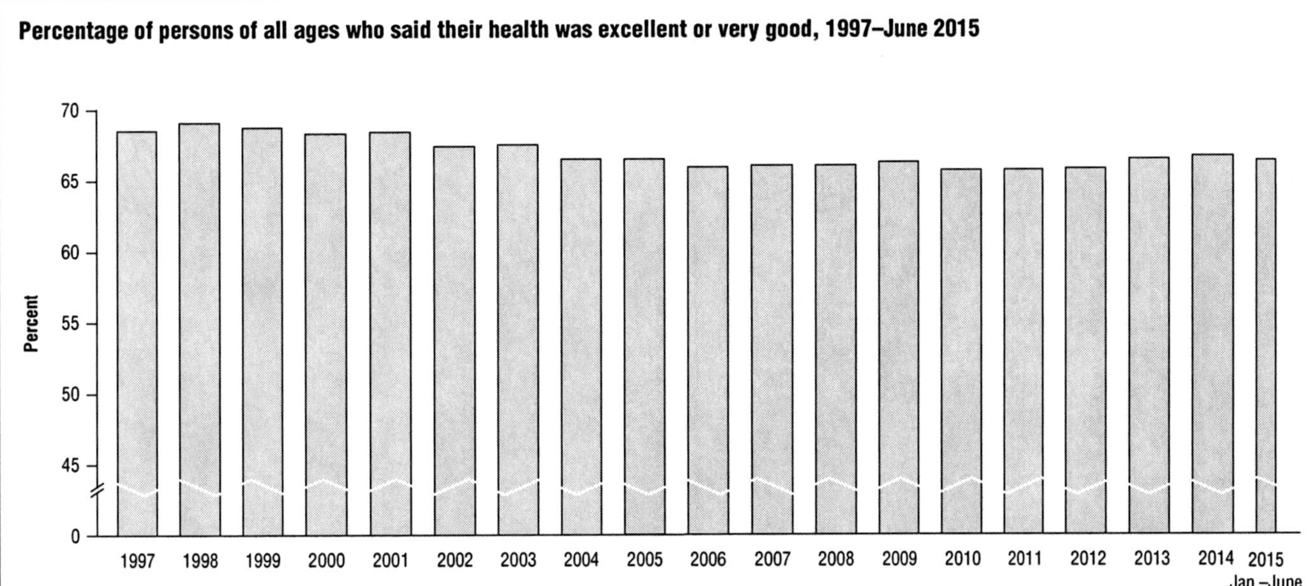

Notes: Data are based on household interviews of a sample of the civilian noninstitutionalized population. Health status data were obtained by asking respondents to assess their own health and that of family members living in the same household as excellent, very good, good, fair, or poor. The analyses excluded persons with unknown health status (about 0.2% of respondents each year).

SOURCE: "Figure 11.1. Percentage of Persons of All Ages Who Had Excellent or Very Good Health: United States, 1997–June 2015," in *Early Release of Selected Estimates Based on Data from the January–June 2015 National Health Interview Survey*, Centers for Disease Control and Prevention, National Center for Health Statistics, November 2015, http://www.cdc.gov/nchs/data/nhis/earlyrelease/earlyrelease201511_11.pdf (accessed December 16, 2015)

FIGURE 1.8

Percentage distribution of respondent-assessed health status, by sex, for all ages, January–June 2015

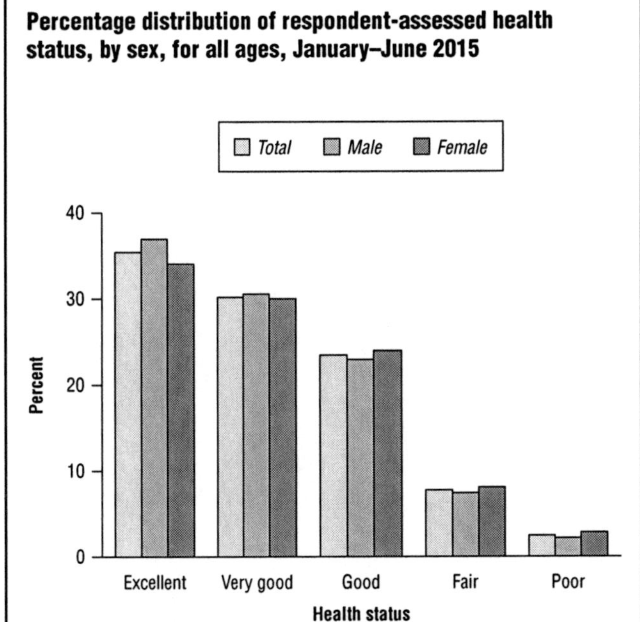

Notes: Data are based on household interviews of a sample of the civilian noninstitutionalized population. Health status data were obtained by asking respondents to assess their own health and that of family members living in the same household as excellent, very good, good, fair, or poor. The analyses excluded the 0.1% of persons with unknown health status.

SOURCE: "Figure 11.2. Percent Distribution of Respondent-Assessed Health Status for All Ages, by Sex: United States, January–June 2015," in *Early Release of Selected Estimates Based on Data from the January–June 2015 National Health Interview Survey*, Centers for Disease Control and Prevention, National Center for Health Statistics, November 2015, http://www.cdc.gov/nchs/data/nhis/earlyrelease/earlyrelease201511_11.pdf (accessed December 16, 2015)

FIGURE 1.9

Percentage of persons of all ages who said their health was excellent or very good, by age group and sex, January–June 2015

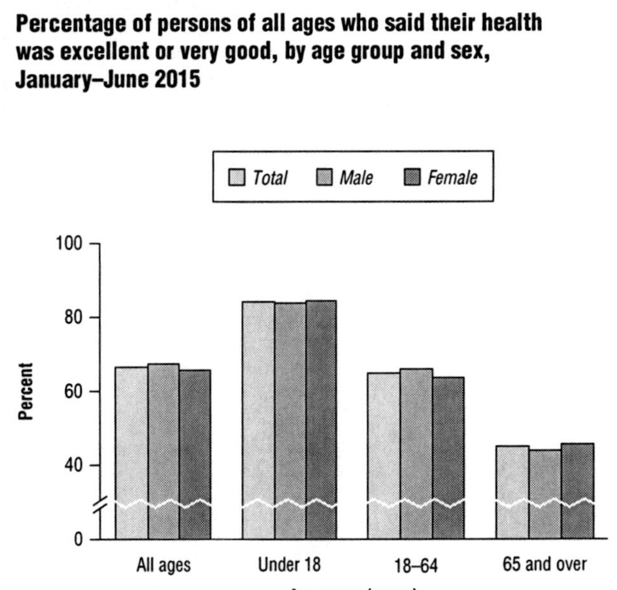

Notes: Data are based on household interviews of a sample of the civilian noninstitutionalized population. Health status data were obtained by asking respondents to assess their own health and that of family members living in the same household as excellent, very good, good, fair, or poor. The analyses excluded the 0.1% of persons with unknown health status.

SOURCE: "Figure 11.3. Percentage of Persons of All Ages Who Had Excellent or Very Good Health, by Age Group and Sex: United States, January–June 2015," in *Early Release of Selected Estimates Based on Data from the January–June 2015 National Health Interview Survey*, Centers for Disease Control and Prevention, National Center for Health Statistics, November 2015, http://www.cdc.gov/nchs/data/nhis/earlyrelease/earlyrelease201511_11.pdf (accessed December 16, 2015)

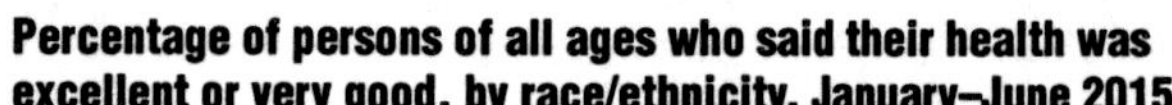

FIGURE 1.10

Percentage of persons of all ages who said their health was excellent or very good, by race/ethnicity, January–June 2015

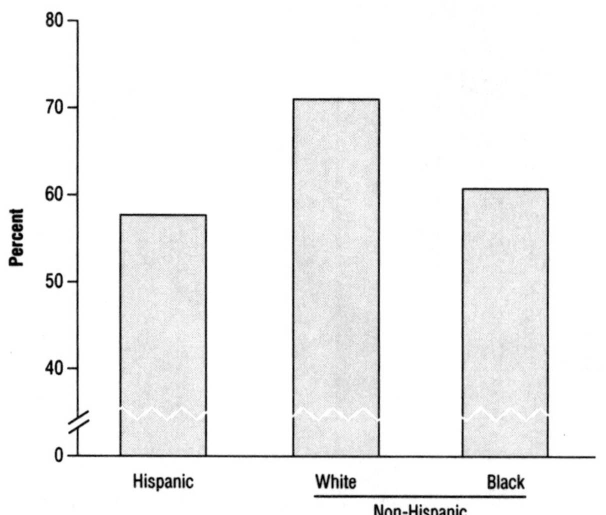

Notes: Data are based on household interviews of a sample of the civilian noninstitutionalized population. Health status data were obtained by asking respondents to assess their own health and that of family members living in the same household as excellent, very good, good, fair, or poor. The analyses excluded the 0.1% of persons with unknown health status. Estimates are age-sex adjusted using the projected 2000 U.S. population as the standard population and using three age groups: under 18, 18–64, and 65 and over.

SOURCE: "Figure 11.4. Age-Sex-Adjusted Percentage of Persons of All Ages Who Had Excellent or Very Good Health, by Race/Ethnicity: United States, January–June 2015," *Early Release of Selected Estimates Based on Data from the January–June 2015 National Health Interview Survey*, Centers for Disease Control and Prevention, National Center for Health Statistics, November 2015, http://www.cdc.gov/nchs/data/nhis/earlyrelease/earlyrelease201511_11.pdf (accessed December 16, 2015)

CHAPTER 2
PREVENTION OF DISEASE

Prevention is better than cure.

—Desiderius Erasmus

Preventing disease involves a wide range of interrelated programs, actions, and activities. Some prevention measures are sweeping global policy initiatives, such as national and state government actions to reduce health risks by limiting air pollution and other toxic exposures or to increase standards to ensure the safety of food and water supplies. Others are focused efforts of public health professionals and agencies, such as the National Institutes of Health's Office of Disease Prevention, the Centers for Disease Control and Prevention (CDC), and the American Cancer Society (ACS), to reduce the incidence (occurrence of new cases) of specific diseases such as heart disease, diabetes (a disease in which the body's inability to produce or effectively use the hormone insulin causes high levels of sugar in the blood), and lung cancer.

The effectiveness of local and global disease prevention programs largely depends on the extent to which individuals take personal responsibility for their own health by avoiding known health risks such as tobacco use, substance abuse (misuse of alcohol and drugs), and unsafe sex. People who have a healthy diet; get adequate exercise and rest; wear seat belts in automobiles and helmets on bicycles, motorcycles, and scooters; successfully manage stress; and maintain a positive outlook on life are on the front line of disease prevention. Similarly, individuals who effectively use health care resources by obtaining recommended immunizations, physical examinations, and health screenings are actively working to prevent disease and disability.

Prevention involves governments, professional organizations, public health professionals, health care practitioners (physicians, nurses, and allied health professionals), and individuals working at three levels to maintain and improve the health of communities. The first level, primary prevention, focuses on inhibiting the development of disease before it occurs. Secondary prevention, also called screening, refers to measures that detect disease before it is symptomatic. Tertiary prevention efforts focus on people who are already affected by disease and attempt to reduce resultant disability and restore functionality.

The Patient Protection and Affordable Care Act (more commonly known as the Affordable Care Act [ACA] or Obamacare) is the landmark health reform legislation signed into law by President Barack Obama (1961–) in March 2010. Besides extending health care coverage to millions of low-income and previously uninsured Americans, the ACA aims to improve access to preventive services, such as blood pressure and cholesterol tests, screening tests for breast and colon cancer, screenings for diabetes and osteoporosis, and vaccines, by requiring that health insurance companies cover these services. Besides expanding covered services for women and older adults, the ACA requires coverage of 26 preventive services for children. (See Table 2.1.)

PRIMARY PREVENTION

Primary prevention measures fall into two categories. The first category includes actions to protect against disease and disability, such as getting immunizations, ensuring the supply of safe drinking water, applying dental sealants to prevent tooth decay, and guarding against accidents. Examples of primary prevention of accidents include government and state requirements for workplace safety to prevent industrial injuries and equipping automobiles with air bags and antilock brakes. Examples of primary prevention of mental health problems include measures to strengthen family and community support systems as well as to teach children communication and interpersonal skills, conflict management, and other relationship and life skills that foster emotional resiliency.

General action to promote health is the other category of primary prevention measures. Health promotion

TABLE 2.1

26 preventive services for children covered by the Affordable Care Act

1. **Alcohol and drug use** assessments for adolescents
2. **Autism** screening for children at 18 and 24 months
3. **Behavioral** assessments for children of all ages: 0 to 11 months, 1 to 4 years, 5 to 10 years, 11 to 14 years, 15 to 17 years.
4. **Blood pressure** screening for children ages: 0 to 11 months, 1 to 4 years, 5 to 10 years, 11 to 14 years, 15 to 17 years.
5. **Cervical dysplasia** screening for sexually active females
6. **Congenital hypothyroidism** screening for newborns
7. **Depression** screening for adolescents
8. **Developmental** screening for children under age 3, and surveillance throughout childhood
9. **Dyslipidemia** screening for children at higher risk of lipid disorders ages: 1 to 4 years, 5 to 10 years, 11 to 14 years, 15 to 17 years.
10. **Fluoride chemoprevention** supplements for children without fluoride in their water source
11. **Gonorrhea** preventive medication for the eyes of all newborns
12. **Hearing** screening for all newborns
13. **Height, weight and body mass index** measurements for children ages: 0 to 11 months, 1 to 4 years, 5 to 10 years, 11 to 14 years, 15 to 17 years.
14. **Hematocrit or hemoglobin** screening for children
15. **Hemoglobinopathies** or sickle cell screening for newborns
16. **HIV** screening for adolescents at higher risk
17. **Immunization** vaccines for children from birth to age 18—doses, recommended ages, and recommended populations vary:
    - Diphtheria, tetanus, pertussis,
    - *Haemophilus influenzae* type b
    - Hepatitis A
    - Hepatitis B
    - Human papillomavirus
    - Inactivated poliovirus
    - Influenza (flu shot)
    - Measles, mumps, rubella
    - Meningococcal
    - Pneumococcal
    - Rotavirus
    - Varicella
18. **Iron** supplements for children ages 6 to 12 months at risk for anemia
19. **Lead** screening for children at risk of exposure
20. **Medical history** for all children throughout development ages: 0 to 11 months, 1 to 4 years, 5 to 10 years, 11 to 14 years, 15 to 17 years.
21. **Obesity** screening and counseling
22. **Oral health** risk assessment for young children ages: 0 to 11 months, 1 to 4 years, 5 to 10 years.
23. **Phenylketonuria (PKU)** screening for this genetic disorder in newborns
24. **Sexually transmitted infection (STI)** prevention counseling and screening for adolescents at higher risk
25. **Tuberculin** testing for children at higher risk of tuberculosis ages: 0 to 11 months, 1 to 4 years, 5 to 10 years, 11 to 14 years, 15 to 17 years.
26. **Vision** screening for all children

SOURCE: "26 Covered Preventive Services for Children," in *Preventive Care for Children*, U.S. Department of Health & Human Services, June 7, 2013, http://www.hhs.gov/healthcare/prevention/children/index.html (accessed December 15, 2015)

includes the basic activities of a healthy lifestyle: good nutrition and hygiene, adequate exercise and rest, and avoidance of environmental and health risks. Limiting exposure to sunlight, using sunscreen, and wearing protective clothing are examples of primary prevention measures to reduce the risk of developing skin cancer.

Health promotion also includes education about the other interdependent dimensions of health known as wellness. Examples of health education programs that are aimed at wellness include stress management, parenting classes, preparation for retirement from the workforce, and cooking classes.

Historically, public health programs in developed countries have emphasized the primary prevention of infectious diseases (illnesses caused by microorganisms) by making environmental changes, such as improving the safety and purity of food and water supplies, and providing immunizations. Figure 2.1 shows the 2015 recommended immunizations for people up to the age of six years, Figure 2.2 shows the 2015 recommended immunizations for people aged seven to 18 years, and Figure 2.3 shows the 2015 recommended immunization schedule for adults aged 19 years and older. Immunization is a key primary prevention measure in the United States and other developed countries.

The most pressing health problems in developed countries in the 21st century are chronic diseases, such as heart disease, cancer, diabetes, and obesity. Primary prevention of chronic diseases is more challenging than primary prevention of infectious diseases because it requires changing health behaviors. Efforts to change deeply rooted and often culturally influenced patterns of behaviors—such as diet, alcohol and tobacco use, and physical inactivity—generally have been less successful than environmental health and immunization programs.

Primary prevention programs are developed in response to actual and potential threats to community public health. Recent primary prevention programs have examined ways to prevent smoking and obesity and to increase physical activity. In 2016 primary prevention programs included encouraging seasonal flu immunizations to reduce the spread and incidence of influenza and initiatives such as First Lady Michelle Obama's (1964–) Let's Move! (http://www.letsmove.gov), which aims to prevent childhood obesity.

Primary Prevention of Childhood Obesity

According to the CDC, in "Childhood Obesity Facts" (June 19, 2015, http://www.cdc.gov/obesity/data/childhood.html), in the United States in 2011–12, 17% (12.7 million) of children and adolescents aged two to 19 years were obese. The percentages were higher among Hispanic (22.4%) and non-Hispanic African American (20.2%) children. During this period an estimated 8.4% of preschoolers (children aged two to five years) were obese.

Obese children are five times as likely as their healthy-weight peers to become overweight or obese as teens and adults. In older children and teens, obesity is associated with several health problems, including high cholesterol, high blood sugar, asthma (inflammation and obstruction of the airways that makes breathing difficult), and poor mental health.

FIGURE 2.1

Recommended immunizations for children from birth to aged 6 years, 2015

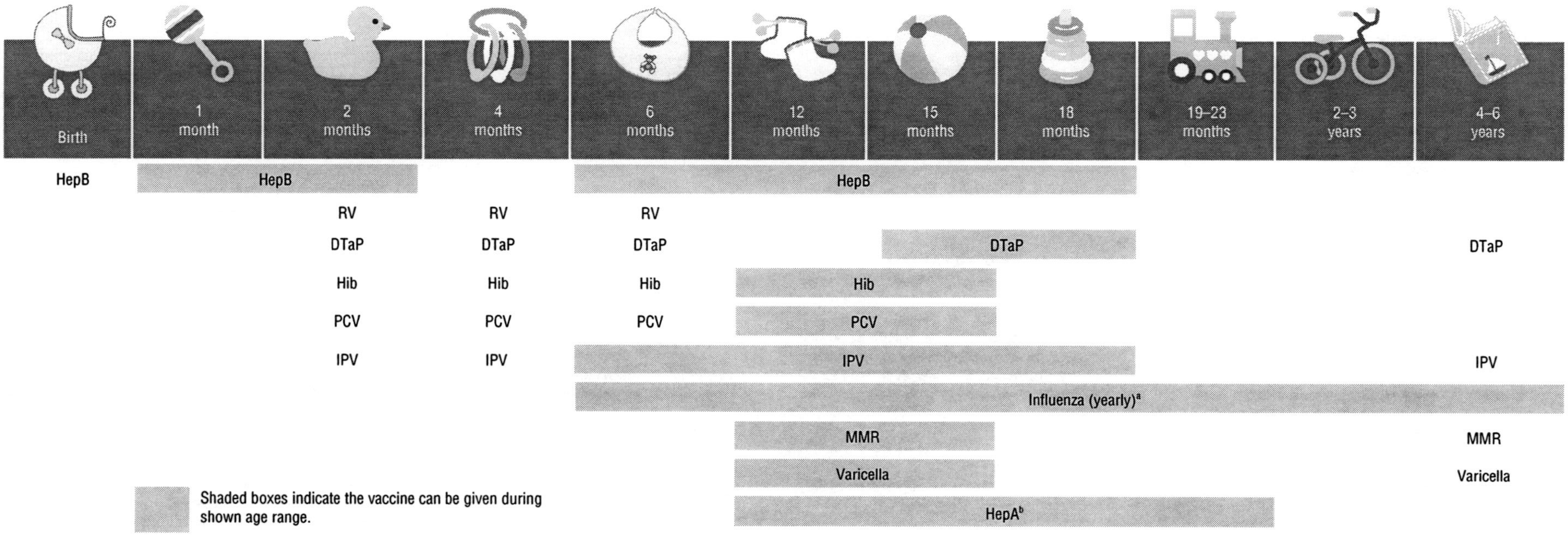

<table>
<tr><th>Birth</th><th>1 month</th><th>2 months</th><th>4 months</th><th>6 months</th><th>12 months</th><th>15 months</th><th>18 months</th><th>19–23 months</th><th>2–3 years</th><th>4–6 years</th></tr>
<tr><td>HepB</td><td colspan="2">HepB</td><td></td><td colspan="4">HepB</td><td></td><td></td><td></td></tr>
<tr><td></td><td></td><td>RV</td><td>RV</td><td>RV</td><td></td><td></td><td></td><td></td><td></td><td></td></tr>
<tr><td></td><td></td><td>DTaP</td><td>DTaP</td><td>DTaP</td><td></td><td colspan="2">DTaP</td><td></td><td></td><td>DTaP</td></tr>
<tr><td></td><td></td><td>Hib</td><td>Hib</td><td>Hib</td><td colspan="2">Hib</td><td></td><td></td><td></td><td></td></tr>
<tr><td></td><td></td><td>PCV</td><td>PCV</td><td>PCV</td><td colspan="2">PCV</td><td></td><td></td><td></td><td></td></tr>
<tr><td></td><td></td><td>IPV</td><td>IPV</td><td colspan="4">IPV</td><td></td><td></td><td>IPV</td></tr>
<tr><td></td><td></td><td></td><td></td><td colspan="7">Influenza (yearly)[a]</td></tr>
<tr><td></td><td></td><td></td><td></td><td></td><td colspan="2">MMR</td><td></td><td></td><td></td><td>MMR</td></tr>
<tr><td></td><td></td><td></td><td></td><td></td><td colspan="2">Varicella</td><td></td><td></td><td></td><td>Varicella</td></tr>
<tr><td></td><td></td><td></td><td></td><td></td><td colspan="4">HepA[b]</td><td></td><td></td></tr>
</table>

Shaded boxes indicate the vaccine can be given during shown age range.

[a]Two doses given at least four weeks apart are recommended for children aged 6 months through 8 years of age who are getting an influenza (flu) vaccine for the first time and for some other children in this age group.
[b]Two doses of HepA vaccine are needed for lasting protection. The first dose of HepA vaccine should be given between 12 months and 23 months of age. The second dose should be given 6 to 18 months later. HepA vaccination may be given to any child 12 months and older to protect against HepA. Children and adolescents who did not receive the HepA vaccine and are at high-risk, should be vaccinated against HepA.

FIGURE 2.1

Recommended immunizations for children from birth to aged 6 years, 2015 [CONTINUED]

Notes:

Disease	Vaccine	Disease spread by	Disease symptoms	Disease complications
Chickenpox	Varicella vaccine protects against chickenpox.	Air, direct contact	Rash, tiredness, headache, fever	Infected blisters, bleeding disorders, encephalitis (brain swelling), pneumonia (infection in the lungs)
Diphtheria	DTaP vaccine protects against diphtheria. DTaP combines protection against diphtheria, tetanus, and pertussis.	Air, direct contact	Sore throat, mild fever, weakness, swollen glands in neck	Swelling of the heart muscle, heart failure, coma, paralysis, death
Hib	Hib vaccine protects against *Haemophilus influenzae* type b.	Air, direct contact	May be no symptoms unless bacteria enter the blood	Meningitis (infection of the covering around the brain and spinal cord), intellectual disability, epiglottitis (life-threatening infection that can block the windpipe and lead to serious breathing problems), pneumonia (infection in the lungs), death
Hepatitis A	HepA vaccine protects against hepatitis A.	Direct contact, contaminated food or water	May be no symptoms, fever, stomach pain, loss of appetite, fatigue, vomiting, jaundice (yellowing of skin and eyes), dark urine	Liver failure, arthralgia (joint pain), kidney, pancreatic, and blood disorders
Hepatitis B	HepB vaccine protects against hepatitis B.	Contact with blood or body fluids	May be no symptoms, fever, headache, weakness, vomiting, jaundice (yellowing of skin and eyes), joint pain	Chronic liver infection, liver failure, liver cancer
Flu	Flu vaccine protects against influenza.	Air, direct contact	Fever , muscle pain, sore throat, cough, extreme fatigue	Pneumonia (infection inthe lungs)
Measles	MMR vaccine protects against measles. MMR combines protection against measles, mumps, and rubella.	Air, direct contact	Rash, fever, cough, runny nose, pinkeye	Encephalitis (brain swelling), pneumonia (infection in the lungs), death
Mumps	MMR vaccine protects against mumps. MMR combines protection against measles, mumps, and rubella.	Air, direct contact	Swollen salivary glands (under the jaw), fever, headache, tiredness, muscle pain	Meningitis (infection of the covering around the brain and spinal cord), encephalitis (brain swelling), inflammation of testicles or ovaries, deafness
Pertussis	DTaP vaccine protects against pertussis (whooping cough). DTaP combines protection against diphtheria, tetanus, and pertussis.	Air, direct contact	Severe cough, runny nose, apnea (a pause in breathing in infants)	Pneumonia (infection in the lungs), death
Polio	IPV vaccine protects against polio.	Air, direct contact, through the mouth	May be no symptoms, sore throat, fever, nausea, headache	Paralysis, death
Pneumococcal	PCV vaccine protects against pneumococcus.	Air, direct contact	May be no symptoms, pneumonia (infection in the lungs)	Bacteremia (blood infection), meningitis (infection of the covering around the brain and spinal cord), death
Rotavirus	RV vaccine protects against rotavirus.	Through the mouth	Diarrhea, fever, vomiting	Severe diarrhea, dehydration
Rubella	MMR vaccine protects against rubella. MMR combines protection against measles, mumps, and rubella.	Air, direct contact	Children infected with rubella virus sometimes have a rash, fever, swollen lymph nodes	Very serious in pregnant women—can lead to miscarriage, stillbirth, premature delivery, birth defects
Tetanus	DTaP vaccine protects against tetanus. DTaP combines protection against diphtheria, tetanus, and pertussis.	Exposure through cuts in skin	Stiffness in neck and abdominal muscles, difficulty swallowing, muscle spasms, fever	Broken bones, breathing difficulty, death

SOURCE: "2015 Recommended Immunizations for Children from Birth through 6 Years Old," in *2015 Child and Adolescent Immunization Schedules*, Centers for Disease Control and Prevention, January 2015, http://www.cdc.gov/vaccines/parents/downloads/parent-ver-sch-0-6yrs.pdf (accessed December 17, 2015)

FIGURE 2.2

Recommended immunizations for children and teens aged 7–18, 2015

☐ *These shaded boxes indicate when the vaccine is recommended for all children unless your doctor tells you that your child cannot safely receive the vaccine.*

☐ *These shaded boxes indicate the vaccine should be given if a child is catching up on missed vaccines.*

☐ *These shaded boxes indicate the vaccine is recommended for children with certain health conditions that put them at high risk for serious diseases. Note that healthy children can get the HepA series[f].*

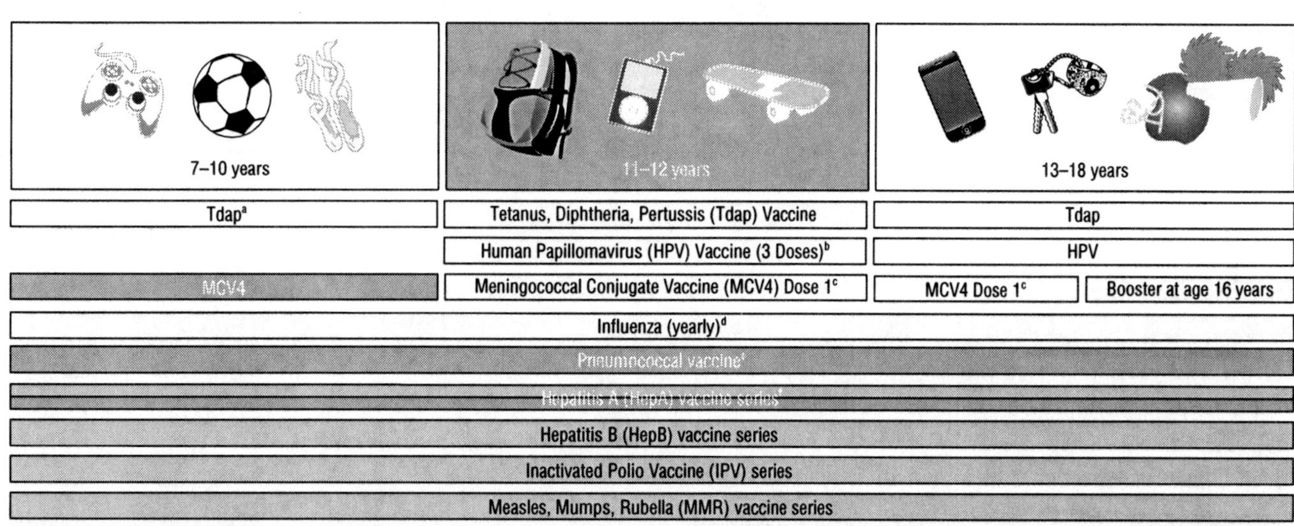

[a]Tdap vaccine is recommended at age 11 or 12 to protect against tetanus, diphtheria and pertussis. If your child has not received any or all of the DTaP vaccine series, or if you don't know if your child has received these shots, your child needs a single dose of Tdap when they are 7–10 years old. Talk to your child's health care provider to find out if they need additional catch-up vaccines.

[b]All 11 or 12 year olds—both girls *and* boys—should receive 3 doses of HPV vaccine to protect against HPV-related disease. The full HPV vaccine series should be given as recommended for best protection.

[c]Meningococcal conjugate vaccine (MCV) is recommended at age 11 or 12. A booster shot is recommended at age 16. Teens who received MCV for the first time at age 13 through 15 years will need a one-time booster dose between the ages of 16 and 18 years. If your teenager missed getting the vaccine altogether, ask their health care provider about getting it now, especially if your teenager is about to move into a college dorm or military barracks.

[d]Everyone 6 months of age and older—including preteens and teens—should get a flu vaccine every year. Children under the age of 9 years may require more than one dose. Talk to your child's health care provider to find out if they need more than one dose.

[e]Pneumococcal Conjugate Vaccine (PCV13) and Pneumococcal Polysaccharide Vaccine (PPSV23) are recommended for some children 6 through 18 years old with certain medical conditions that place them at high risk. Talk to your healthcare provider about pneumococcal vaccines and what factors may place your child at high risk for pneumococcal disease.

[f]Hepatitis A vaccination is recommended for older children with certain medical conditions that place them at high risk. HepA vaccine is licensed, safe, and effective for all children for all ages. Even if your child is not at high risk, you may decide you want your child protected against HepA. Talk to your healthcare provider about HepA vaccine and what factors may place your child at high risk for HepA.

SOURCE: "2015 Recommended Immunizations for Children from 7 through 18 Years Old," in *2013 Child and Adolescent Immunization Schedules*, Centers for Disease Control and Prevention, January 2015, http://www.cdc.gov/vaccines/who/teens/downloads/parent-version-schedule-7-18yrs.pdf (accessed December 17, 2015)

In "Progress on Childhood Obesity: Many States Show Declines" (August 2013, http://www.cdc.gov/VitalSigns/ChildhoodObesity/), the CDC describes primary prevention efforts state and local governments can take to prevent childhood obesity, including:

- Improving access to healthy, affordable foods and beverages
- Ensuring the availability of safe, free drinking water in parks, recreation areas, child care centers, and schools
- Helping schools to open gyms, playgrounds, and athletic fields during nonschool hours so children have safe places to play
- Helping child care providers improve children's nutrition and physical activity and limit computer and television time
- Forging partnerships with civic leaders, child care providers, and others to create communities that promote healthy eating and physical activity

Table 2.2 describes preventive measures the federal government, state and local officials, physicians and nurses, child care providers, and parents are taking to promote healthy eating and physical activity and prevent obesity.

The Institute of Medicine outlines in "Indicators for Measuring Progress in Obesity Prevention" (August 2013,

FIGURE 2.3

Adult immunization schedule, 2015

For all persons in this category who meet the age requirements and who lack documentation of vaccination or have no evidence of previous infection; zoster vaccine recommended regardless of prior episode of zoster

Recommended if some other risk factor is present (e.g., on the basis of medical, occupational, lifestyle, or other indication)

No recommendation

<table>
<tr><th>Vaccine ▼ Age group ▶</th><th>19–21 years</th><th>22–26 years</th><th>27–49 years</th><th>50–59 years</th><th>60–64 years</th><th>≥65 years</th></tr>
<tr><td>Influenza*</td><td colspan="6">1 dose annually</td></tr>
<tr><td>Tetanus, diphtheria, pertussis (Td/Tdap)*</td><td colspan="6">Substitute 1-time dose of Tdap for Td booster; then boost with Td every 10 years</td></tr>
<tr><td>Varicella*</td><td colspan="6">2 doses</td></tr>
<tr><td>Human papillomavirus (HPV) Female*</td><td colspan="2">3 doses</td><td></td><td></td><td></td><td></td></tr>
<tr><td>Human papillomavirus (HPV) Male*</td><td colspan="2">3 doses</td><td></td><td></td><td></td><td></td></tr>
<tr><td>Zoster</td><td></td><td></td><td></td><td></td><td colspan="2">1 dose</td></tr>
<tr><td>Measles, mumps, rubella (MMR)*</td><td colspan="4">1 or 2 doses</td><td></td><td></td></tr>
<tr><td>Pneumococcal 13-valent conjugate (PCV13)*</td><td colspan="6">1 time dose</td></tr>
<tr><td>Pneumococcal polysaccharide (PPSV23)</td><td colspan="5">1 or 2 doses</td><td>1 dose</td></tr>
<tr><td>Meningococcal*</td><td colspan="6">1 or more doses</td></tr>
<tr><td>Hepatitis A*</td><td colspan="6">2 doses</td></tr>
<tr><td>Hepatitis B*</td><td colspan="6">3 doses</td></tr>
<tr><td>Haemophilus influenzae type b (Hib)*</td><td colspan="6">1 or 3 doses</td></tr>
</table>

*Covered by the Vaccine Injury Compensation Program.

SOURCE: "Recommended Adult Immunization Schedule—United States—2015," in *Immunization Schedules*, Centers for Disease Control and Prevention, 2015, http://www.cdc.gov/vaccines/schedules/downloads/adult/adult-schedule-bw.pdf (accessed December 17, 2015)

http://www.iom.edu/~/media/Files/Report%20Files/2013/Evaluating-Obesity-Prevention-Efforts/ObesityChart.pdf) prevention strategies for schools, including increasing the proportion of:

- Students who participate in daily school physical education
- Schools that require daily physical education for all students
- School districts that require the availability of fruits or vegetables whenever other food is offered or sold
- School districts that offer a school breakfast program
- Students who consume foods and beverages at school recommended by the *Dietary Guidelines for Americans, 2010* (December 2010, http://www.health.gov/dietaryguidelines/dga2010/DietaryGuidelines2010.pdf)

The CDC reports that between 2008 and 2011 obesity rates among preschoolers decreased in 19 states and territories and increased in just three states. Although it is not yet possible to determine whether this downward trend is directly attributable to primary prevention efforts, childhood obesity steadily increased between 1998 and 2003. In "Prevalence of Obesity among Adults and Youth: United States, 2011—2014" (November 2015, http://www.cdc.gov/nchs/data/databriefs/db219.pdf), Cynthia L. Ogden et al. report that between 2011 and 2014 the prevalence of obesity among preschoolers (aged two to five years; 8.9%) was lower than among school-aged children (six to 11 years; 17.5%) and adolescents (12 to 19 years; 20.5%). Although obesity increased among adults and children between 1999–2000 and 2013–14, there was no change in prevalence among children between 2003–04 and 2013–14. Figure 2.4 shows obesity trends in adults and youth between 1999 to 2014.

SECONDARY PREVENTION

The goal of secondary prevention is to identify and detect disease in its earliest stages, before noticeable symptoms develop, when it is most likely to be treated successfully. With early detection and diagnosis, it may be possible to cure a disease, slow its progression, prevent or minimize complications, and limit disability.

Another goal of secondary prevention is to prevent the spread of communicable diseases (illnesses that can be transmitted from one person to another). In the community,

TABLE 2.2

Actions to prevent childhood obesity

Federal government is:

- Funding states and communities to implement programs that promote healthy eating and physical activity.
- Measuring trends in childhood obesity and its risk factors.
- Funding research to investigate the causes and effects of childhood obesity and to identify effective interventions.
- Providing training and resources for parents, child care centers and communities to help prevent childhood obesity through initiatives such as We Can! and the First Lady's Let's Move! initiative.
- Helping low-income families to get affordable, nutritious foods through programs such as the Supplemental Nutrition Program for Women, Infants, and Children (WIC) and the Child and Adult Care Feeding Program.

State and local officials can:

- Create partnerships with community members such as civic leaders and child care providers to make community changes that promote healthy eating and active living.
- Make it easier for families with children to buy healthy, affordable foods and beverages nearby.
- Help provide access to safe, free drinking water in places such as community parks, recreation areas, child care centers, and schools.
- Help local schools open up gyms, playgrounds, and sports fields during nonschool hours so more children can safely play.
- Help child care providers use best practices for improving nutrition, increasing physical activity, and decreasing computer and television time.

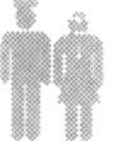

Doctors and nurses can:

- Measure children's weight, height and body mass index routinely.
- Counsel parents about nutrition and physical activity for their children.
- Connect families with community resources such as nutrition education and breastfeeding support services.

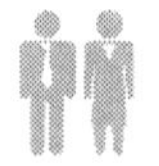

Child care providers and parents can:

- Serve fruits and vegetables and other nutritious foods for meals and snacks.
- Be role models by eating healthy meals and snacks with preschoolers.
- Make water easily available throughout the day.
- Limit the time preschoolers watch TV or use the computer in child care and the home.
- Support and encourage preschoolers to be physically active every day.

SOURCE: "What Can Be Done," in "Progress on Childhood Obesity," *CDC Vitalsigns*, Centers for Disease Control and Prevention, August 2013, http://www.cdc.gov/vitalsigns/pdf/2013-08-vitalsigns.pdf (accessed December 17, 2015)

early identification and treatment of people with communicable diseases, such as sexually transmitted infections, provides not only secondary prevention for those who are infected but also primary prevention for people who come in contact with infected individuals.

Like primary prevention, individual health care practitioners and public health agencies and organizations perform secondary prevention. An example of secondary prevention that is conducted by many different professionals (physicians, nurses, and allied health professionals) in a variety of settings (medical offices, clinics, and health fairs) is blood pressure screening to identify people with hypertension (high blood pressure). An example of mental health secondary prevention is the effort to identify young children with behavior problems to intervene early and prevent development of, or progression to, more serious mental disorders.

The U.S. Preventive Services Task Force (USPSTF; January 2016, http://www.uspreventiveservicestaskforce.org/Page/Name/about-the-uspstf) was convened in 1984 by the U.S. Public Health Service to evaluate clinical research in order to assess the merits of preventive measures, including screening tests, counseling, immunizations, and preventive medications. Consisting of an independent panel of experts, the task force "works to improve the health of all Americans by making evidence-based recommendations about clinical preventive services such as screenings, counseling services, and preventive medications." It also stipulates the preventive measures that should be taken by healthy adult men, women, pregnant women, and children. Figure 2.5 shows the process the USPSTF uses as it researches, weighs the evidence, and develops and disseminates recommendations. Table 2.3 lists the preventive services that are recommended by the USPSTF. The recommendations include screening to detect and identify a wide range of conditions, including high blood pressure, depression, obesity, and sexually transmitted infections such as chlamydia and syphilis infection.

Secondary prevention plays an important role in diseases such as diabetes, glaucoma (a disorder caused by too much fluid pressure inside the eyeball), breast cancer, and cancer of the cervix (the opening of the uterus). State and local health departments, voluntary health agencies, hospitals, medical clinics, schools, and physicians often conduct screenings for these conditions during which people with no signs or symptoms are tested to uncover these diseases in their earliest stages.

USPSTF Updates Screening Guidelines for Breast Cancer and Skin Cancer

The USPSTF issued updated recommendations for breast cancer screening in January 2016. In "Breast Cancer Screening Final Recommendation" (2016, http://screeningforbreastcancer.org), the USPSTF recommends that mammography screening begin at age 50 and be conducted biennially (every two years) to age 74. (See Table 2.4.) Women at higher than average risk, such as those with a parent, sibling, or child with breast cancer, may benefit from beginning screening between the ages of 40 and 49 years. The USPSTF concludes that the current evidence is insufficient to assess the balance of benefits and harms of screening mammography in women aged 75 years and older.

The USPSTF also evaluates the risks and benefits of screening for skin cancer. The task force advises in "Draft Recommendation Statement Skin Cancer: Screening" (November 2015, http://www.uspreventiveservicestaskforce.org/Page/Document/draft-recommendation-statement168/skin-cancer-screening2) that "the evidence is insufficient to reliably conclude that early detection of skin cancer through visual examination by a clinician reduces morbidity or mortality." This recommendation only applies to adults who do

FIGURE 2.4

Trends in adult and youth obesity, 1999–2014

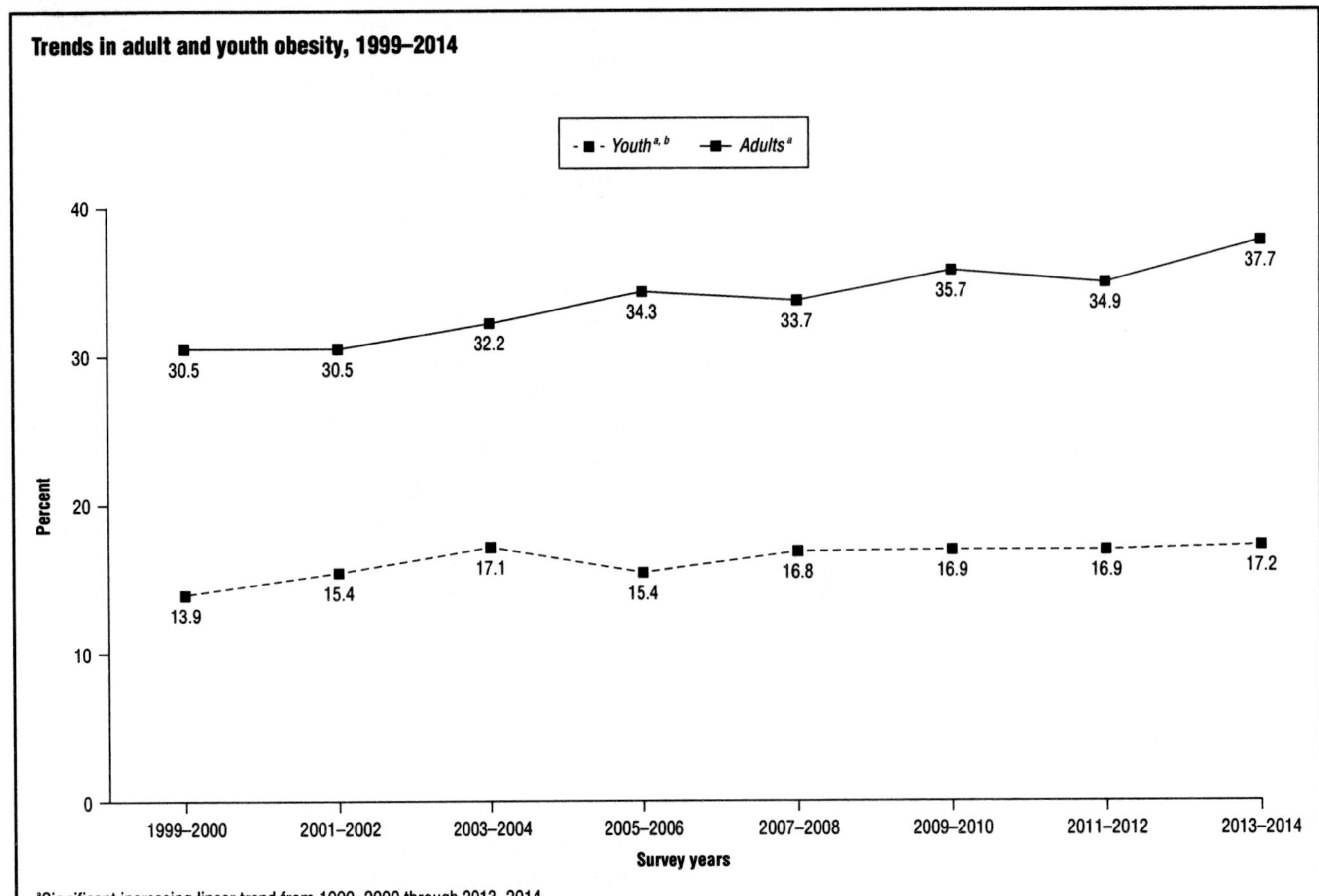

[a]Significant increasing linear trend from 1999–2000 through 2013–2014.
[b]Test for linear trend for 2003–2004 through 2013–2014 not significant.
Note: All adult estimates are age-adjusted by the direct method to the 2000 U.S. census population using the age groups 20–39, 40–59, and 60 and over.

SOURCE: Cynthia L. Ogden et al., "Figure 5. Trends in Obesity Prevalence among Adults Aged 20 and over (Age-Adjusted) and Youth Aged 2–19 Years: United States, 1999–2000 through 2013–2014," in "Prevalence of Obesity among Adults and Youth: United States, 2011–2014," *NCHS Data Brief*, no. 219, November 2015, http://www.cdc.gov/nchs/data/databriefs/db219.pdf (accessed December 17, 2015)

not have any symptoms of skin cancer or a history of precancerous or malignant (cancerous) skin lesions.

BREAST CANCER SCREENING RECOMMENDATIONS GENERATE DEBATE. In November 2009 the USPSTF updated its breast cancer screening recommendations from doing annual mammography starting at the age of 40 to doing biennial mammography starting at the age of 50. The guidelines also advised against teaching breast self-examination. The USPSTF determined that the risks of this practice—in terms of unnecessary diagnostic tests and procedures such as fine-needle aspiration and biopsies (invasive procedures that remove some breast tissue cells for examination)—outweigh the benefits.

Many health practitioners, professional associations, and breast cancer survivors assert that women's health will be harmed by adherence to the new recommendations. Others question whether the new guidelines justify rationing preventive services. Still others flatly reject the new guidelines. For example, the ACS advises annual screening using mammography for all women who want it beginning at the age of 40 years. In "American Cancer Society Guidelines for the Early Detection of Cancer" (October 20, 2015, http://www.cancer.org/healthy/findcancerearly/cancerscreeningguidelines/american-cancer-society-guidelines-for-the-early-detection-of-cancer), the ACS states, "Women ages 40 to 44 should have the choice to start annual breast cancer screening with mammograms (x-rays of the breast) if they wish to do so. Women age 45 to 54 should get mammograms every year. Women 55 and older should switch to mammograms every 2 years, or can continue yearly screening. Screening should continue as long as a woman is in good health and is expected to live 10 more years or longer."

Carlie K. Thompson, Martin Eklund, and Laura J. Esserman explain in "Putting the 'Great Mammography Debate' to Rest" (*American Journal of Hematology/Oncology*, 2015) that there are supporters and opponents of annual breast cancer screening in the medical community. For example, many radiologists argue that

FIGURE 2.5

How the U.S. Preventive Services Task Force develops recommendations

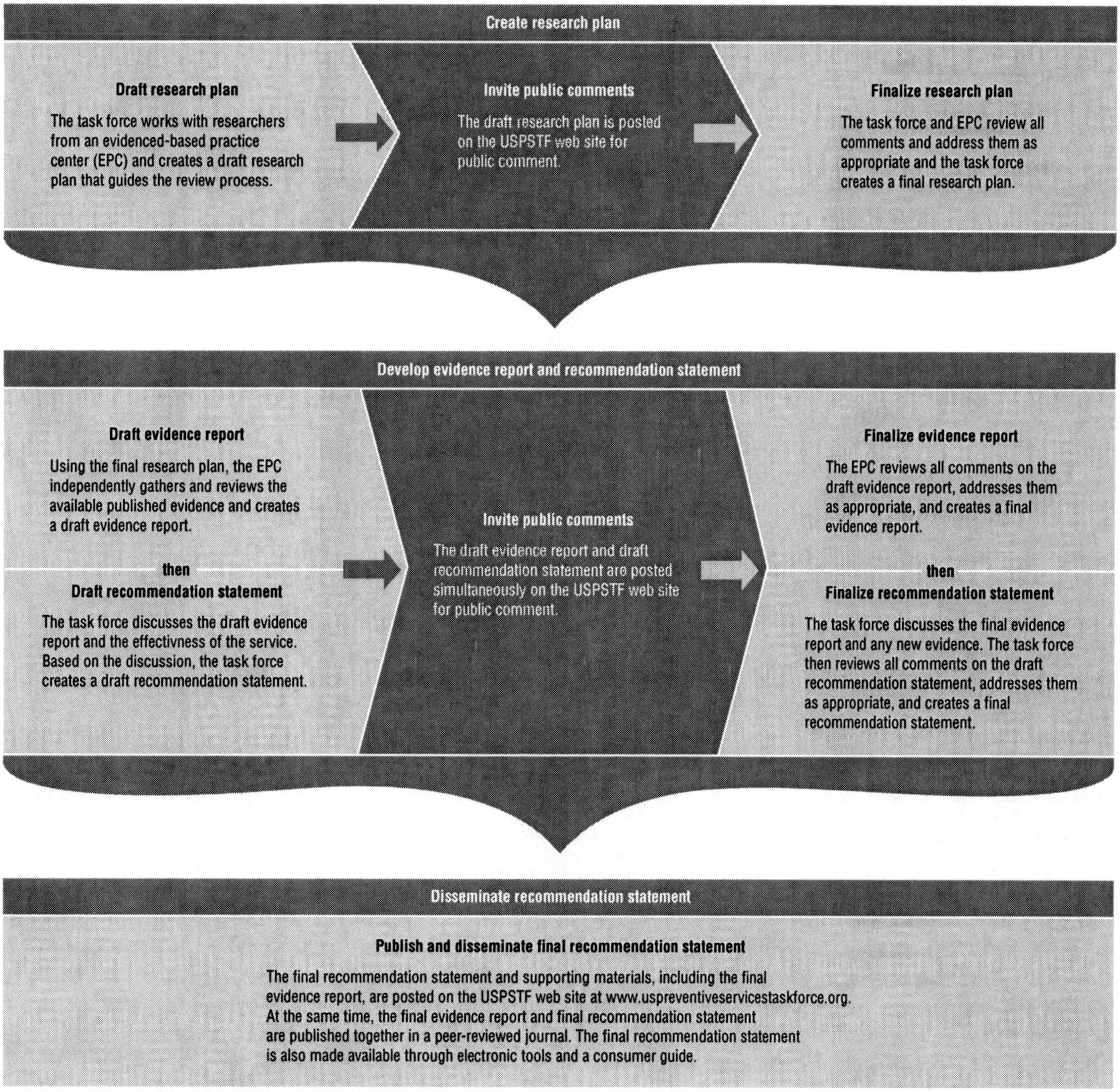

SOURCE: "Stages of Development," in *Topics in Progress*, U.S. Preventive Services Task Force, October 2015, http://www.uspreventiveservicestaskforce.org/Page/Name/home (accessed December 17, 2015)

annual mammograms reduce the occurrence of interval cancer (breast cancer diagnosed in the interval between scheduled screening episodes). Proponents of annual screening mammography cite a 21% reduction in breast cancer mortality based on data from screening performed during the 1970s and 1980s. Detractors assert that the rates of false-positive results and follow-up can cause long-lasting psychological distress that can make women unwilling to be screened for breast cancer in the future.

TESTICULAR CANCER SCREENING RECOMMENDATIONS GENERATE NO DEBATE. In contrast to the fiery debate that was generated by the breast cancer screening recommendations, the USPSTF's recommendations advising against screening for testicular cancer went almost entirely unnoticed by the media in 2011. In "Testicular Cancer: Screening" (April 2011, http://www.uspreventiveservicestaskforce.org/Page/Document/RecommendationStatementFinal/testicular-cancer-screening), the task force observes that testicular cancer is relatively rare—5.4 cases

TABLE 2.3

Recommended preventive services, 2014

Recommendation	Adults		Special populations	
	Men	**Women**	**Pregnant women**	**Children**
Abdominal aortic aneurysm, screening[a]	X			
Alcohol misuse screening and behavioral counseling	X	X	X	
Aspirin for the prevention of cardiovascular disease[b]	X	X		
Bacteriuria, screening[c]			X	
BRCA-related cancer in women, screening[d]		X		
Breast cancer, preventive medications[e]		X		
Breast cancer, screening[f]		X		
Breastfeeding, counseling[g]		X	X	
Cervical cancer, screening[h]		X		
Chlamydial infection, screening[i]		X	X	
Colorectal cancer, screening[j]	X	X		
Congenital hypothyroidism, screening[k]				X
Depression in adults, screening[l]	X	X		
Diabetes mellitus, screening[m]	X	X		
Falls in older adults, counseling, preventive medication, and other interventions[n]	X	X		
Folic acid supplementation to prevent neural tube defects, preventive medication[o]		X		
Gestational diabetes mellitus, screening[p]			X	
Gonococcal ophthalmia neonatorum, preventive medication[q]				X
Gonorrhea, screening[r]		X	X	
Hearing loss in newborns, screening[s]				X
Hepatitis B virus in pregnant women, screening[t]			X	
Hepatitis C virus infection in adults, screening[u]				
High blood pressure in adults, screening	X	X		
HIV infection, screening[v]	X	X	X	X
Intimate partner violence and elderly abuse, screening[w]		X		
Iron deficiency anemia, prevention[x]				X
Iron deficiency anemia, screening[y]			X	
Lipid disorders in adults, screening[z]	X	X		
Lung cancer, screening[aa]	X	X		
Major depressive disorder in children and adolescents, screening[bb]				X
Obesity in adults, screening[cc]	X	X		
Obesity in children and adolescents, screening[dd]				X
Osteoporosis, screening[ee]		X		
Phenylketonuria (PKU), screening[ff]				X
Sexually transmitted infections, counseling[gg]	X	X		X
Sickle cell disease in newborns, screening[hh]				X
Skin cancer, counseling[ii]	X	X	X	X
Syphilis infection (pregnant women), screening			X	
Tobacco use in adults, counseling and interventions[jj]	X	X	X	
Tobacco use in children and adolescents, primary care interventions[kk]				X
Visual impairment in children ages 1 to 5, screening[ll]				X

per 100,000 males—and that patients or their partners discover most cases. The USPSTF concludes that "there is inadequate evidence that screening by clinician examination or patient self-examination has a higher yield or greater accuracy for detecting testicular cancer at earlier (and more curable) stages.... Based on the low incidence of this condition and favorable outcomes of treatment, even in cases of advanced disease, there is adequate evidence that the benefits of screening for testicular cancer are small to none."

Screening and Early Detection of Breast and Cervical Cancers

The ACS estimates in *Breast Cancer Facts and Figures 2015–2016* (2015, http://www.cancer.org/acs/groups/content/@research/documents/document/acspc-046381.pdf) that in 2015, 292,130 women were diagnosed with breast cancer and 40,290 died of the disease. In *Cancer Facts and Figures 2015* (2015, http://www.cancer.org/acs/groups/content/@editorial/documents/document/acspc-044552.pdf), the ACS estimates that 12,900 new cases of cervical cancer were diagnosed in 2015 and that 4,100 women died of the disease. As with many other cancers, treatment for these types of cancer is most likely to be successful when the disease begins, before the cancer has metastasized (spread from its original site to other parts of the body).

In November 2009 the American College of Obstetricians and Gynecologists released new cervical cancer screening guidelines for the Papanicolaou test (also called Pap smear or Pap test). The Pap test is a screening examination for cancer of the cervix that can prevent practically all deaths from cervical cancer by detecting cervical cancer at an early stage, when it is most curable, or even preventing the disease if precancerous lesions found during the test are treated. The incidence of cervical cancer has decreased dramatically over the past 40 years largely because of screening and early treatment. The guidelines indicate that women should have their first Pap test at age 21 and then should be screened every two years until age 30 as opposed to annually. Women aged 30 years and older should be screened every three years.

TABLE 2.3

Recommended preventive services, 2014 [CONTINUED]

[a]One-time screening by ultrasonography in men aged 65 to 75 who have ever smoked.
[b]When the potential harm of an increase in gastrointestinal hemorrhage is outweighed by a potential benefit of a reduction in myocardial infarctions (men aged 45–79 years) or in ischemic strokes (women aged 55–79 years).
[c]Pregnant women at 12–16 weeks gestation or at first prenatal visit, if later.
[d]Refer women whose family history is associated with an increased risk for deleterious mutations in *BRCA1* or *BRCA2 genes for genetic counseling and evaluation for BRCA testing.*
[e]Engage in shared, informed decision making and offer to prescribe risk-reducing medications, if appropriate, to women aged ≥35 years without prior breast cancer diagnosis who are at increased risk.
[f]Biennial screening mammography for women aged 50 to 74 years.
[g]Interventions during pregnancy and after birth to promote and support breastfeeding.
[h]Screen with cytology every 3 years (women ages 21 to 65) or co-test (cytology/HPV testing) every 5 years (women ages 30–65).
[i]Sexually active women 24 and younger and other asymptomatic women at increased risk for infection. Asymptomatic pregnant women 24 and younger and others at increased risk.
[j]Adults aged 50–75 using fecal occult blood testing, sigmoidoscopy, or colonoscopy.
[k]Newborns.
[l]When staff-assisted depression care supports are in place to assure accurate diagnosis, effective treatment, and follow-up.
[m]Asymptomatic adults with sustained blood pressure greater than 135/80 mg Hg.
[n]Provide intervention (exercise or physical therapy and/or vitamin D supplementation) to community-dwelling adults ≥65 years at increased risk for falls.
[o]All women planning or capable of pregnancy take a daily supplement containing 0.4 to 0.8 mg (400 to 800 μg) of folic acid.
[p]Asymptomatic pregnant women after 24 weeks of gestation.
[q]Newborns.
[r]Sexually active women, including pregnant women 25 and younger, or at increased risk for infection.
[s]Newborns.
[t]Screen at first prenatal visit.
[u]Persons at high risk for infection and adults born between 1945 and 1965.
[v]All adolescents and adults ages 15 to 65 years and others who are at increased risk for HIV infection and all pregnant women.
[w]Asymptomatic women of childbearing age; provide or refer women who screen positive to intervention services.
[x]Routine iron supplementation for asymptomatic children aged 6 to 12 months who are at increased risk for iron deficiency anemia.
[y]Routine screening in asymptomatic pregnant women.
[z]Men aged 20–35 and women over age 20 who are at increased risk for coronary heart disease; all men aged 35 and older.
[aa]Asymptomatic adults aged 55 to 80 years who have a 30 pack-year smoking history and currently smoke or have quit smoking within the past 15 years.
[bb]Adolescents (age 12–18) when systems are in place to ensure accurate diagnosis, psychotherapy, and follow-up.
[cc]Patients with a body mass index of 30 kg/m^2 or higher should be offered or referred to intensive, multicomponent behavioral interventions.
[dd]Screen children aged 6 years and older; offer or refer for intensive counseling and behavioral interventions.
[ee]Women aged 65 years and older and women under age 65 whose 10-year fracture risk is equal to or greater than that of a 65-year-old white woman without additional risk factors.
[ff]Newborns.
[gg]All sexually active adolescents and adults at increased risk for STIs.
[hh]Newborns.
[ii]Children, adolescents, and young adults aged 10 to 24 years.
[jj]Ask all adults about tobacco use and provide tobacco cessation interventions for those who use tobacco; provide augmented, pregnancy-tailored counseling for those pregnant women who smoke.
[kk]Provide interventions to prevent initiation of tobacco use in school-aged children and adolescents.
[ll]Screen children ages 3 to 5 years.
Note: The Department of Health and Human Services, in implementing the Affordable Care Act, follows the 2002 USPSTF recommendation for screening mammography, with or without clinical breast examination, every 1–2 years for women aged 40 and older.

SOURCE: "Section 1. Preventive Services Recommended by the USPSTF," in *Guide to Clinical Preventive Services, 2014*, Agency for Healthcare Research and Quality, June 2014, http://www.ahrq.gov/professionals/clinicians-providers/guidelines-recommendations/guide/section1.html (accessed December 18, 2015)

According to Saundra Young, in "New Cervical Cancer Screening Guidelines Released" (CNN.com, November 20, 2009), this change in cervical cancer screening frequency did not generate the kind of controversy that surrounded the new mammography screening guidelines because Pap tests detect precancers that can take from 10 to 20 years to develop into cancers. Furthermore, this change was welcomed by professional associations such as the ACS, which "supports the guidelines and said it is reviewing new data and updating its own recommendations."

Although a vaccine to immunize women against contracting the strain of human papillomavirus (HPV) that causes cervical cancer has been available since 2006, it is only effective for people who have not yet become sexually active and contracted the virus. For this reason, cervical cancer screening will continue to be important for several generations after widespread immunization has occurred.

Initially, the vaccine was only recommended for girls and young women. In late 2011, however, the Advisory Committee on Immunization Practices, which advises the CDC, voted unanimously to recommend routine use of Gardasil in 11- and 12-year-old boys. By immunizing boys, it is hoped that transmission of the virus will be reduced and, ultimately, eliminated. Immunization also protects boys from genital warts and HPV-related cancers of the mouth, penis, and anus.

Because immunization against HPV must be done before young people become sexually active, the vaccine is recommended for preteens aged 11 years and older. The CDC explains in "Human Papillomavirus (HPV): Questions and Answers" (December 8, 2015, http://www.cdc.gov/hpv/parents/questions-answers.html) that the vaccine is not licensed for people over the age of 26 years because it has not been demonstrated to prevent HPV-related health problems in a general population of women and men older than age 26. Nonetheless, the CDC and physicians' professional organizations, including the American Academy of Pediatrics and the American Academy of Family Physicians, strongly support vaccination, and many communities and school districts require it.

TABLE 2.4

U.S. Preventive Services Task Force breast cancer screening recommendations, 2015

Population	Recommendation
Women ages 50 to 74 years	The USPSTF recommends biennial screening mammography for women ages 50 to 74 years.
Women ages 40 to 49 years	The decision to start screening mammography in women prior to age 50 years should be an individual one. Women who place a higher value on the potential benefit than the potential harms may choose to begin biennial screening between the ages of 40 and 49 years. • For women at average risk for breast cancer, most of the benefit of mammography will result from biennial screening during ages 50 to 74 years. Of all age groups, women ages 60 to 69 years are most likely to avoid a breast cancer death through mammography screening. Screening mammography in women ages 40 to 49 years may reduce the risk of dying of breast cancer, but the number of deaths averted is much smaller than in older women and the number of false-positive tests and unnecessary biopsies are larger. • All women undergoing regular screening mammography are at risk for the diagnosis and treatment of noninvasive and invasive breast cancer that would otherwise not have become a threat to her health, or even apparent, during her lifetime (known as "overdiagnosis"). This risk is predicted to be increased when beginning regular mammography before age 50 years. • Women with a parent, sibling, or child with breast cancer may benefit more than average-risk women from beginning screening between the ages of 40 and 49 years.
Women age 75 years and older	The USPSTF concludes that the current evidence is insufficient to assess the balance of benefits and harms of screening mammography in women age 75 years and older.
All women	The USPSTF concludes that the current evidence is insufficient to assess the benefits and harms of tomosynthesis (3-D mammography) as a screening modality for breast cancer.
Women with dense breasts	The USPSTF concludes that the current evidence is insufficient to assess the balance of benefits and harms of adjunctive screening for breast cancer using breast ultrasound, magnetic resonance imaging (MRI), tomosynthesis, or other modalities in women identified to have dense breasts on an otherwise negative screening mammogram.

Notes: This recommendation applies to asymptomatic women age 40 years and older who do not have pre-existing breast cancer or a previously diagnosed high-risk breast lesion and who are not at high risk for breast cancer because of a known underlying genetic mutation (such as a BRCA mutation or other familial breast cancer syndrome) or a history of chest radiation at a young age.

SOURCE: Adapted from "Draft: Recommendation Summary," in *Draft Recommendation Statement Breast Cancer: Screening*, U.S. Preventive Services Task Force, May 2015, http://www.uspreventiveservicestaskforce.org/Page/Document/UpdateSummaryFinal/breast-cancer-screening1 (accessed December 18, 2015), and "Grade Definitions after July 2012," in *Grade Definitions*, U.S. Preventive Services Task Force, October 2014, http://www.uspreventiveservicestaskforce.org/Page/Name/grade-definitions#grade-definitions-after-july-2012 (accessed December 18, 2015)

However, the HPV vaccine has also been controversial. During a September 13, 2011, appearance on the *Today Show*, Michele Bachmann (1956–), who served as a member of the U.S. House of Representatives from Minnesota from 2007 to 2015, suggested that the HPV vaccine could cause mental retardation. In "The Digital Distribution of Public Health News surrounding the Human Papillomavirus Vaccination: A Longitudinal Infodemiology Study" (*JMIR Public Health Surveillance*, vol. 1, no 1, January–June 2015), L. Meghan Mahoney et al. observe that Bachmann's comment fueled the spread of misinformation about the safety of the HPV vaccine.

Michelle Vichnin et al. confirm in "An Overview of Quadrivalent Human Papillomavirus Vaccine Safety" (*Pediatric Infectious Disease Journal*, vol. 34, no. 9, September 2015) the safety of the HPV vaccine. The researchers state, "In the 9 years of post-licensure vaccine safety monitoring and evaluation conducted following the initial licensure of HPV4 in the US, no serious safety concerns have been identified in any study conducted worldwide." They note that the vaccine has been shown to be highly effective and has caused marked reductions in the prevalence of HPV vaccine-type–related infection and disease. Vichnin et al. also indicate that key policy, medical, and regulatory organizations throughout the world independently reviewed the data and "continue to recommend routine HPV vaccination."

In 1990 Congress passed the Breast and Cervical Cancer Mortality Prevention Act, which established the CDC's National Breast and Cervical Cancer Early Detection Program (NBCCEDP). The NBCCEDP provides breast and pelvic examinations, screening mammography, and Pap tests to women who are at greater risk of death from breast or cervical cancer—racial and ethnic minorities, those who live below the poverty level, older women, and women with less than a high school education.

Between July 2009 and June 2014 the NBCCEDP (March 15, 2016, http://www.cdc.gov/cancer/nbccedp/data/summaries/national_aggregate.htm) had screened more than 1.7 million women and detected 17,482 breast cancers and 24,237 precancerous cervical lesions or cervical cancers. Figure 2.6 shows the number of women who were served by the NBCCEDP for each program year between 2010 and 2014. A significant component of the NBCCEDP effort is community education and outreach. Health educators must not only communicate the lifesaving benefits of screening and early identification of disease but also overcome barriers to access to care, such as the lack of transportation or child care.

The NBCCEDP also funds follow-up care for women who have abnormal screening results to enable them to receive needed services. These may include a biopsy (surgical removal of a sample of cells for microscopic

FIGURE 2.6

Numbers of women served in National Breast and Cervical Cancer Early Detection Program, 2010–14

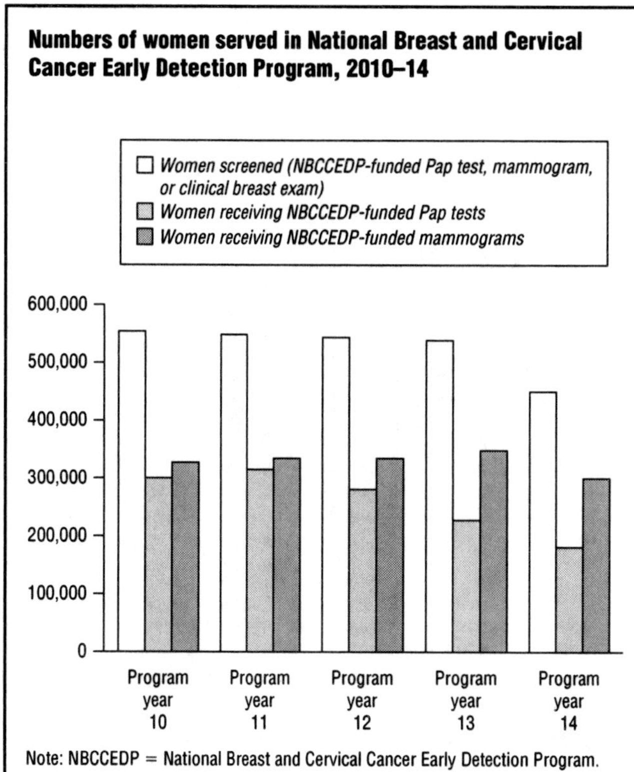

Note: NBCCEDP = National Breast and Cervical Cancer Early Detection Program.

SOURCE: "Screening Totals by Year: Number of Women Screened by Year," in *National Breast and Cervical Cancer Early Detection Program (NBCCEDP): National Aggregate*, Centers for Disease Control and Prevention, September 17, 2015, http://www.cdc.gov/cancer/nbccedp/data/summaries/national_aggregate.htm (accessed December 18, 2015)

examination) to confirm the diagnosis and visits with surgeons and other medical specialists to receive timely treatment. The provision of follow-up care and treatment is a fundamental principle underlying screening programs.

Screening programs that do not provide facilities for diagnosis and treatment are unlikely to be effective and many public health professionals believe it is unethical to offer screening without plans and provisions to care for diseases that have been identified through the screening process.

TERTIARY PREVENTION

Tertiary prevention programs aim to improve the quality of life for people with various diseases by limiting complications and disabilities, reducing the severity and progression of disease, and providing rehabilitation (therapy to restore functionality and self-sufficiency). Unlike primary and secondary prevention, tertiary prevention involves actual treatment for the disease and is conducted primarily by health care practitioners, rather than by public health agencies.

Tertiary prevention efforts demonstrate that it is possible to slow the natural course of some progressive diseases and prevent or delay many of the complications that are associated with chronic diseases such as arthritis (inflammation of the joints that causes pain, swelling, and stiffness), asthma, heart disease, and diabetes.

Tertiary Prevention of Diabetes

Insulin is a hormone produced by the pancreas to control the amount of glucose (sugar) in the blood. Diabetes mellitus is a disease in which high blood glucose levels result from insufficient insulin production or action. When there is not enough insulin produced, the body is unable to use, regulate, and store glucose, and it remains in the blood.

Type 1 diabetes mellitus (also called insulin-dependent diabetes or juvenile-onset diabetes) occurs when pancreatic beta cells, the cells that make insulin, are destroyed by the body's own immune system. It usually develops in children and young adults. Because people with diabetes do not have enough insulin, they must inject themselves with insulin several times a day or receive insulin via a pump. In "Basics about Diabetes" (March 31, 2015, http://www.cdc.gov/diabetes/basics/diabetes.html), the CDC states that about 5% of all diagnosed cases of diabetes are type 1.

Type 2 diabetes mellitus (also called noninsulin-dependent diabetes or adult-onset diabetes) occurs when the body becomes resistant to insulin. As a result of the cells being unable to use insulin effectively, the amount of glucose they can take up is sharply reduced and high levels of glucose accumulate in the blood. The CDC notes that approximately 95% of all diagnosed cases of diabetes are type 2 diabetes.

Many people with type 2 diabetes are able to control their blood sugar by losing excess weight, maintaining proper nutrition, and exercising regularly. Others require insulin injections or orally administered (taken by mouth) drugs to lower their blood sugar.

Other types of diabetes can occur as a result of pregnancy (gestational diabetes) or physiologic stress such as surgery, trauma, malnutrition, infections, and other illnesses.

Data from the 2015 National Health Interview Survey reveal the increasing prevalence of diagnosed diabetes from 5.1% in 1997 to 9.6% in 2015. (See Figure 2.7.) Because as many as 37% (86 million) of adults have prediabetes (a condition in which blood sugar is high but not yet in the diabetic range), the USPSTF recommends in "Abnormal Blood Glucose and Type 2 Diabetes Mellitus: Screening" (October 2015, http://www.uspreventiveservicestaskforce.org/Page/Document/RecommendationStatementFinal/screening-for-abnormal-blood-glucose-and-type-2-diabetes) that physicians screen all overweight and obese adults aged 40 to 70 years for

FIGURE 2.7

Prevalence of diagnosed diabetes in adults, 1997–2015

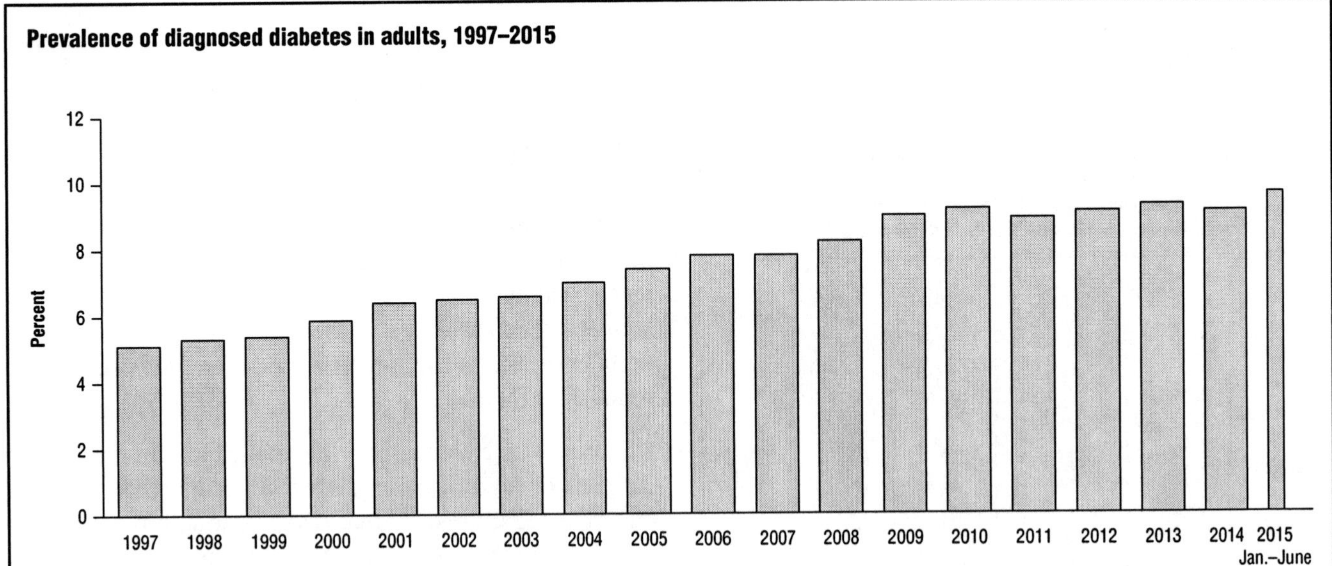

Notes: Data are based on household interviews of a sample of the civilian noninstitutionalized population. Prevalence of diagnosed diabetes is based on self-report of ever having been diagnosed with diabetes by a doctor or other health professional. Persons reporting "borderline" diabetes status and women reporting diabetes only during pregnancy were not coded as having diabetes in the analyses. The analyses excluded persons with unknown diabetes status (about 0.1% of respondents each year).

SOURCE: "Data Table for Figure 14.1. Prevalence of Diagnosed Diabetes among Adults Aged 18 and over: United States, 1997–June 2015," in *Early Release of Selected Estimates Based on Data from the January–June 2015 National Health Interview Survey*, Centers for Disease Control and Prevention, National Center for Health Statistics, November 2015, http://www.cdc.gov/nchs/data/nhis/earlyrelease/earlyrelease201511_14.pdf (accessed December 16, 2015)

abnormal blood sugar levels and type 2 diabetes. The USPSTF also advises that patients with abnormal blood glucose be referred to intensive behavioral counseling to promote a healthful diet and physical activity.

COMPLICATIONS OF DIABETES. According to the National Institute of Diabetes and Digestive and Kidney Diseases (NIDDK), in *National Diabetes Statistics Report, 2014* (2014, http://www.cdc.gov/diabetes/pubs/statsreport14/national-diabetes-report-web.pdf), adults with diabetes suffer from heart disease at much higher rates—in fact, heart disease is the number-one cause of death among people with diabetes. Similarly, adults with diabetes have an increased risk for stroke (damage to the brain that occurs when its blood supply is cut off, frequently because of blockage in an artery that supplies the brain) and hypertension (71% of adults with diabetes have high blood pressure). Other serious complications of this disease include:

- Diabetic retinopathy—this is a condition that can cause blindness
- Diabetic neuropathy—this condition causes damage to the nervous system that may produce pain or loss of sensation in the hands or feet and other nerve problems
- Kidney disease—diabetes accounts for almost half of all new end-stage renal disease cases that require dialysis (mechanical cleansing of the blood of impurities) or kidney transplant
- Amputation—diabetes is responsible for 60% of all lower-limb amputations (surgical removal of toes, feet, and the leg below the knee) performed in the United States
- Dental disease—gum diseases are common among people with diabetes, and nearly one-third of all people with diabetes have severe periodontal (tooth and gum) diseases
- Problems with pregnancy—diabetes may cause birth defects, miscarriage (spontaneous abortion), and excessively large babies that may create additional health risks for expectant mothers
- Increased risk of infection—people with diabetes are more susceptible to infection and do not recover as quickly as people without diabetes

Furthermore, poorly controlled or uncontrolled diabetes may produce life-threatening medical emergencies, such as diabetic ketoacidosis (excessive ketones; chemicals in the blood resulting from insufficient insulin and an excessive amount of counterregulatory hormones such as glucagon) or hyperosmolar coma (extremely high blood glucose, leading to dehydration).

Achieving optimal control of blood glucose levels can prevent many of the complications of diabetes and decrease the risk of death that is associated with the disease. Optimal control involves aggressive treatment of diabetes with close attention to the roles of diet,

FIGURE 2.8

Percentage of adults with diabetes that reported receiving preventive services, 2012

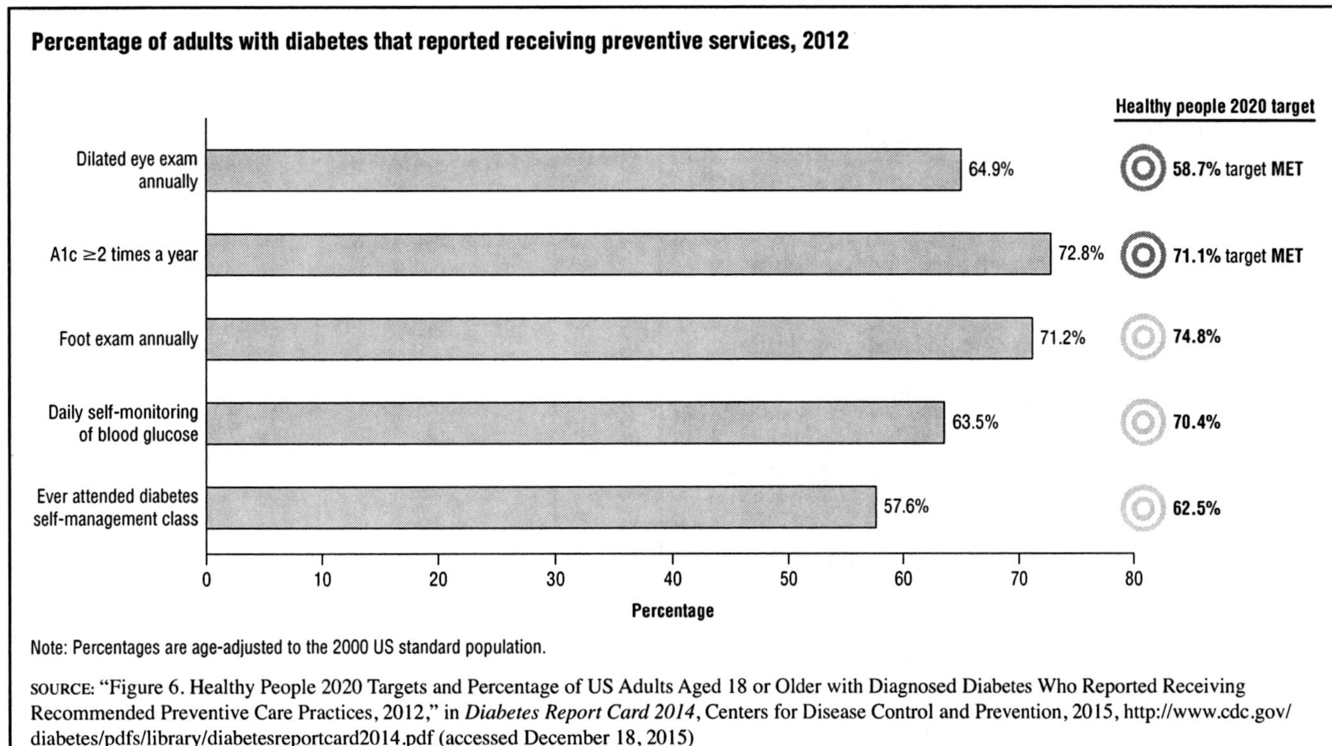

Note: Percentages are age-adjusted to the 2000 US standard population.

SOURCE: "Figure 6. Healthy People 2020 Targets and Percentage of US Adults Aged 18 or Older with Diagnosed Diabetes Who Reported Receiving Recommended Preventive Care Practices, 2012," in *Diabetes Report Card 2014*, Centers for Disease Control and Prevention, 2015, http://www.cdc.gov/diabetes/pdfs/library/diabetesreportcard2014.pdf (accessed December 18, 2015)

exercise, weight management, and pharmacology (proper use of insulin and other medication) in the self-management of the disease. Figure 2.8 shows the percentage of adults with diabetes who reported receiving preventive services in 2012.

PREVENTING COMPLICATIONS OF DIABETES. The NIDDK explains that even modest improvement in controlling blood glucose acts to help prevent diabetic retinopathy, neuropathy, and kidney disease. Reducing blood pressure can decrease cardiovascular complications (heart disease and stroke) by as much as 50% and can reduce the risk of retinopathy, neuropathy, and kidney disease by 33%. Lowering blood cholesterol (a waxy substance produced by the body and found in animal products), low-density lipoproteins (LDL), and triglycerides also reduces, by as much as 50%, the cardiovascular complications of diabetes. (Cholesterol, LDL, and triglycerides are lipids that may be measured in the blood.)

The CDC reports that early detection and treatment of diabetic eye disease can reduce the possibility of blindness or serious loss of vision by more than 60%. Similarly, early detection and treatment of kidney disease sharply reduces the risk of developing kidney failure, and careful attention to foot care reduces the risk of amputation by as much as 85%.

To help increase early detection of diabetes (secondary prevention) and reduce the morbidity (illnesses) and mortality (deaths) associated with it (tertiary prevention), the CDC and the NIDDK launched the National Diabetes Education Program (NDEP) in 1997. The NDEP's objectives are to increase public awareness of diabetes, improve self-management of people with diabetes, enhance health care providers' knowledge and treatment of diabetes, and promote health policies that improve access, availability, and quality of diabetes care. To meet these educational objectives, the NDEP, in working with a variety of other health organizations, develops and distributes teaching tools and resources.

The NDEP enumerates in *Guiding Principles for the Care of People with or at Risk for Diabetes* (September 2014, http://www.niddk.nih.gov/health-information/health-communication-programs/ndep/health-care-professionals/guiding-principles/Documents/Guiding_Principles_508.pdf) self-management strategies to help people with diabetes prevent its complications. Diabetes educators and others in the health care team can help people with or at risk for diabetes to:

- Understand the diabetes disease process and the risks and benefits of treatment options.
- Incorporate healthy eating behaviors into their lifestyles.
- Incorporate physical activity into their lifestyles.
- Understand how to use medications safely and for their best effect.

- Perform self-monitoring of blood pressure when prescribed.
- Perform self-monitoring of blood glucose when prescribed and demonstrate how to interpret and use the results for self-management decision making.
- Understand how to prevent, detect, and treat high and low blood glucose.
- Understand self-management needs during illness or medical procedures.
- Prevent, detect, and treat chronic diabetes complications.
- Develop personal strategies to address psychosocial issues and concerns.
- Develop personal strategies to promote health and behavior change.

PREVENTION PROGRAMS REDUCE COMPLICATIONS. Tertiary prevention programs help prevent complications of diabetes. In *Diabetes Report Card 2014* (2015, http://www.cdc.gov/diabetes/pdfs/library/diabetesreportcard2014.pdf), the CDC notes that over the past two decades death rates from hyperglycemic crises have declined, as have rates of lower-limb amputations and kidney failure (end-stage renal disease). (See Figure 2.9.)

FIGURE 2.9

Trends in rates of diabetes complications among adults with diagnosed diabetes, 1990–2010

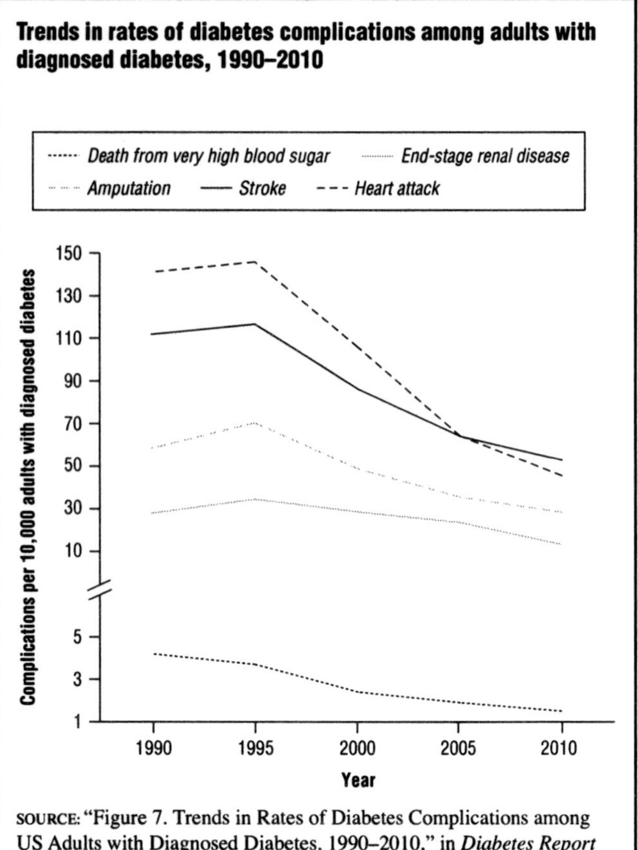

SOURCE: "Figure 7. Trends in Rates of Diabetes Complications among US Adults with Diagnosed Diabetes, 1990–2010," in *Diabetes Report Card 2014*, Centers for Disease Control and Prevention, 2015, http://www.cdc.gov/diabetes/pdfs/library/diabetesreportcard2014.pdf (accessed December 18, 2015)

Tertiary Prevention to Reduce Heart Attack and Stroke

In 2015 the CDC launched a new tertiary prevention program that aims to identify and celebrate medical practices that achieve high rates (70% or greater) of blood pressure control of their patients with high blood pressure. In the press release "Million Hearts Launches Annual Blood Pressure Control Challenge" (August 18, 2015, http://www.cdc.gov/media/releases/2015/p0818-million-hearts.html), Thomas R. Frieden (1960–), the director of the CDC, explains, "Many heart attacks and strokes—and needless early deaths—can be prevented if we get better control of high blood pressure. We applaud the many medical practices which have made hypertension control a daily priority with all of their patients. We look forward to recognizing their achievements and learning from top performing practices."

EXEMPLARY MENTAL HEALTH PREVENTION PROGRAMS

This section presents a national mental health and suicide risk screening program for youth that was first described in *Achieving the Promise: Transforming Mental Health Care in America* (July 2003, http://govinfo.library.unt.edu/mentalhealthcommission/reports/FinalReport/downloads/FinalReport.pdf) by the President's New Freedom Commission on Mental Health. It also offers descriptions of interventions that are considered to be effective at preventing suicide from *Reducing Suicide: A National Imperative* (2002, http://www.nap.edu/books/0309083214/html/), which was edited by Sara K. Goldsmith et al.

Goldsmith et al. characterize current mental health prevention programs as rooted in the "universal, selective, and indicated prevention model." This model considers three defined populations: the entire population is included in universal programs, specific high-risk groups are targeted by selective programs, and indicated programs address specific high-risk individuals. Universal programming assumes a basically healthy population and generally aims at protection against developing a disorder by offering, for example, enhanced coping skills and resiliency training. Examples of universal programs are educational programs that heighten awareness of a problem and mass-media campaigns that are intended to increase understanding of and improve attitudes about a particular issue.

Population-based programs often produce greater gains than programs that target individuals because there are higher rates of program participation. For example, all the students in a given grade will be exposed to school-based drug prevention programs. Selective programs target subsets of populations that have been identified as at risk but are not yet diagnosed with a specific problem or disorder—people who have a greater-than-average likelihood of developing mental disorders, such as adolescents with truancy or suspected substance abuse problems. Indicated programs are aimed at specific high-risk individuals who have presented early signs or symptoms of mental disorders, such as children diagnosed with attention-deficit/hyperactivity disorder, who may be at a greater risk of developing conduct disorders, or students who have engaged in disruptive or other disturbed behavior at school.

By recounting the histories, benefits, and scientific evaluation of mental health prevention programs, *Achieving the Promise* and *Reducing Suicide* offer a framework for developing and implementing mental health prevention programs and policies in a wide range of settings, including primary medical care practices and clinics, maternal and infant health and mental health programs, child care centers, school-based health centers, vocational training programs, social service agencies, parent education programs, and the media. Furthermore, these reports disseminate the methods and results of effective programs that have demonstrated efficacy (the ability of an intervention to produce the intended diagnostic or therapeutic effect in optimal circumstances), enabling mental health service providers throughout the country to replicate these results.

Adolescent Intervention Programs

One recommendation from *Achieving the Promise* is to "improve and expand school mental health programs." The commission cites research demonstrating that approximately 42% of students with serious emotional disturbances graduate from high school, compared with 57% of students with other disabilities. The commission believes this could be changed, because it finds ample evidence that school mental health programs improved academic achievement—with improved test scores, fewer absences, and fewer discipline problems—by detecting mental health problems early and providing timely referral to appropriate treatment.

The commission observes that the concerted effort needed to deliver quality mental health services in schools entails collaboration with parents and local providers of mental health care to support screening, assessment, and early intervention. It also asserts that mental health services must be integral parts of school health centers and that federal funds must be available to support the programs.

Screening increases the likelihood that students who are at risk for suicidal behavior will get into treatment. Madelyn S. Gould et al. indicate in "Service Use by At-Risk Youths after School-Based Suicide Screening" (*Journal of the American Academy of Child and Adolescent Psychiatry*, vol. 48, no. 12, December 2009) that school-based mental health assessments effectively identify adolescents who are at risk for suicidal behavior and help ensure high rates of follow-up treatment. The researchers note that nearly 70% of the adolescents who were identified by a school-based suicide screening effort followed through on referrals to treatment within one year.

In "Services for Adolescents with Psychiatric Disorders: 12-Month Data from the National Comorbidity Survey—Adolescent" (*Psychiatric Services*, vol. 65, no. 3, March 1, 2014), Elizabeth Jane Costello et al. analyze adolescents' rates of service use for mental, emotional, and behavioral disorders. The researchers find that only a minority of adolescents with psychiatric disorders receives any kind of treatment at all. Such findings highlight the urgent need for new mechanisms to identify, track, and monitor people with mental illness to prevent them from leaving treatment and becoming a danger to themselves and others.

Are Mental Health Prevention Programs Working?

Irwin Sandler et al. review in "Overview of Meta-analyses of the Prevention of Mental Health, Substance Use and Conduct Problems" (*Annual Review of Clinical Psychology*, vol. 10, March 28, 2014) 48 meta-analyses (analyses of the results of many studies) to determine the impact of programs aimed at preventing mental, emotional, and behavioral problems of children, youth, and young adults (to age 26). The researchers looked at programs targeting depression, anxiety, antisocial behavior (including delinquency and violence), and substance use. They considered school-based and after-school programs; mentoring programs intended to promote positive outcomes via relationships between people aged 18 years and younger and nonparental adults or older youth who act in a nonprofessional helping capacity; parent training programs; and preschool/home visiting programs that target family disruptions such as divorce.

Sandler et al. find that most programs had "small but significant effects to prevent each problem area that was included in this review, depression, anxiety, anti-social behavior and substance use." The researchers also find long-term and lasting effects of many prevention programs, with benefits after one year or longer. They note that interactive programs to promote the use of behaviors and skills were more effective than programs that were not interactive. Sandler et al. observe that not unexpectedly children and youth at higher risk for problem outcomes generally received more benefits from participation in prevention programs than those at lower risk.

PREVENTING SUICIDE

In the landmark report *Mental Health: A Report of the Surgeon General* (1999, http://www.surgeongeneral.gov/library/mentalhealth/home.html), the Office of the

TABLE 2.5

Suicide risk factors, protective factors, and national prevention strategy

- National Strategy for Suicide Prevention: AIM
  - **A**wareness: promote public awareness of suicide as a public health problem
  - **I**ntervention: enhance services and programs
  - **M**ethodology: advance the science of suicide prevention
- Risk factors
  - Male gender
  - Mental disorders, particularly depression and substance abuse
  - Prior suicide attempts
  - Unwillingness to seek help because of stigma
  - Barriers to accessing mental health treatment
  - Stressful life event/loss
  - Easy access to lethal methods such as guns
- Protective factors
  - Effective and appropriate clinical care for underlying disorders
  - Easy access to care
  - Support from family, community, and health and mental health care staff

SOURCE: Adapted from "Figure 4-1. Surgeon General's Call to Action to Prevent Suicide—1999," in *Mental Health: A Report of the Surgeon General*, U.S. Department of Health and Human Services, Substance Abuse and Mental Health Services Administration, Center for Mental Health Services, with the National Institute of Mental Health, 1999, http://www.surgeongeneral.gov/library/mentalhealth/toc.html#chapter4 (accessed December 15, 2015)

Surgeon General states that suicide is a serious public health problem and recommends a three-pronged national strategy to prevent suicide, which includes programs that educate, heighten understanding, intervene, and advance the science of suicide prevention. Table 2.5 shows the components of AIM (awareness, intervention, and methodology)—the national strategy for suicide prevention—as well as the risk factors and protective factors for suicide.

According to the National Institutes of Health, in "Suicide Prevention" (April 2015, https://www.nimh.nih.gov/health/topics/suicide-prevention/index.shtml), there are more than 41,000 suicides in the United States annually and suicide is the second-leading cause of death for people aged 15 to 34 years. Laura Kann et al. indicate in "Youth Risk Behavior Surveillance—United States, 2013" (*Morbidity and Mortality Weekly Report*, vol. 63, no. 4, June 13, 2014) that in 2013, 17% of high school students (grades nine to 12) said they had seriously considered suicide in the previous 12 months, 8% of students reported trying to commit suicide at least once in the previous 12 months, and 2.7% of students had tried to commit suicide in a way that resulted in an injury, poisoning, or overdose that required medical attention.

In *Preventing Suicide: Program Activities Guide* (October 2010, http://www.cdc.gov/violenceprevention/pdf/PreventingSuicide-a.pdf), the CDC describes activities in key prevention areas, including surveillance, research, capacity building, communication, partnership, and leadership. The CDC's violence prevention activities emphasize primary prevention by advancing the science of prevention, translating scientific advances into practical applications, and building on existing efforts to address community needs or gaps in preventive services. Ongoing activities include:

- Monitoring, tracking, and researching the problem. State and local agencies work together to gather data that enable policy and community leaders to make informed decisions about violence prevention programs and strategies. Other CDC research focuses on the relationship between different forms of violent behavior and suicide among adolescent and school-associated violent deaths.
- Supporting and enhancing prevention programs that are university- and school-based as well as multistate and national prevention and education initiatives that promote awareness of suicide as a preventable public health problem.
- Providing prevention resources, such as a toll-free hotline, a website, or a fax-on-demand service that supplies prevention information and print publications.
- Encouraging research and development on violence, injury, and suicide prevention in specific populations such as adolescents making the transition to early adulthood, urban youth, and youth identified as at risk for suicidal behavior by screening programs.

ACTIVE MILITARY AND VETERANS ARE AT RISK FOR SUICIDE

According to Craig J. Bryan et al., in "Combat Exposure and Suicide Risk in Two Samples of Military Personnel" (*Journal of Clinical Psychology*, vol. 69, no. 1, January 2013), suicide is the second-leading cause of death in the U.S. military, accounting for between 9 and 15 deaths per 100,000 service members. Escalating suicide rates among military personnel between 2005 and 2011 and increasing suicide attempts by military personnel and veterans are cause for concern.

Thomas Joiner, Ingrid Lim, and Ted Bender observe in *Optimizing Screening and Risk Assessment for Suicide Risk in the U.S. Military* (March 2015, http://www.dtic.mil/get-tr-doc/pdf?Location=U2&doc=GetTRDoc.pdf&AD=ADA614421) that military suicide has increased over the past decade. They note that one way to understand suicide in the military is through the use of the Interpersonal-Psychological Theory of Suicide. This theory posits that three factors are needed to complete suicide: feelings that one does not belong with other people, feelings that one is a burden on others or society, and an acquired capability to overcome the fear and pain associated with suicide. The researchers opine that acquired capability may be the most affected by military experience, in that combat exposure and training may condition military personnel to be less fearful of painful experiences, including suicide. Joiner, Lim, and Bender assert that regular screening of military personnel for suicidal symptoms may serve to assess risk and prevent suicide.

Identifying Troops and Veterans Who Are at Risk for Suicide

The U.S. Department of Veterans Affairs (VA) identifies in "How to Recognize When to Ask for Help" (June 3, 2015, http://www.mentalhealth.va.gov/suicide_prevention/whentoaskforhelp.asp) veteran-specific risks for suicide, including:

- Frequent deployments
- Deployments to hostile environments
- Exposure to extreme stress
- Physical/sexual assault while in the service (not limited to women)
- Length of deployments
- Service-related injury

The VA also instructs health professionals about how to identify and respond to risk for suicide. Table 2.6 enumerates the warning signs for suicide risk.

Jitender Sareen and Shay-Lee Belik note in "The Need for Outreach in Preventing Suicide among Young Veterans" (*PLoS Medicine*, vol. 6, no. 3, March 3, 2009) that most service members with mental health problems do not seek or receive treatment. One study finds that just one out of five veterans who committed suicide had any contact with a mental health professional. Sareen and Belik describe five major areas of suicide prevention:

TABLE 2.6

Warning signs for suicide risk

Look for the warning signs

- Threatening to hurt or kill self
- Looking for ways to kill self
- Seeking access to pills, weapons or other means
- Talking or writing about death, dying or suicide

Presence of any of the above warning signs requires immediate attention and referral. Consider hospitalization for safety until complete assessment may be made.

Additional warning signs

- Hopelessness
- Rage, anger, seeking revenge
- Acting reckless or engaging in risky activities, seemingly without thinking
- Feeling trapped—like there is no way out
- Increasing alcohol or drug abuse
- Withdrawing from friends, family and society
- Anxiety, agitation, unable to sleep or sleeping all the time
- Dramatic changes in mood
- No reason for living, no sense of purpose in life

For any of the above refer for mental health treatment or assure that follow-up appointment is made.

SOURCE: "Warning Signs," in *Suicide Prevention*, U.S. Department of Veterans Affairs, 2015, http://www.mentalhealth.va.gov/suicide_prevention/index.asp (accessed December 18, 2015)

- Education and awareness programs for the general public and professionals
- Screening methods for high-risk people
- Treatment of psychiatric disorders
- Restricting access to lethal means
- Safe media reporting of suicide to minimize the risk of so-called copycat suicides, especially in youth

In "Risk Factors Associated with Suicide in Current and Former US Military Personnel" (*Journal of the American Medical Association*, vol. 310, no. 5, August 7, 2013), Cynthia A. LeardMann et al. identify risk factors that are associated with suicide in current and former U.S. military personnel, including demographic, mental health, behavioral, and deployment characteristics. The researchers find that suicide risk is associated with being male and with mental health problems but is not associated with any military-specific factors such as deployment characteristics. LeardMann et al. conclude that "knowing the psychiatric history, screening for mental and substance use disorders, and early recognition of associated suicidal behaviors combined with high-quality treatment are likely to provide the best potential for mitigating suicide risk."

The VA Suicide Prevention Program Expands

The VA's veterans' crisis line is available 24 hours per day, seven days per week, and is staffed by trained mental health counselors. In "About the Veterans Crisis Line" (2016, http://www.veteranscrisisline.net/About/AboutVeteransCrisisLine.aspx), the VA states that since 2007 the line "has answered nearly 2 million calls and initiated the dispatch of emergency services to callers in crisis over 53,000 times."

In 2009 the VA launched an online chat service that provides a forum where veterans, their families, and friends can chat anonymously with a trained VA counselor. Should the counselor identify the person's problem as a crisis or emergency, he or she can provide immediate assistance by connecting the person online to the Veterans Crisis Line for counseling and crisis intervention services. The online service, which has logged more than 250,000 chats, is an outreach program that is intended to communicate with and inform all veterans—not only those enrolled in the VA health care system—and offer them immediate online access to peer support and trained counselors who can provide anonymous suicide prevention services. In 2011 the VA added a text messaging option for veterans in need of confidential support and by 2016 counselors had responded to more than 44,000 texts.

The U.S. Air Force Suicide Prevention Program

The suicide prevention program initiated by the U.S. Air Force is comprehensive and acts to increase knowledge and change attitudes within a community, dispel barriers to treatment, and improve access to support and intervention. According to Kerry L. Knox et al., in "The US Air Force Suicide Prevention Program: Implications for Public Health Policy" (*American Journal of Public Health*, vol. 100, no. 12, December 2010), the program is effective. Since its launch in 1997, the program has helped decrease suicides from an average of 3 per 100,000 people per quarter to 2 per 100,000 people per quarter.

The Air Force Suicide Prevention Program is a population-based, community approach to suicide risk prevention and behavioral health promotion. It integrates human, medical, and mental health services by uniting a coalition of community agencies from within and outside the health care delivery system to significantly reduce suicide among air force personnel, which had risen to an all-time high during the mid-1990s.

The program attempts to reduce risk factors such as problems with finances, intimate relationships, mental health, job performance, substance abuse, social isolation, and poor coping skills. It simultaneously seeks to strengthen protective factors such as effective coping skills, a sense of social connectedness, and policies and norms that encourage effective help-seeking behaviors. To stimulate help-seeking behaviors, the program stresses the urgent need for air force leaders, supervisors, and frontline workers to support one another during times of heightened life stress. It exhorts members of the air force to seek help from mental health clinics and observes that seeking help early is likely to enhance careers rather than hinder them. The program instructs commanders and supervisors to support and protect those who seek mental health care and eliminates policies that previously served as barriers to seeking and obtaining mental health care.

To improve surveillance, a Web-based database is used to capture demographic, risk factor, and protective factor information about individuals who attempted or completed suicide. This extremely secure tool protects privacy and permits timely detection of changes in patterns in suicidal behavior that can be used to strengthen policies and enhance practices throughout the air force community. To improve crisis management, critical incident stress management teams are assembled and sent to installations that are hit hard by potentially traumatizing events such as combat deployments, serious aircraft accidents, natural disasters, and suicides within the units.

The air force experience is not necessarily applicable to the general population, because the air force is a tightly controlled and relatively homogenous community with identifiable leaders readily able to influence community norms and priorities. Regardless, it can still serve as a model for comparable hierarchical organizations and offer insight into prevention program planning. The program's overarching principles, such as engaging community leaders to change cultural norms, improving coordination of diverse human and health services, and providing educational programs to community members, can inform national efforts and may be replicable in other populations.

PREVENTION RESEARCH AND GOALS

In 1986 Congress funded the first Prevention Research Centers. In "Prevention Research Centers—Building the Public Health Research Base with Community Partners: At a Glance 2015" (November 2, 2015, http://www.cdc.gov/chronicdisease/resources/publications/AAG/prc.htm), the CDC indicates that 26 such centers are affiliated with medical schools or schools of public health. The centers explore and research a wide range of public health problems and test strategies to address these issues. Funded projects examine programs that address myriad prevention efforts such as reducing childhood obesity, decreasing tobacco use, promoting healthy aging, and enhancing workplace safety.

Primary prevention research and programming in the past aimed to prevent illness by more effectively encouraging people to avoid behaviors (such as smoking, abusing drugs, engaging in unsafe sexual practices, or overeating) that were linked to health risk. By 2015 prevention research and education also emphasized preventing falls among older adults, helping teens to delay sexual behavior, and reducing environmental exposures (such as sun, water pollution, radon, ozone, pesticides, and hazardous chemicals) that increase health risk.

In 2015 the CDC awarded $11 million to six academic institutions (Emory University; Johns Hopkins University; University of Illinois, Chicago; University of Iowa; University of Maryland, Baltimore; and University of Utah) to advance research to prevent infectious diseases and the spread of infection in health care facilities. In the press release "CDC Names Six New Medical Research Centers to Accelerate Health Care Innovations" (October 5, 2015, http://www.cdc.gov/media/releases/2015/p1005-medical-research-centers.html), the CDC states that the new prevention research will identify new ways to protect patients and hospital personnel from high-risk disease threats such as Ebola (an infectious, often fatal viral illness).

SATISFYING WORK, SOCIAL ACTIVITIES, AND PERSONAL RELATIONSHIPS ARE KEY TO HEALTH AND WELLNESS

Family, friends, active interests, and community involvement may do more than simply help people enjoy their life. Social activities and relationships may actually enable people to live longer by preventing or delaying the development of many diseases, including dementia. During the past three decades research has demonstrated that social experiences, activities, relationships, and work stress are related to health, well-being, and longevity. The kind of work stress that causes the greatest harm to physical and mental health is effort-reward imbalance—when great effort is made and the effort is neither recognized nor rewarded. Although women appear more vulnerable to work stress, men's health seems more dependent on the availability of social relationships and emotional support.

Several studies, such as the landmark Rand Corporation's "Health, Marriage, and Longer Life for Men" (1998, http://www.rand.org/pubs/research_briefs/RB5018/index1.html), show that marriage or living with a partner has greater health benefits for men than for women, because traditionally women are caregivers. More recent findings, such as a comparison of blood pressure and mental health among people who are happily married, unhappily married, and single, question whether the nurturing qualities of women are solely responsible for married men's improved health. Julianne Holt-Lunstad, Wendy Birmingham, and Brandon Q. Jones find in "Is There Something Unique about Marriage? The Relative Impact of Marital Status, Relationship Quality, and Network Social Support on Ambulatory Blood Pressure and Mental Health" (*Annals of Behavioral Medicine*, vol. 35, no. 2, April 2008) that both marital status and marital quality influence health status. Married people reported greater satisfaction with life and lower blood pressure than single individuals. Among married people, those who deemed their marital quality "higher" had lower blood pressure, lower stress, less depression, and reported higher levels of overall satisfaction with life. Holt-Lunstad, Birmingham, and Jones also observe that men and women living alone had better health than those with unsatisfactory relationships with their partner.

Cheryl A. Frye of the University at Albany, State University of New York, finds in "Neurosteroids' Effects and Mechanisms for Social, Cognitive, Emotional, and Physical Functions" (*Psychoneuroendocrinology*, vol. 34, suppl. 1, December 2009) that social supports—their presence or absence—may influence the course of age-related changes in physical, mental, and emotional health and well-being. The loss of close relationships, especially among older adults, is one of the greatest risk factors for mental and physical decline. Emerging research suggests that these changes may be hormonally mediated, and Frye indicates that "further understanding of these neurobiological and/or behavioral factors may lead to findings that ultimately can promote health and prevent disease."

Along with personal relationships, social activities also seem to protect against disease and increase longevity, even when the activities do not involve physical exercise. In "The Quality of Dyadic Relationships, Leisure Activities and Health among Older Women" (*Health Care for Women International*, vol. 30, no. 12, December 2009), Tanya R. Fitzpatrick of McGill University examines the influence of social relationships and leisure activities on the health of older women and finds that the quality of interpersonal relationships "has a strong influence on mental health measured by spirit, happiness, and an interesting life." Furthermore, Fitzpatrick observes that leisure activities not only predict but also improve physical health as measured by self-report and the number of chronic health conditions. There is also evidence that close relationships can substitute for other close relationships. This is a key concern because the death of a spouse or a close friend may increase the survivor's risk for social isolation. The observation that strong connections with children, relatives, and friends can substitute for relationships with spouses or partners is especially significant for widowed, divorced, or never-married older adults.

There is mounting evidence of the health benefits of socialization. Yumiko Kamiya et al. note in "Back to Basics or into a Brave New World? The Potential and Pitfalls of Biomarkers in Explaining the Pathways between Social Engagement and Health" (*Applied Demography and Public Health*, vol. 3, 2013) that the protective influence of social relationships on health is widely recognized. Findings from multiple studies consistently demonstrate the beneficial effects of social relationships on health. These include reduced overall mortality, reduced rates of physical and mental illness, and improved ability to perform the activities of daily living. People who are socially integrated—those with adequate or high levels of social relationships—are less likely to have heart attacks and less likely to develop respiratory illnesses when exposed to the common cold virus. They are more likely to survive breast cancer and less likely to suffer from cognitive decline (loss of the ability to think and reason) even when there is evidence of Alzheimer's disease (a progressive neurological disease that attacks brain cells causing memory loss and problems with thinking). Furthermore, the health risks associated with low levels of social integration are as harmful as those associated with smoking, high blood pressure, and excessive alcohol consumption.

In "Trajectories of Social Engagement and Limitations in Late Life" (*Journal of Health and Social Behavior*, vol. 52, no. 4, December 2011), Patricia A. Thomas of the University of Texas, Austin, confirms the observation that maintaining high levels of social interaction and engagement exerts a protective effect on the health of older adults. Thomas looked at how changing frequency and intensity of social interaction influenced the physical health and cognitive abilities of older adults. Survey participants were asked how often they attended religious services, visited with friends and family, and participated in volunteer activities, organizations, or special-interest clubs. Thomas posits that social interaction and engagement may act to prevent cognitive and physical decline by giving older adults a sense of purpose in their life and motivating them to engage in healthy behaviors.

Pets Are More Than Best Friends

Research conducted during the late 1990s found that pet ownership was associated with better health. At first, it was believed that the effects were simply increased well-being—the obvious delight of hospital and nursing home patients petting puppies, watching kittens play, or viewing fish in an aquarium clearly demonstrated pets' abilities to enhance mood and stimulate social interactions.

In 1999, however, Parminder Raina et al. reported in "Influence of Companion Animals on the Physical and Psychological Health of Older People: An Analysis of a One-Year Longitudinal Study" (*Journal of the American Geriatrics Society*, vol. 47, no. 3) that attachment to a companion animal was linked to maintaining or slightly improving the physical and psychological well-being of older adults. The researchers followed 1,054 older adults for one year and found that pet owners were better able to perform the activities of daily living and were more satisfied with their physical health, mental health, family relationships, living arrangements, finances, and friends. These findings were confirmed by Karen Allen, Jim Blascovich, and Wendy B. Mendes in "Cardiovascular Reactivity and the Presence of Pets, Friends, and Spouses: The Truth about Cats and Dogs" (*Psychosomatic Medicine*, vol. 64, no. 5, September 1, 2002).

In "Pet Ownership and Physical Health" (*Current Opinion in Psychiatry*, vol. 28, no. 5, 2015), Robert L. Matchock of Pennsylvania State University, Altoona, explains that today pet ownership is considered a "healthy preventive behavior" and that animal-assisted therapy is recognized as an effective social support, serving to relieve loneliness and ease emotional distress. Matchock reports that many studies find correlation between pet ownership and positive physical health such as improved cardiovascular health.

There are specific health benefits of human interaction with animals. Erika Friedmann et al. examine in "Relation between Pet Ownership and Heart Rate Variability in Patients with Healed Myocardial Infarcts" (*American Journal of Cardiology*, vol. 91, no. 6, March 2003) the differences in survival between pet owners and nonowners who suffered heart attacks over a two-year period. The researchers find that subjects without pets had reduced heart rate variability, which was associated with an increased risk of cardiac disease and mortality. Several researchers observe that petting dogs and cats actually lowers blood pressure. The physiologic mechanisms responsible for these health benefits are as yet unidentified; however, some researchers think that pets connect people to the natural world, enabling them to focus on others, rather than simply on themselves. Other researchers observe that dog owners walk more than people without dogs and credit pet owners' improved health to exercise. Nearly all agree that the nonjudgmental affection pets offer boosts health and wellness.

In "The Human-Companion Animal Bond: How Humans Benefit" (*Veterinary Clinics of North America Small Animal Practice*, vol. 39, no. 2, March 2009), Erika Friedmann and Heesook Son assert that pet ownership, or just the presence of a companion animal, is associated with health benefits, including improvements in mental, social, and physiologic health status. Sandra B. Barker and Aaron R. Wolen conclude in "The Benefits of Human–Companion Animal Interaction: A Review" (*Journal of Veterinary Medical Education*, vol. 35, no. 4, Winter 2008), a review of research published since 1980 about the benefits of human-companion animal bonds, that many studies support the health benefits of interacting with companion animals.

According to Allen R. McConnell et al., in "Friends with Benefits: On the Positive Consequences of Pet Ownership" (*Journal of Personality and Social Psychology*, vol. 101, no. 6, December 2011), the emotional benefits of pet ownership rival those of human friendship. The researchers observe that "pet owners had greater self-esteem, were more physically fit, tended to be less lonely, were more conscientious, were more extroverted, tended to be less fearful and tended to be less preoccupied than non-owners" and find "considerable evidence that pets benefit the lives of their owners, both psychologically and physically, by serving as an important source of social support."

In "Pet Ownership and Cardiovascular Risk: A Scientific Statement from the American Heart Association" (*Circulation*, vol. 127, no. 23, June 11, 2013), Glenn N. Levine et al. report that many studies find that pet ownership confers beneficial effects, including increased physical activity, favorable lipid profiles (low levels of cholesterol and triglycerides, which are associated with heart health), lower blood pressure, and improved survival after a sudden loss of blood flow to the heart. The researchers note that the strongest relationship between pet ownership and health benefits appears to be among dog owners, possibly because these relationships are studied more frequently or because dogs increase their owners' physical activity levels.

Healthy People 2020

Since 1979 the U.S. Department of Health and Human Services has been compiling scientific insights and advances in medicine from each decade to develop 10-year national objectives for promoting health and preventing disease. The department explains in "Leading Health Indicators Development and Framework" (March 14, 2016, http://www.healthypeople.gov/2020/

FIGURE 2.10

Healthy People 2020 goals

[Action model to achieve Healthy People 2020 overarching goals]

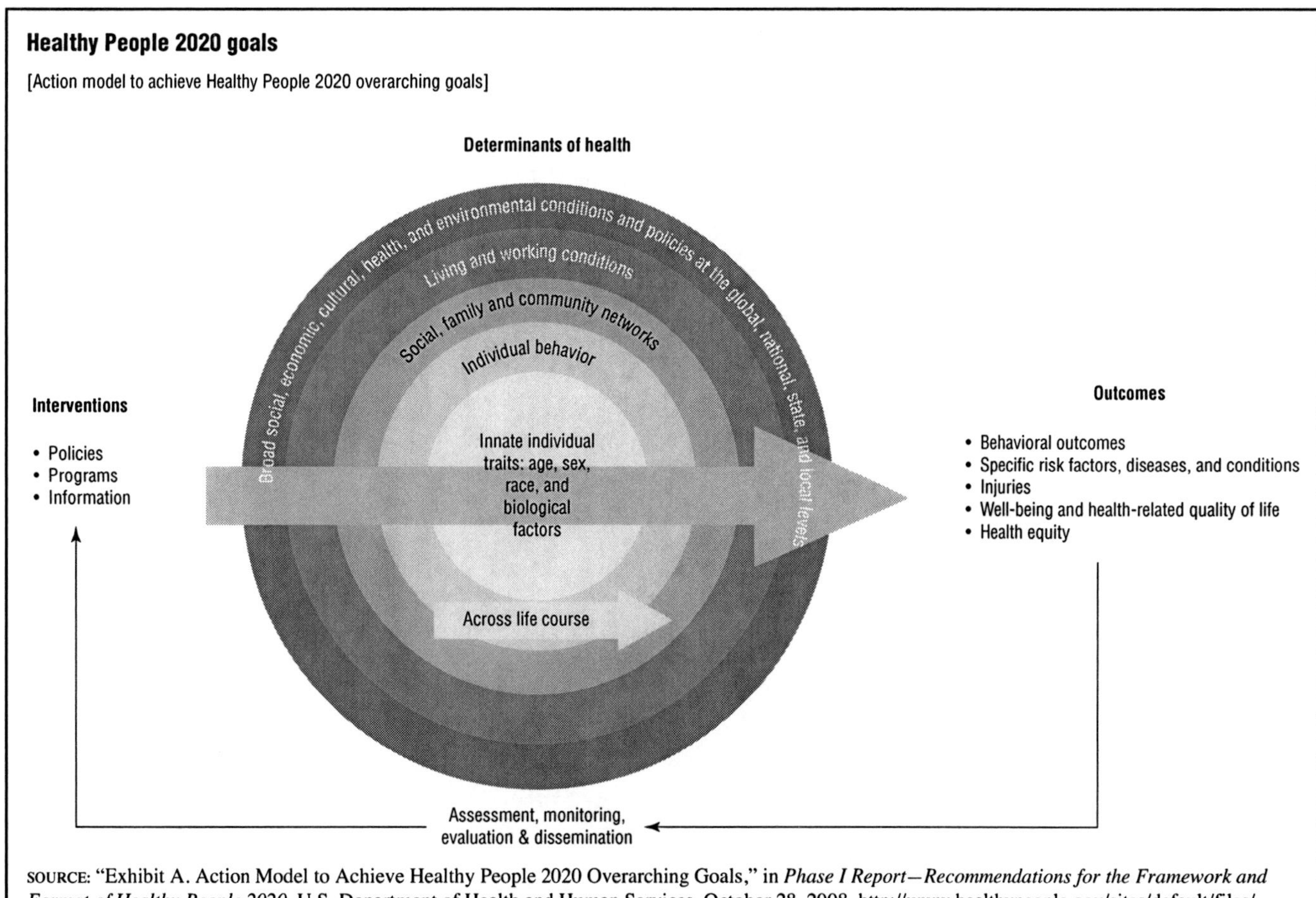

SOURCE: "Exhibit A. Action Model to Achieve Healthy People 2020 Overarching Goals," in *Phase I Report—Recommendations for the Framework and Format of Healthy People 2020*, U.S. Department of Health and Human Services, October 28, 2008, http://www.healthypeople.gov/sites/default/files/PhaseI_0.pdf (accessed December 18, 2015)

leading-health-indicators/Leading-Health-Indicators-Development-and-Framework) that Healthy People 2020 builds on previous public health objectives and aims to "draw attention to both individual and societal determinants that affect the public's health and contribute to health disparities from infancy through old age, thereby highlighting strategic opportunities to promote health and improve quality of life for all Americans." Health People 2020's (March 14, 2016, https://www.healthypeople.gov/2020/About-Healthy-People) overarching goals are to:

- Attain high-quality, longer lives free of preventable disease, disability, injury, and premature death.
- Achieve health equity, eliminate disparities, and improve the health of all groups.
- Create social and physical environments that promote good health for all.
- Promote quality of life, healthy development, and healthy behaviors across all life stages.

Nearly all the Healthy People 2020 goals and objectives involve one or more of the three levels of prevention that were discussed in this chapter. Figure 2.10 displays a graphic framework of the determinants of health and the overarching goals of Healthy People 2020.

CHAPTER 3

DIAGNOSING DISEASE: THE PROCESS OF DETECTING AND IDENTIFYING ILLNESS

"Diagnosis" means finding the cause of a disorder, not just giving it a name.

—Sydney Walker III, *A Dose of Sanity: Mind, Medicine, and Misdiagnosis* (1996)

The practice of medicine is often considered to be both science and art because identifying the underlying causes of disease and establishing a diagnosis require that health care practitioners (physicians, nurses, and allied health professionals) use a combination of scientific method, intuition, and interpersonal (communication and human relations) skills. Diagnosis relies on the powers of observation; listening and communication skills; analytical ability; knowledge of human anatomy (structure and parts of the human body) and physiology (the functions and life processes of body systems); and an understanding of the natural course of illness.

The editors of the 18th edition of *Harrison's Principles of Internal Medicine* (2011) explain that diagnosis requires a logical approach to problem solving that involves analysis and synthesis. In other words, health care practitioners must systematically break down the information they obtain from a patient's medical history, physical examination, and laboratory test results and then reassemble it into a pattern that fits a well-defined syndrome (a group of symptoms that collectively describe a disease).

MEDICAL HISTORIES

Obtaining a complete and accurate medical history is the first step in the diagnostic process. In fact, many health care practitioners believe that the patient's medical history is the key to diagnosis and that the physical examination and results of any diagnostic testing (laboratory analyses of blood or urine, x-rays, or other imaging studies) simply serve to confirm the diagnosis that is made on the basis of the medical history.

A medical history is developed using data that are collected during the health care practitioner's interview with the patient. The medical history may also include data from a health history form or health questionnaire that is completed by the patient before the visit with the practitioner. The objectives of taking a medical history are to:

- Obtain, develop, and document (in writing) a clear, accurate, and chronological account of the individual's medical history (including a family history, employment history, social history, and other relevant information) and current medical problems
- List, describe, and assign priority to each symptom, complaint, and problem presented
- Observe the patient's emotional state as reflected in voice, posture, and demeanor
- Establish and enhance communication, trust, understanding, and comfort in the physician-patient (or nurse-patient) relationship

Besides eliciting a history of all the patient's previous medical problems and illnesses, the health care practitioner asks questions to learn about the history of the present illness or complaint—how and when it began, the nature of symptoms, aggravating and relieving factors, its effect on function, and any self-care measures the patient has taken.

The medical history also includes a review of physiological systems—such as the cardiovascular (related to heart and circulation), gastrointestinal (digestive disorders), psychiatric (mental and emotional health), and neurologic (brain and nerve disorders) systems—through which the patient may experience symptoms of disease. The review of physiological systems frequently helps the practitioner assess the severity of the present problem and confirm the diagnosis.

Because it relies on the patient's assessment of the severity, duration, and other characteristics of symptoms, as well as the patient's memories and interpretation of past illnesses, the medical history provides the practitioner with subjective information. With the objective findings of the physical examination and other diagnostic tests, it helps the practitioner to identify disease correctly.

PHYSICAL EXAMINATION

The National Institutes of Health's U.S. National Library of Medicine notes in "Physical Examination" (March 2, 2016, http://www.nlm.nih.gov/medlineplus/ency/article/002274.htm) that during a physical examination "a health care provider studies your body to determine if you do or do not have a physical problem." This examination includes inspection (looking), palpation (feeling), auscultation (listening), and percussion (tapping to produce sounds).

Vital Signs

In a clinic or office-based medical practice, the physical examination may begin with a nurse or medical assistant measuring the patient's vital signs: temperature, respiration, pulse, and blood pressure. Temperature is measured using a thermometer. Normal oral temperature (measured by mouth) is 98.6 degrees Fahrenheit (37 degrees C). Temperature may also be measured rectally, under the arm (axillary), or aurally with an electronic thermometer placed in the ear.

Respiration is measured by observing the patient's rate of breathing. Besides determining the rate of respiration (the average adult takes 12 to 20 breaths per minute), the practitioner also notes any difficulties in breathing.

Pulse rate and rhythm are assessed by compressing the resting patient's radial artery at the wrist. The normal resting pulse rate is between 60 and 100 beats per minute, and the rhythm should be regular, with even spaces between beats. Pulse rates higher than 100 beats per minute are called tachycardia, and rates lower than 60 beats per minute are called bradycardia. Some variations in pulse rates are considered normal and do not signify disease. Athletes who engage in high levels of physical conditioning often have pulse rates of less than 60 beats per minute at rest. Similarly, pulse rates increase naturally in response to exercise or emotional stress.

Blood pressure is measured using an inflatable blood pressure cuff, also known as a sphygmomanometer. Blood pressure is measured in millimeters of mercury (mm Hg). Two readings are recorded: systolic pressure and diastolic pressure. Systolic pressure is the top number of a blood pressure reading and represents the pressure at which beats are first heard in the artery; diastolic pressure is the bottom number and is the pressure at which the beat can no longer be heard. As with pulse rates, blood pressure varies in response to exercise and emotional stress. Normally, the systolic blood pressure of an adult is less than 140 mm Hg and diastolic blood pressure is less than 90 mm Hg. Repeated blood pressure readings higher than 140/90 mm Hg may lead to a diagnosis of hypertension (high blood pressure).

In October 2015 the U.S. Preventive Services Task Force (http://www.uspreventiveservicestaskforce.org/Page/Document/RecommendationStatementFinal/high-blood-pressure-in-adults-screening) recommended that before initiating treatment, high blood pressure should be confirmed at home or outside of the doctor's office given that many people experience "white-coat hypertension" (elevated blood pressure at the doctor's office in response to stress).

Head and Neck

Physical examination of the head and neck involves inspection of the head (including the skin and hair), ears, nose, throat, and neck. An instrument called an otoscope is used to examine the ear canal and tympanic membrane for swelling, redness, lesions, drainage, discharge, or deformity. When examining the throat, the practitioner looks for abnormalities and, by depressing the tongue, can inspect the mouth, oropharynx, and tonsils.

The practitioner notes any scars, asymmetry, or masses (lumps or thickenings) in the neck and systematically palpates (presses) to examine the chains of lymph nodes (also called lymph glands, which are clusters of cells that filter fluid known as lymph) that run in front and behind the ear, near the jaw, and at the base of the neck. The practitioner also inspects and palpates the thyroid gland (the largest gland in the endocrine system, located where the larynx and trachea meet).

Eye Examination

An eye examination consists of a vision test and visual inspection of the eye and surrounding areas for abnormalities, deformities, and signs of infection. Two numbers describe visual acuity (vision). The first number is the distance (in feet) that the patient is standing from the test chart, and the second number is the distance that the eye can read a line of letters from the test chart. Because 20/20 is considered normal vision, a person with 20/60 vision can read a line of letters from 20 feet (6.1 m) away that a person with normal vision can read from a distance of 60 feet (18.3 m) away from the test chart. Using an ophthalmoscope, the practitioner examines the inner structures of the eye by looking through the pupil.

Chest and Lungs

The examination of the chest and lungs focuses on identifying disorders of breathing, which consists of inspiration and expiration (inhaling and exhaling). Changes in the length of either action could be a sign of disease. For example, prolonged expiration may be the result of an obstruction in the airway due to asthma.

Percussion is a tapping technique used to produce sounds on the chest wall that may be distinguished as normal, dull, or hyperresonant. Dull sounds may indicate the presence of pneumonia (infection of the lungs), whereas hyperresonant sounds may be signs of pneumothorax (collapsed lung) or emphysema (a disease in which the alveoli [microscopic air sacs] of the lung are destroyed).

The practitioner listens to breath sounds with a stethoscope. Listening with the stethoscope is called auscultation. Decreased breath sounds may be signs of emphysema or pneumothorax, whereas high-pitched wheezes are associated with asthma. Another device that is used to monitor the breathing of patients with asthma is a peak flow meter. After taking a deep breath, the patient exhales into the peak flow meter, which measures the velocity of exhaled breath.

Back and Extremities

The examination of the back and extremities (arms and legs) focuses on the anatomy of the musculoskeletal system. Major muscle groups and all joints are examined, and pulses on the arms, legs, and feet (radial, posterior tibial, and dorsalis pedis, respectively) are checked to be certain that blood flow to the extremities is adequate. Monitoring capillary refill time is another way to assess the adequacy of blood flow. To do this, the practitioner presses the patient's fingernail or toenail until it pales and then observes how long it takes to regain color once the pressure is released. Longer capillary refill time may be a sign of peripheral vascular disease or blocked arteries.

Cardiovascular System

The examination of the cardiovascular system focuses on the rate and rhythm of the radial and carotid artery pulses (located at the wrist and neck), blood pressure, and the sounds that are associated with blood flow through the carotid arteries and the heart. After measuring and recording the rate and rhythm of the radial and carotid pulses, the practitioner may listen with a stethoscope for abnormal sounds in the carotid arteries. Rushing sounds, called bruits, may indicate a narrowing of the arteries and an increased risk for stroke.

Examination also entails assessment of jugular vein pressure and listening with a stethoscope to heart sounds. Heart murmurs, clicks, and extra sounds are abnormal heart sounds that are associated with the functioning of heart valves. Some murmurs are considered innocent (normal variations), whereas others are indicators of serious malfunctioning of heart valves.

Abdominal Examination

Inspection of the abdomen focuses on the shape of the abdomen and the presence of scars, lesions, rashes, and hernias (protrusion of an organ through a wall that usually encloses it). Using a stethoscope, the practitioner listens to the arteries that supply blood to the kidneys, listens to the aorta (the main artery that supplies blood to all the organs except the lungs), and listens for bowel sounds.

Percussion of the abdomen that produces a dull sound may indicate an abnormality, such as an abdominal mass. Percussion is also used to determine the size of the liver (the largest gland in the body, which produces bile to aid in the digestion of fats) that measures 2.5 to 5 inches (6 to 12.7 cm) in a healthy adult. An expanse of dullness around the liver or spleen (an organ on the left side of the body, below the diaphragm, that filters and stores blood) may indicate that these organs are enlarged.

Breast and Pelvic Examination

Visual inspection of the breast focuses on symmetry, dimpling, swelling, or discoloration of the skin and position of the nipple. Manual breast examination is performed by methodically palpating breast tissue in overlapping vertical strips using small circular movements from the midline to the axilla (armpit). The practitioner presses the nipple to observe whether there is any discharge (fluid) and palpates the axilla for the presence of lymph nodes.

A pelvic examination may be performed after the breast examination, during a woman's physical examination. At this time, a sample of tissue may be obtained for a Papanicolaou (Pap) test, which is examined microscopically by the cytology laboratory for cervical cancer cells.

Neurologic and Mental Status Examinations

Neurologic examination considers mental status, cranial nerves (the 12 cranial nerves are abducens, accessory, acoustic, facial, glossopharyngeal, hypoglossal, oculomotor, olfactory, optic, trigeminal, trochlear, and vagus), muscle strength, coordination and gait, reflexes, and the senses. Figure 3.1 shows the nervous system and describes each of the four types of nerves. The cranial nerves connect the brain to the eyes, mouth, ears, and other parts of the head. The central nerves are in the brain and spinal cord. The peripheral nerves go from the spinal cord to the arms, hands, legs, and feet. The autonomic nerves go from the spinal cord to internal organs—lungs, heart, stomach, intestines, bladder, and sex organs.

Generally, the cranial nerves are assessed by observation as the health care practitioner asks the patient to demonstrate their use. For example, the facial nerve may be tested by watching patients open their mouth and clench their teeth. The practitioner also tests sensation

FIGURE 3.1

The nervous system

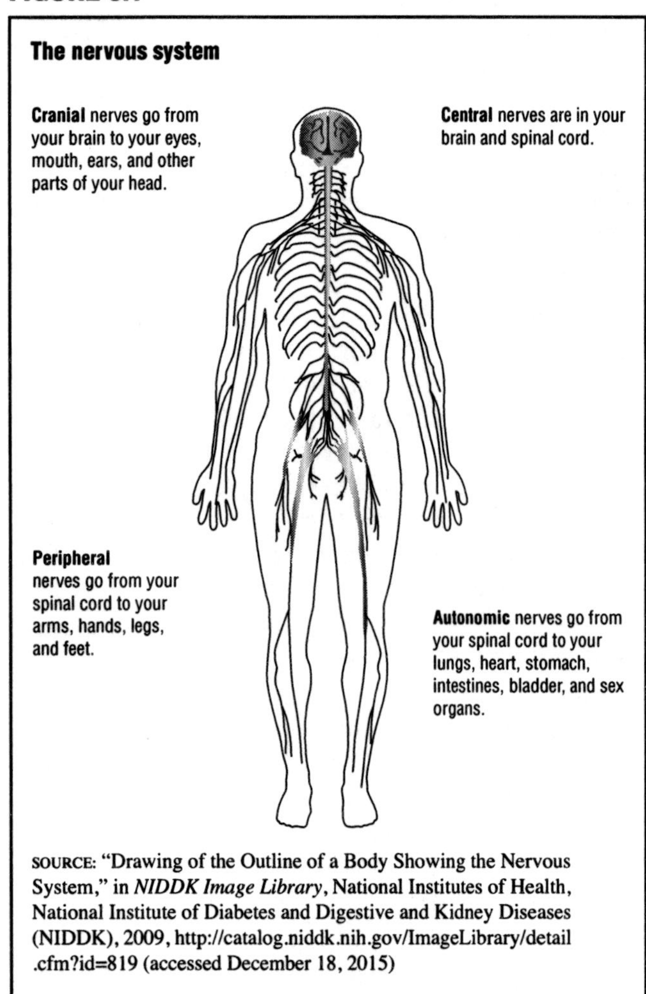

SOURCE: "Drawing of the Outline of a Body Showing the Nervous System," in *NIDDK Image Library*, National Institutes of Health, National Institute of Diabetes and Digestive and Kidney Diseases (NIDDK), 2009, http://catalog.niddk.nih.gov/ImageLibrary/detail.cfm?id=819 (accessed December 18, 2015)

to the parts of the face that are supplied by branches of the trigeminal nerve by applying sharp and dull objects to these areas and asking the patient to distinguish between them. Finally, the practitioner touches the patient's cornea lightly to observe whether the corneal reflex is functioning properly; if it is, the patient will blink.

Evaluating the motor system involves the assessment of muscle symmetry, tone, strength, gait, and coordination. Patients are observed performing different skills and walking. Reflexes are tested and graded as normal, hypoactive, or hyperactive. An example of reflex testing is when the practitioner strikes the patellar tendon just below the kneecap to observe contraction of the quadriceps muscle in the thigh and extension of the knee.

The sensory system test determines whether there is a loss of sensation in any body part. The practitioner may use the vibrations from a tuning fork or hot, cold, or sharp objects to evaluate the patient's ability to perceive sensation accurately. The practitioner may also test discrimination (the ability to accurately interpret touch and position) by tracing a number on the patient's palm and asking the patient to name the number.

A preliminary evaluation of mental status aims to determine the patient's orientation, immediate and short-term memory, and ability to follow simple verbal and written commands. Patients are considered "oriented" if they can identify time, place, and person accurately. Immediate and short-term memories are tested when the practitioner poses simple questions for the patient to answer, and the ability to follow commands is assessed by observing the patient perform tasks in response to verbal or written instructions.

Weighing the Value of Annual Physicals

In recent years the American Medical Association and other medical professional societies have downplayed the importance of traditional "head-to-toe" annual physical examinations. Instead, they favor a periodic health examination—an individualized screening and examination that is based on the patient's age, health status, lifestyle, and risk factors.

In the October 15, 2015, issue of the *New England Journal of Medicine* (vol. 373, no. 16), Allan H. Goroll of the Massachusetts General Hospital, Boston, opines in "Toward Trusting Therapeutic Relationships—In Favor of the Annual Physical" that the annual physical is an opportunity to cultivate and reaffirm a trusted, meaningful doctor-patient relationship. In the same issue Ateev Mehrotra and Allan Prochazka observe in "Improving Value in Health Care—Against the Annual Physical" that annual physicals do not improve how patients fare in terms of illness or death rates. They concede that annual exams may be associated with reduced patient worry and increased use of preventive care but note that annual exams also have the potential to be harmful, as when diagnostic testing produces false-positive results, which generate additional testing and patient worry. Mehrotra and Prochazka assert that reducing the number of physicals (roughly one-third of Americans receive annual exams) would save billions of dollars and free up primary care providers' time. Instead of annual physicals, they advise "shifting our approach to preventive care delivery, and creating and reimbursing for a visit whose sole goal is to establish primary care relationships."

DIAGNOSTIC TESTING

Once the history and physical examination have been completed, the health care practitioner is often relatively certain about the cause of illness and the diagnosis. However, occasions occur when the history and physical examination point to more than one possible diagnosis. In such instances, the practitioner develops a differential diagnosis (a list of several likely diagnoses). The practitioner may then order specific diagnostic tests to narrow the list of possibilities. The results of these tests are evaluated in the context of the patient's history and physical examination.

There are scores of diagnostic tests—including blood tests, x-rays, computed tomography (CT) scans, ultrasounds, and magnetic resonance imaging (MRI) scans—to help the health care practitioner identify the cause of disease. It is important for practitioners to choose tests that not only improve their understanding of the disease but also affect treatment decisions. The decision to order a specific diagnostic test takes into account the test's reliability, validity, sensitivity, and specificity besides its risks to the patient and costs in terms of time and dollars.

The Reliability and Validity of Diagnostic Tests

The reliability of diagnostic testing refers to the test's ability to be repeated and to produce equivalent results in comparable circumstances. A reliable test is consistent and measures the same way each time it is used with the same patients in the same circumstances. For example, a well-calibrated balance scale is a reliable instrument for measuring body weight.

Validity is the accuracy of the diagnostic test. It is the degree to which the diagnostic test measures the disease, blood level, or other quality or characteristic it is intended to detect. A valid diagnostic test is one that can distinguish between those who have the disease from those who do not. There are two components of validity: sensitivity and specificity.

THE SENSITIVITY AND SPECIFICITY OF DIAGNOSTIC TESTS. Sensitivity refers to a test's ability to identify people who have the disease. By contrast, specificity refers to a test's ability to identify people who do not have the disease. Ideally, diagnostic tests should be highly sensitive and highly specific, thereby accurately classifying all people tested as either positive or negative. In practice, however, sensitivity and specificity are frequently inversely related—most tests with high levels of sensitivity have low specificity, and the reverse is also true.

The likelihood that a test result will be incorrect can be gauged based on the sensitivity and specificity of the test. For example, if a test's sensitivity is 95%, then when 100 patients with the disease are tested, 95 will test positive and five will test "false negative"—they have the disease but the test has failed to detect it. If a test is 90% specific, when 100 healthy, disease-free people are tested, 90 will receive negative test results and 10 will be given "false-positive" results—they do not have the disease but the test has inaccurately classified them as positive.

The advantages of highly sensitive tests are that they produce few false-negative results, and people who test negative are almost certain to be truly negative. Highly sensitive tests may be useful as preliminary screening measures for diseases where early detection is vitally important, such as the enzyme-linked immunosorbent assay screening test for the human immunodeficiency virus (HIV), the virus that produces acquired immunodeficiency syndrome (AIDS).

In contrast, highly specific tests produce few false-positive results and those who test positive are nearly certain to be positive. Highly specific tests are useful when confirming a diagnosis and in cases where the risks of treatment are high, such as the Western blot test to confirm the presence of HIV after it has been detected by the highly sensitive, but less specific, enzyme-linked immunosorbent assay test.

Laboratory Tests

The editors of *Harrison's Principles of Internal Medicine* observe that the growing number and availability of laboratory tests has encouraged physicians and other health care practitioners to become increasingly reliant on them as diagnostic tools. Laboratory tests are easy and convenient screening measures because multiple tests may be performed on a single sample of blood, urine, or other tissue and abnormal test results can provide valuable clues for diagnosis.

For screening purposes (to detect disease at its earliest stage, before it produces symptoms), the health care practitioner may order a complete blood count (a measurement of the size, number, and maturity of the different blood cells in a specific volume of blood), as well as a variety of other blood tests, including:

- Fasting blood glucose—this is a screening and diagnostic test for diabetes; values consistently greater than 126 milligrams per deciliter (mg/dl) indicate diabetes. Fasting blood glucose levels between 100 mg/dl and 125 mg/dl are considered impaired and are called prediabetes.
- Calcium—blood levels of calcium can be elevated as a result of hyperactive parathyroid glands.
- Lipids—elevated cholesterol, triglycerides, and low-density lipoproteins are associated with an increased risk of heart disease.
- Thyroid stimulating hormone (TSH)—high levels of TSH indicate hypothyroidism (underactivity of the thyroid gland), and abnormally low levels indicate hyperthyroidism (overly active thyroid gland).
- Venereal Disease Research Laboratory or rapid plasma reagin—these tests screen for syphilis, a sexually transmitted infection.
- HIV—it is important to screen for the presence of this virus.
- Stool occult blood (also called fecal occult blood test)—this tests for the presence of blood in the stool, which could be an indicator of colon cancer.

Diagnostic Imaging Techniques

Imaging studies are another form of diagnostic testing. In the past all diagnostic imaging studies were obtained using ionizing radiation (x-rays) and recorded on transparent film. Modern imaging studies, such as ultrasound and MRI, use nonionizing radiation and can be recorded digitally, viewed on computer monitors, sent via e-mail, and stored on compact discs, digital tape, or transparent film. Most imaging studies are painless and pose little risk to patients apart from minimal exposure to radiation.

X-RAYS AND ULTRASOUND. The images produced by x-rays are the result of varying radiation absorption rates of different body tissues—the calcium in bone has the highest x-ray absorption, soft tissue such as fat absorbs less, and air absorbs the least. Chest x-rays, which offer images of the lungs, ribs, heart, and diaphragm, are among the most frequently ordered imaging studies.

To view tissues that are normally invisible on x-ray, contrast agents, such as barium and iodine, may be introduced into the body. For example, contrast agents are often used for imaging studies of the gastrointestinal tract to diagnose digestive disorders.

Another common use of diagnostic x-rays is the measurement of bone density. Bone mass measurement (also called bone mineral density) is performed to evaluate the risk of bone fractures. Bone density is usually measured in the spine, hip, and/or wrist because these are the most common sites of fractures resulting from osteoporosis (a disease in which bones become weak, thin, fragile, and more likely to break).

Mammography also relies on x-ray technology to detect and pinpoint changes or abnormalities in the breast tissue that are too small to be felt by hand. Another imaging technique for breast examination is ultrasound, which can accurately distinguish solid tumors (lumps or masses) from fluid-filled cysts.

Ultrasound images are produced using the heat that is reflected from body tissues in response to high-frequency sound waves. Whereas x-ray is ideal for examining bone, ultrasound is used to examine soft tissue, such as the ovaries, uterus, breast, and prostate. It is not suitable for looking at bones, because calcium-containing tissues such as bone absorb, rather than reflect, sound waves.

COMPUTED TOMOGRAPHY, MAGNETIC RESONANCE IMAGING, AND POSITRON EMISSION TOMOGRAPHY. For conventional flat x-rays, the patient, x-ray source, and camera remain fixed and immobile. CT scans use a mobile x-ray source and generate a series of cross-section pictures, or slices, that are assembled by computer into images. Because CT distinguishes differences in soft tissue more effectively and with higher resolution than conventional x-rays, it is often used to examine internal organs in the abdomen, such as the liver, pancreas, spleen, kidneys, and adrenal gland, and the aorta and vena cava (large blood vessels that pass through the abdomen).

MRI scans generate images that are based on the interaction between a large magnet, radio waves, and hydrogen atoms in the body. Stimulated by ordinary radio waves within the powerful magnetic field, these atoms give off weak signals that a computer builds into images. MRI is frequently used to create images of the brain, spinal cord, heart, abdomen, bone marrow, and knee.

A variety of specialized MRI techniques are also available, including:

- Diffusion MRI—this technique, which is principally used to image the brain, reveals the movement of water molecules in tissue and the microstructure of the tissue. It also detects swelling in tissues.
- Dynamic contrast enhanced MRI—this technique, which is often used to assess blood flow to a tumor, creates a series of images before, during, and after injection of a contrast agent.
- Fluid attenuated inversion recovery—this technique removes the effect of fluid from MRI images, enabling differentiation of brain and spine lesions. It is used to assess stroke (when blood flow to the brain is reduced below the threshold for irreversible cell death) and degenerative neurological diseases such as multiple sclerosis.
- Functional MRI—this technique measures changes in blood flow in the brain and produces high-resolution images that help assess the activity of different parts of the brain.
- Magnetic resonance angiography—this technique enables examination of blood vessels and is frequently used to look at the arteries in or near the heart, brain, abdomen, or legs. The use of a contrast agent helps produce a clear image of the blood vessels.
- Magnetic resonance spectroscopy (MRS)—this technique detects chemical activity in cells. Because tumors contain high levels of specific chemicals, MRS may be used to identify and characterize a tumor.
- Perfusion MRI—this technique, which is generally used to assess problems in the brain such as tumors or stroke, detects capillary blood flow—both the amount and transit time of blood flow in the smallest blood vessels in the body. The use of a contrast agent helps identify blood flow in the capillaries and enables the identification of regions of brain tissue with diminished blood flow.

CT and MRI scans generate images of the body's structure (anatomy), whereas positron emission tomography (PET) scans offer insight into body function or processes (physiology). To create PET images, positron-emitting atoms are injected into the body, where they travel and strike other electrons, producing gamma rays. The gamma rays are then interpreted into images by a computer. Unlike CT and MRI scans, PET scans are rarely used for screening or diagnostic purposes. Instead, they are used to track the progress and treatment of patients with diagnosed diseases such as cancer.

Diagnostic Procedures

Other diagnostic tests that are commonly performed to screen for the presence of disease include:

- Throat culture—this test is used to determine whether streptococcus pyrogenes (commonly called strep) bacteria are the cause of a sore throat. To obtain a sample of the mucus in the throat, the health care practitioner swabs the back of the throat and places the swab in a tube. The swab is transferred into a culture in the laboratory, where it is examined for bacterial growth. The results of this test are available in two to three days. A rapid strep test that produces results in minutes is also available.
- Urinalysis and urine culture—chemical and microscopic examination of urine allow the identification of infection, diabetes, and the presence of blood in the urine.
- Colonoscopy—using a long tube that is fitted with a lens, the health care practitioner is able to look at the entire colon; identify and remove polyps; detect cancer; and diagnose other causes of blood in the stool, abdominal pain, and digestive disorders. To prepare for a colonoscopy, patients must empty their intestines completely before the examination.
- Flexible sigmoidoscopy—this test is similar to the colonoscopy, in that it uses a tube that is fitted with a camera to examine the colon. However, because the instrument is shorter than a colonoscope, it does not enable views of the entire colon. Through the flexible sigmoidoscope, the practitioner can examine only the sigmoid (lower portion) of the colon to detect polyps and cancers.
- Electrocardiogram—this test assesses the electrical function of the heart, detects abnormal heart rhythms, and aids in the diagnosis of myocardial infarction (heart attack) and other heart diseases.

Prenatal Diagnostic Testing

Ultrasound is routinely used to monitor the progress of pregnancy; evaluate the size, health, and position of the fetus; and detect some birth defects. Fetal ultrasound assists in the prediction of multiple births (more than one fetus) and sometimes provides information about the gender of the unborn child. Table 3.1 describes how and why ultrasound and other common prenatal tests are performed.

Chorionic villus sampling (CVS) enables obstetricians and perinatologists (physicians specializing in the evaluation and care of high-risk expectant mothers and babies) to assess the progress of pregnancy during the first trimester (the first three months). A physician passes a small, flexible tube called a catheter through the cervix to extract chorionic villi tissue—cells that will become the placenta and are genetically identical to the fetus's cells. The cells are examined in the laboratory for indications of genetic disorders such as cystic fibrosis (an inherited disease that is characterized by chronic respiratory and digestive problems), Down syndrome (a genetic condition that is caused by having an extra copy of chromosome 21), Tay-Sachs disease (a fatal disease that generally affects children of east European Jewish ancestry), and thalassemia (an inherited disorder of hemoglobin in red blood cells). The results of the testing are available within seven to 14 days. CVS provides the same diagnostic information as amniocentesis; however, the risks (miscarriage, infection, vaginal bleeding, and birth defects) that are associated with CVS are slightly higher.

Amniocentesis involves analyzing a sample of the amniotic fluid that surrounds the fetus in the uterus. The fluid is obtained when a physician inserts a hollow needle through the abdominal wall and the uterine wall. Like CVS, amniocentesis samples and analyzes cells that are derived from the fetus to enable parents to learn of chromosomal abnormalities and the gender of the unborn child. Results are usually available about two weeks after the test is performed.

Blood tests are also available to help diagnose fetal abnormalities. The enhanced alpha-fetoprotein test (also called a triple screen) measures the levels of protein and hormones that are produced by the fetus and can identify some birth defects, such as Down syndrome and neural tube defects. Two of the most common neural tube defects are anencephaly (absence of the majority of the brain) and spina bifida (incomplete development of the back and spine). Test results are available within two to three days. Women with abnormal results are often advised to undergo additional diagnostic testing, such as CVS or amniocentesis.

DIAGNOSING MENTAL ILLNESS

Unlike physical health problems and medical conditions, there are no laboratory tests such as blood and urine analyses or x-rays to assist practitioners to definitively diagnose mental illnesses. Instead, practitioners generally rely on listening carefully to patients' complaints and observing

TABLE 3.1

Common prenatal tests

Test	What it is	How it is done
Amniocentesis (AM-nee-oh-sen-TEE-suhss)	This test can diagnosis certain birth defects, including: • Down syndrome • Cystic fibrosis • Spina bifida It is performed at 14 to 20 weeks. It may be suggested for couples at higher risk for genetic disorders. It also provides DNA for paternity testing.	A thin needle is used to draw out a small amount of amniotic fluid and cells from the sac surrounding the fetus. The sample is sent to a lab for testing.
Biophysical profile (BPP)	This test is used in the third trimester to monitor the overall health of the baby and to help decide if the baby should be delivered early.	BPP involves an ultrasound exam along with a nonstress test. The BPP looks at the baby's breathing, movement, muscle tone, heart rate, and the amount of amniotic fluid.
Chorionic villus (KOR-ee-ON-ihk VIL-uhss) sampling (CVS)	A test done at 10 to 13 weeks to diagnose certain birth defects, including: • Chromosomal disorders, including Down syndrome • Genetic disorders, such as cystic fibrosis CVS may be suggested for couples at higher risk for genetic disorders. It also provides DNA for paternity testing.	A needle removes a small sample of cells from the placenta to be tested.
First trimester screen	A screening test done at 11 to 14 weeks to detect higher risk of: • Chromosomal disorders, including Down syndrome and trisomy 18 • Other problems, such as heart defects It also can reveal multiple births. Based on test results, your doctor may suggest other tests to diagnose a disorder.	This test involves both a blood test and an ultrasound exam called nuchal translucency (NOO-kuhl trans-LOO-sent-see) screening. The blood test measures the levels of certain substances in the mother's blood. The ultrasound exam measures the thickness at the back of the baby's neck. This information, combined with the mother's age, help doctors determine risk to the fetus.
Glucose challenge screening	A screening test done at 26 to 28 weeks to determine the mother's risk of gestational diabetes. Based on test results, your doctor may suggest a glucose tolerance test.	First, you consume a special sugary drink from your doctor. A blood sample is taken one hour later to look for high blood sugar levels.
Glucose tolerance test	This test is done at 26 to 28 weeks to diagnose gestational diabetes.	Your doctor will tell you what to eat a few days before the test. Then, you cannot eat or drink anything but sips of water for 14 hours before the test. Your blood is drawn to test your "fasting blood glucose level." Then, you will consume a sugary drink. Your blood will be tested every hour for three hours to see how well your body processes sugar.
Group B streptococcus (STREP-tuh-KOK-uhss) infection	This test is done at 36 to 37 weeks to look for bacteria that can cause pneumonia or serious infection in newborn.	A swab is used to take cells from your vagina and rectum to be tested.
Maternal serum screen (also called quad screen, triple test, triple screen, multiple markerscreen, or AFP)	A screening test done at 15 to 20 weeks to detect higher risk of: • Chromosomal disorders, including Down syndrome and trisomy 18 • Neural tube defects, such as spina bifida Based on test results, your doctor may suggest other tests to diagnose a disorder.	Blood is drawn to measure the levels of certain substances in the mother's blood.
Nonstress test (NST)	This test is performed after 28 weeks to monitor your baby's health. It can show signs of fetal distress, such as your baby not getting enough oxygen.	A belt is placed around the mother's belly to measure the baby's heart rate in response to its own movements.
Ultrasound exam	An ultrasound exam can be performed at any point during the pregnancy. Ultrasound exams are not routine. But it is not uncommon for women to have a standard ultrasound exam between 18 and 20 weeks to look for signs of problems with the baby's organs and body systems and confirm the age of the fetus and proper growth. It also might be able to tell the sex of your baby. Ultrasound exam is also used as part of the first trimester screen and biophysical profile (BPP). Based on exam results, your doctor may suggest other tests or other types of ultrasound to help detect a problem.	Ultrasound uses sound waves to create a "picture" of your baby on a monitor. With a standard ultrasound, a gel is spread on your abdomen. A special tool is moved over your abdomen, which allows your doctor and you to view the baby on a monitor.

TABLE 3.1
Common prenatal tests [CONTINUED]

Test	What it is	How it is done
Urine test	A urine sample can look for signs of health problems, such as: • Urinary tract infection • Diabetes • Preeclampsia If your doctor suspects a problem, the sample might be sent to a lab for more in-depth testing.	You will collect a small sample of clean, midstream urine in a sterile plastic cup. Testing strips that look for certain substances in your urine are dipped in the sample. The sample also can be looked at under a microscope.

SOURCE: "Common Prenatal Tests," in *Pregnancy: Prenatal Care and Tests*, U.S. Department of Health and Human Services, Office on Women's Health in the Office of the Assistant Secretary for Health, September 27, 2010, http://www.womenshealth.gov/pregnancy/you-are-pregnant/prenatal-care-tests.html#c (accessed December 18, 2015)

their behavior to assess their mood, motivation, and thinking. Sometimes mental health disorders may accompany physical complaints or medical conditions. The presence of more than one disease or disorder is called comorbidity.

Although there are varying opinions about the personality traits and characteristics that taken together constitute optimal mental health, historically it has been somewhat easier to define and identify mental illness—deviations from, or the absence of, mental health. Within the broad diagnosis of mental illness, there is more consensus about the origins, nature, and symptoms of mental disorders—serious and often long-term conditions in which changes in cognition (thought processes), behavior, or mood impair functioning—than exists about mental health problems—shorter term, less intense conditions that often resolve spontaneously and without treatment.

Because many mental health disorders are identified by primary-care physicians (general practitioners, family practitioners, internists, and pediatricians), the World Health Organization (WHO) developed educational materials and guidelines to assist practitioners in general medical settings—as opposed to psychiatric or other mental health settings—to assess and treat the mental health problems and disorders of patients in their care. The guidelines call for an assessment interview, during which a series of screening questions are asked. If a patient provides predominantly positive answers, the patient has an "identified mental disorder." If a patient responds positively to many questions but not enough to fulfill the diagnostic criteria for a disorder, the patient has a "subthreshold disorder." These disorders are defined by the WHO's 10th revision of the *International Classification of Diseases: Classification of Mental and Behavioural Disorders* (*ICD-10*), the European guide for the diagnosis of mental disorders. In North America the fifth edition of the *Diagnostic and Statistical Manual of Mental Disorders* (*DSM-V*), which was released in May 2013 by the American Psychiatric Association, is used for the same purpose as the *ICD-10*. It is the encyclopedia of diagnostic criteria for mental disorders. This definitive guide, which expands on the *ICD-10*, catalogs more than 300 mental disorders. Practitioners are encouraged to ask open-ended questions that enable patients to freely express their emotions, to ensure confidentiality, to acknowledge patients' responses, and to closely observe their body language and tone of voice.

Changing Criteria for Mental Illness

There are many controversies in mental health diagnosis, beginning with the definitions and classification of mental illnesses. Which criteria distinguish conditions as mental illness rather than as normal variations in thinking and behavior? Should conditions such as attention-deficit/hyperactivity disorder be classified as a learning problem or a mental disorder? Should practitioners distinguish between neurological conditions that cause brain dysfunction and cognitive impairment such as Alzheimer's disease (a type of dementia that causes confusion, memory failure, speech disturbances, and an inability to function) and mental illness involving brain dysfunction such as depression that may result from an imbalance of chemicals in the brain?

An examination of past versions of the *DSM* reveals that the definitions of mental illnesses have changed dramatically from one edition to another. People diagnosed with a specific mental disorder based on diagnostic criteria in one edition might no longer be considered mentally ill according to the next edition. Critics of the *DSM*, which has expanded more than 10-fold since its inception in 1952, claim that diseases are added arbitrarily by the American Psychiatric Association and that although some entries represent changing ideas about mental health and illness, others are politically motivated. For example, homosexuality was once considered a mental illness, but in the 21st century, largely in response to changing societal attitudes, it is no longer considered an illness.

Skeptics also question the sharp increase in the number of diagnoses and the number of Americans receiving these diagnoses. Does the increasing number of diagnoses reflect rapid advances in mental health diagnostic techniques? Have mental health professionals (psychiatrists, psychologists, clinical social workers, marriage and family therapists, and other mental health practitioners) simply improved their diagnostic skills? Are the stresses of 21st-century life precipitating an epidemic of mental illness in the United States? Or are mental health professionals simply labeling more behaviors and aspects of everyday life as pathological (diseased)?

Furthermore, there is dissent even within the mental health field about diagnosis that is rooted in the ongoing debate about the origins of mental illness. After taking into account all the relevant medical research, the Office of the Surgeon General concludes in the landmark report *Mental Health: A Report of the Surgeon General* (1999, http://www.surgeongeneral.gov/library/mentalhealth/home.html) that for most mental illnesses there is no demonstrable physiological cause. This means there is no laboratory test, imaging study (x-ray, MRI, or PET), or abnormality in brain tissue that has been definitively identified as causing mental illness. As of March 2016, there were no published studies refuting this contention. As such, the majority of people suffering from mental illness apparently have normal brains, and those with abnormal brain structure or function are diagnosed with neurological disorders rather than with mental illnesses.

DSM-V

According to Christine S. Moyer, in "DSM-5 Finally Debuts, Markedly Changed from Earlier Editions" (AMedNews.com, June 3, 2013), the fifth edition of the *DSM* includes new diagnoses, such as binge eating disorder and hoarding disorder, and a single diagnostic category, autism spectrum disorders, that encompasses a variety of diagnoses currently in use, such as Asperger's disorder (which affects the ability to socialize and communicate with others), childhood disintegrative disorder (a serious loss or absence of social, communication, and other skills), and pervasive developmental disorder (a group of disorders that are characterized by delays in the development of socialization and communication skills).

Changing Views of Mental Illness

Finally, there are those who view mental illness as a social condition rather than as one requiring medical diagnosis. They observe that even the surgeon general's report, which favors biological explanations of the origin, diagnosis, and treatment of mental illness, concedes that mental health is poorly understood and defined differently across cultures. If mental health and illness are rooted in cultural mores and values, then they are likely socioeconomic and political in origin. The proponents of societal causes of mental illness contend that mental illness is in part defined as a functional impairment. In 2014, 18.1% (43.6 million) of the U.S. adult population had some type of mental illness. (See Figure 3.2.) Given the prevalence of mental illness, perhaps it is not the individual who is ailing, but the society.

Despite the challenges of diagnosing mental illnesses, the Substance Abuse and Mental Health Services Administration of the U.S. Department of Health and Human Services indicates in *Results from the 2013 National Survey on Drug Use and Health: Mental Health Findings* (November 2014, http://www.samhsa.gov/data/sites/default/files/NSDUHmhfr2013/NSDUHmhfr2013.pdf) that 68.5% of adults in the United States with a serious mental illness received treatment for a mental health problem in 2013. (See Figure 3.3.)There are public health implications for those who do not receive treatment or who delay treatment. Untreated psychiatric disorders can lead to more frequent and more severe episodes and are more likely to become resistant to treatment. In addition, early onset mental disorders that are left untreated are associated with school failure, teenage pregnancy, unstable employment, early marriage, marital instability, and violence.

TOO FEW CHILDREN WITH MENTAL HEALTH DISORDERS RECEIVE EFFECTIVE TREATMENT. Ann F. Garland et al. assert in "Improving Community-Based Mental Health Care for Children: Translating Knowledge into Action" (*Administration and Policy in Mental Health and Mental Health Services Research*, vol. 40, no. 1, January 2013) that there is an urgent need to improve mental health care for children. The researchers observe that in addition to problems accessing mental health services, children who receive community-based mental health services do not show improvement because the usual mental health care for children is generally ineffective.

Garland et al. note that fewer than half of children in need of mental health services receive services and call for efforts to improve not only access but also engagement (attendance and participation in treatment programs) because 40% to 60% of children receiving outpatient mental health services attend a few sessions and drop out prematurely. The researchers emphasize the delivery of evidence-based practices (intervention and treatment that are delivered with the appropriate intensity and frequency), and call for transparency, accountability, and instituting mechanisms to assess the quality and effectiveness of care and treatment.

Technological Advances Improve Diagnostic Accuracy

Technology is advancing diagnostic testing in many ways. For example, in "Digitizing Diagnosis: A Review of Mobile Applications in the Diagnostic Process" (*Diagnosis*, vol. 2, no. 2, June 2015), Annemarie Jutel and Deborah Lupton of Victoria University of Wellington, New Zealand, describe the use of smartphone and software applications (apps) to assist with diagnoses. The researchers note that apps intended for use by medical professionals include digital versions of medical textbooks and dictionaries, training videos, and drug prescribing information. Furthermore, there are apps that monitor and measure blood glucose, blood pressure, and

FIGURE 3.2

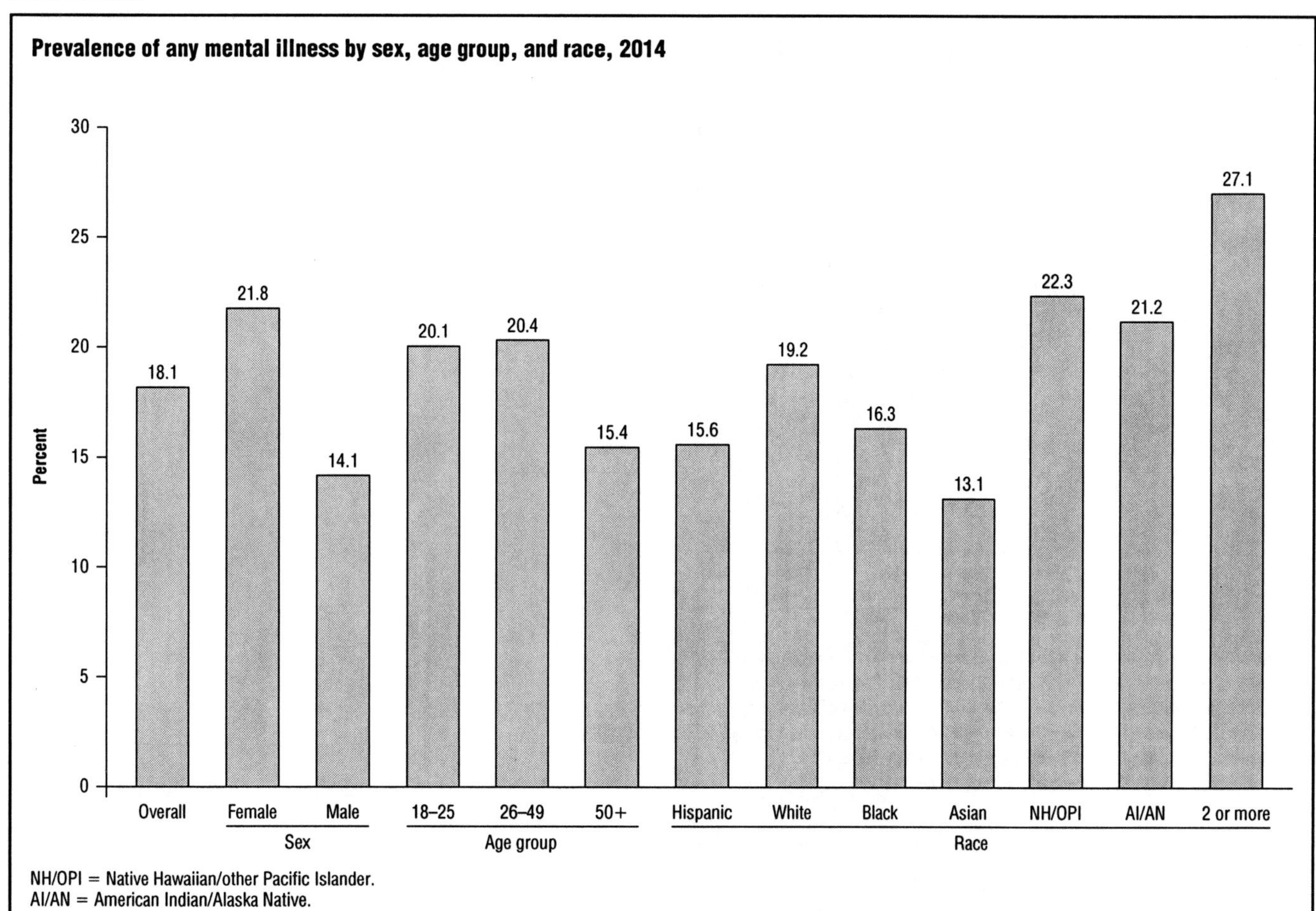

Prevalence of any mental illness by sex, age group, and race, 2014

NH/OPI = Native Hawaiian/other Pacific Islander.
AI/AN = American Indian/Alaska Native.

SOURCE: "Prevalence of Any Mental Illness among U.S. Adults (2014)," in *Any Mental Illness (AMI) among U.S. Adults*, National Institute of Mental Health, 2015, http://www.nimh.nih.gov/health/statistics/prevalence/nsduh-ami-2014-graph-final_150330.pdf (accessed December 18, 2015)

heart, kidney, and lung function via wearable electronics and other add-ons to smartphones, which enable them to serve as medical devices. Many more apps are marketed to lay people to help them self-monitor body weight, blood pressure, energy expended, and steps taken and to help patients manage chronic diseases such as diabetes and asthma. Other apps help patients store and access their medical records and treatment regimens, track medical appointments, access clinical trials, participate in patient support networks, and share information about their condition with friends and family.

Another promising new technology is nanodiagnostics, which involves the use of nanosensors (nanoscale probes and meters) to detect minute particles or miniscule quantities of abnormal cells or bacteria before symptoms of disease are apparent. James McIntosh describes in "Nanosensors: The Future of Diagnostic Medicine?" (MedicalNewsToday.com, January 14, 2016) the potential of nanosensors to detect a wide range of diseases, from recurrence of breast cancer to infection of an artificial joint such as a knee or hip replacement.

FIGURE 3.3

Receipt of mental health services among adults by level of mental illness, 2013

[Adults 18 and older]

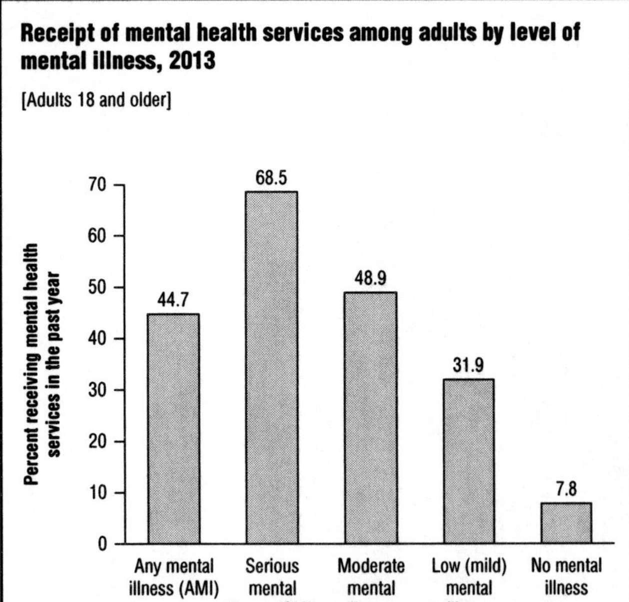

SOURCE: "Figure 2.7 Receipt of Mental Health Services among Adults Aged 18 or Older, by Level of Mental Illness: 2013," in *Results from the 2013 National Survey on Drug Use and Health: Mental Health Findings*, Substance Abuse and Mental Health Services Administration, November 2014, http://www.samhsa.gov/data/sites/default/files/NSDUHmhfr2013/NSDUHmhfr2013.pdf (accessed December 18, 2015)

CHAPTER 4

GENETICS AND HEALTH

Even at birth the whole individual is destined to die, and perhaps his organic disposition may already contain the indication of what he is to die from.

—Sigmund Freud, "The Dissolution of the Oedipus Complex" (1924)

Genetics, which is the branch of biology that studies heredity, concerns the biochemical instructions that convey information from generation to generation. To appreciate the role of genetics in health and illness, it is important to understand the interaction of genes, chromosomes, and genomes and to learn how deoxyribonucleic acid (DNA) functions as the information molecule of living organisms.

Genes are units of hereditary information that are made of DNA and located on chromosomes, which are separate strands of DNA wrapped in a double helix (two intertwined three-dimensional spirals) around a core of proteins contained in the nuclei of cells. Genes contain the instructions for the production of proteins, which make up the structure of cells and direct their activities. They exist in corresponding pairs, and a genome is a complete set of paired genes for an organism. The Human Genome Project explains in "The Science behind the Human Genome Project: Understanding the Basics" (August 19, 2013, http://www.ornl.gov/sci/techresources/Human_Genome/project/info.shtml) that humans have 46 chromosomes arranged in 23 pairs and that the human genome contains between 20,000 and 25,000 genes and 3 billion base pairs of DNA. Changes in the number, size, shape, or structure of chromosomes can result in a variety of physical and mental abnormalities and diseases.

GENETIC INHERITANCE

The inheritance of simple genetic traits involves two inherited copies of the gene that determines the phenotype (the observable characteristic) for that trait. When genes for a particular trait, such as eye color or hair color, exist in two or more different forms that may differ between individuals and populations, they are called alleles. For every gene, the offspring receives two alleles, one from each parent. The specific combination of inherited alleles is known as the genotype of the organism, and its expression, which can be observed, is its phenotype.

For many traits the phenotype results from an interaction between the genotype and environmental influences. For example, many readily apparent traits in humans, such as height, weight, and skin color, result from interactions between genetic and environmental factors. Height and weight are strongly influenced by nutrition as well as by genetic predisposition, and skin color may be influenced by exposure to ultraviolet radiation from sunlight. Along with these easily observed traits, there are other complex phenotypes that involve multiple gene-encoded proteins and the alleles of these particular genes that are influenced by a subtle and intricate interplay of genetic and environmental factors. So even though the presence of specific genes indicates a susceptibility or a likelihood to develop a certain trait, it does not guarantee expression of the trait.

For a specific trait, some alleles may be dominant whereas others are recessive. The phenotype of a dominant allele is always expressed, but the phenotype of a recessive allele is expressed only when both alleles are recessive. Recessive genes are passed from one generation to the next, and they can only be expressed in individuals who do not inherit a copy of the dominant gene for the specific trait.

In some instances, known as incomplete dominance, one allele does not completely dominate over the other, and the resulting phenotype is a blend of both traits. For example, skin color is a trait often governed by incomplete dominance, with offspring appearing to be a blend of the skin tones of each parent. Furthermore, some traits are multigenic or polygenic, which means that they are determined by a combination of several genes, and the resulting phenotype is determined by the final combination of alleles of all the genes that govern the particular trait.

Some multigenic traits are governed by many genes, and each contributes equally to the expression of the trait. In cases such as these, a defect in a single gene pair may have little impact on the expression of the trait. Other multigenic traits are predominantly directed by one major gene pair and only mildly influenced by the effects of other gene pairs. For these traits, the impact of a defective gene pair depends on whether it is the major pair governing expression of the trait or one of the minor pairs influencing its expression.

Genetic inheritance can be quite complex, and a broad array of other factors enters into whether a trait will appear and the extent to which it is expressed. For example, different individuals may express a trait with different levels of intensity or severity. When this occurs, it is known as variable expressivity.

The Influence of Heredity on Health

It has long been understood that heredity exerts a profound influence on health. Genetic inheritance explains how and why certain traits such as the propensity to obesity, eye color, and blood types run in families. Genomics (the study of more than single genes) considers the functions and interactions of all the genes in the genome. Genomics is a relatively recent discipline, because it has only been about two decades since the human genome was fully elaborated, but it already has important applications in advancing an understanding of health and disease.

Genomics relies on knowledge of and access to the entire genome and has already been applied to understanding the causes of many serious and increasingly prevalent diseases such as breast and colorectal cancer, Parkinson's disease (a disease affecting the part of the brain that is associated with movement), and Alzheimer's disease (a type of dementia that causes confusion, memory failure, speech disturbances, and an inability to function). Furthermore, genomics has also played a key role in understanding susceptibility to, and treatment of, infectious diseases, which were, until recently, thought to be caused exclusively by environmental factors. Examples of infectious diseases in which multiple genes and environmental exposures influence the risk of developing the disease include infection with the human immunodeficiency virus (HIV; the virus that produces acquired immunodeficiency syndrome [AIDS]) and tuberculosis. Genetic variations may confer protection against disease or may have a causative role in the expression of disease.

Although most conditions involve an interplay in which genetics and environmental factors make important, though not necessarily equal, contributions, it is nonetheless conventional to classify diseases as primarily genetic in origin or largely attributable to environmental causes. As understanding of genomics advances and scientists identify genes involved in more diseases, the distinction between these two classes of disorders is blurring. This chapter considers genetic testing, some of the disorders that are believed to be predominantly genetic in origin, and some that are the result of genes acted on by environmental factors.

GENETIC DISORDERS

There are two types of genes: dominant and recessive. When a dominant gene is passed on to offspring, the feature or trait it determines will appear independent of the characteristics of the corresponding gene on the chromosome that is inherited from the other parent. If the gene is recessive, the feature it determines cannot appear in the offspring unless both of the parents' chromosomes contain the recessive gene for that characteristic. Similarly, among diseases and conditions that are primarily attributable to a single gene or multiple genes, there are autosomal (a non-sex-related chromosome) dominant disorders and autosomal recessive disorders. Figure 4.1 shows how X-linked recessive inheritance occurs. Duchenne muscular dystrophy (DMD; a disorder that involves progressive muscle weakening) and hemophilia (a rare blood clotting disorder) are examples of diseases with X-linked recessive inheritance.

Another way to characterize genetic disorders is by their pattern of inheritance, as single gene, multifactorial, chromosomal, or mitochondrial. Single-gene disorders (also called Mendelian or monogenic) are caused by mutations in the DNA sequence of one gene. According to the U.S. National Library of Medicine, in "Genetics" (March 2, 2016, http://www.nlm.nih.gov/medlineplus/ency/article/002048.htm), there are approximately 4,000 known single-gene disorders. Examples are cystic fibrosis (CF; an inherited disease that is characterized by chronic respiratory and digestive problems), sickle-cell anemia (an inherited disease that produces abnormal hemoglobin in the blood), Huntington disease (HD; an inherited disease that affects the functioning of both the body and brain), and hereditary hemochromatosis. Hemochromatosis is a disorder in which the body absorbs too much iron from food. Instead of excreting the excess iron, the body stores it throughout the body, and this buildup of iron eventually damages the pancreas, liver, skin, and other tissues. Single-gene disorders are the result of either autosomal dominant, autosomal recessive, or X-linked inheritance (involving a gene on the X chromosome that is passed down through the family).

Multifactorial disorders (also called polygenic disorders) involve a complex interaction of environmental factors and mutations in multiple genes. For example, different genes that influence breast cancer susceptibility

FIGURE 4.1

An example of X-linked recessive inheritance

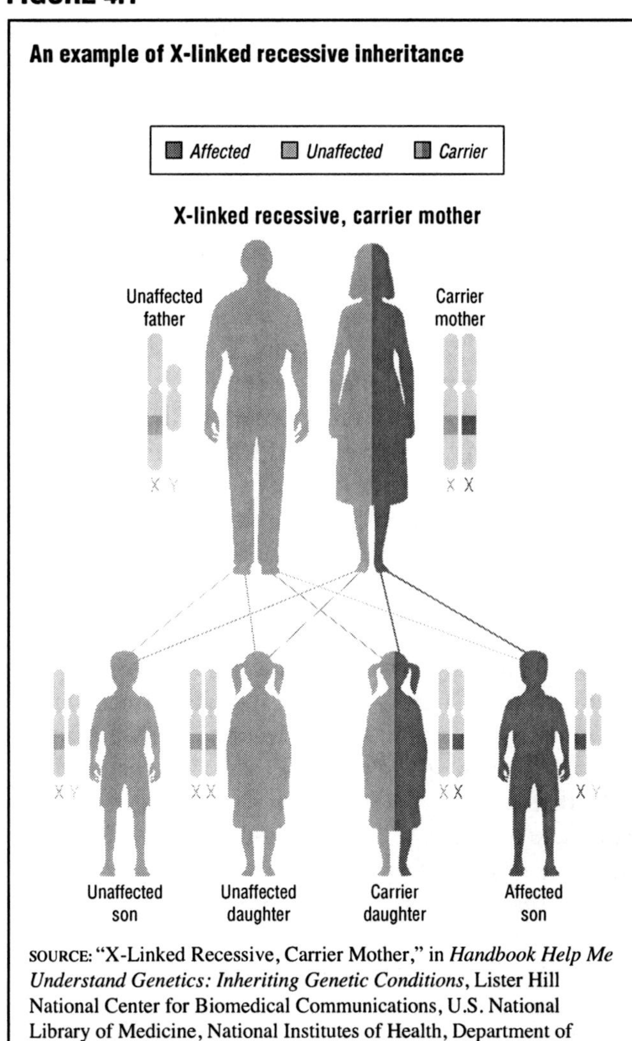

SOURCE: "X-Linked Recessive, Carrier Mother," in *Handbook Help Me Understand Genetics: Inheriting Genetic Conditions*, Lister Hill National Center for Biomedical Communications, U.S. National Library of Medicine, National Institutes of Health, Department of Health & Human Services, December 15, 2015, http://ghr.nlm.nih.gov/handbook/inheritance.pdf (accessed December 19, 2015)

have been found on different chromosomes, rendering it more difficult to analyze than single-gene or chromosomal disorders. Many common chronic diseases such as heart disease, Alzheimer's disease, arthritis, diabetes, and cancer are multifactorial in origin.

Chromosomal disorders result from abnormalities in chromosome structure, missing or extra copies of chromosomes, or errors such as the movement of a chromosome section from one chromosome to another, which is called translocation. Down syndrome is a chromosomal disorder that results when an individual has an extra copy, or a total of three copies, of chromosome 21. Mitochondrial disorders, which occur infrequently compared with other inherited disorders, result from mutations in the nonchromosomal DNA of mitochondria, which are organelles involved in cellular respiration.

The possibility of preventing and changing genetic legacies appears to be within the reach of modern medical science in the 21st century. Genomic medicine has the capacity to predict the risk of disease—from disorders that are highly probable as in the case of some of the well-established single-gene disorders to those in which increased susceptibility may be triggered by environmental factors. The promise of genomic medicine is to make preventive medicine more powerful and to individualize and customize treatment for each individual. Such treatment takes into account an individual's genetic susceptibilities and the characteristics of the specific disease or disorder.

GENETIC TESTING

A genetic test analyzes DNA, ribonucleic acid (RNA), chromosomes, and proteins to detect heritable diseases for the purposes of diagnosis, treatment, and other clinical decision making. A simple blood sample, which allows the extraction of the DNA from white blood cells, enables most genetic tests to be performed, but other body fluids and tissues may also be used for genetic testing. Genetic tests are used to screen for and diagnose genetic disease in newborns, children, and adults; to identify future health risks; to predict drug responses; and to assess the risk of disease in future generations.

Genetic tests that are performed to establish a diagnosis are different from those that are used to screen for a disease. Diagnostic tests are intended to definitively determine whether a patient has a particular problem. Such tests are generally quite complex and often require sophisticated analysis and interpretation. Because they are complex, require highly trained personnel to interpret them, and may be expensive, they are usually performed only on people who are believed to be at risk, such as patients who already have symptoms of a specific disease.

By contrast, screening is performed on healthy people with no symptoms of disease and may often be applied to the entire population or to people who are considered to be at risk of developing a specific disorder. By definition, a good screening test is relatively inexpensive, easy to use and interpret, and assists to identify which individuals in the population are at higher risk for a specific disease. Screening tests identify people who require further testing or people who should take special preventive measures or precautions. For example, people who are deemed especially susceptible to genetic conditions with specific environmental triggers, such as people with life-threatening allergic sensitivities, are advised to avoid specific environmental triggers.

Commonly used genetic tests include screening people of Ashkenazi Jewish heritage (the east European Jewish population primarily from Germany, Poland, and Russia, as opposed to the Sephardic Jewish population, which is primarily from Spain, parts of France, Italy, and North Africa) for Tay-Sachs disease (TSD); screening African Americans for sickle-cell disease (SCD); and screening expectant mothers over the age of 35 years whose fetuses are at an increased risk for Down syndrome. Table 4.1 lists some of the commonly used genomic tests that are currently available and the scenarios in which they are used.

The most common form of genetic testing is the screening of newborn infants for genetic abnormalities. This screening is accomplished by testing blood that is obtained from a prick of the newborn's heel within the first few days of being born. Newborn infants are screened for specific genetic disorders such as phenylketonuria, an inherited error of metabolism resulting from a deficiency of an enzyme called phenylalanine hydroxylase. If left undiagnosed and untreated, the deficiency of this enzyme can cause mental retardation, organ damage, and postural problems.

TABLE 4.1

Commonly used genomic tests

Test/application	Scenario
Newborn screening panel of 31 core conditions	Screening all newborns at birth through public health programs
BRCA genetic counseling/BRCA genetic testing	Referral to genetic counseling of women with specific family history patterns of breast or ovarian cancer
Lynch syndrome testing	Screening newly diagnosed cases of colorectal cancer for Lynch syndrome and cascade testing of relatives of affected Lynch syndrome cases
Familial hypercholesterolemia	Cascade cholesterol testing with/without DNA analysis among relatives of affected persons with familial hypercholesterolemia
HLA testing for abacavir sensitivity	Testing HIV patients before starting abacavir to reduce adverse effects and inform drug choice
HER2 mutation testing in breast cancer	Routine testing for HER2 mutations in patients with invasive breast cancer to target therapy
EGFR mutation tumor analysis in non-small cell lung cancer	Testing for EGFR-positive mutation in patients with non-small cell lung cancer (NSCLC) to target tyrosine kinase inhibitor (TKI) therapy
KRAS mutation analysis in patients with mCRC being considered for anti-EGFR therapy	Pharmacogenomic; prediction of non-response to cetuximaband panitumumab
First-degree family history of breast cancer	To inform discussion of chemoprevention for breast cancer for women; consider with age and other risk factors to identify high risk for breast cancer and low risk for adverse effects
Family history of cardiovascular disease before age 50 years in male relatives and age 60 years in female relatives	To inform earlier start to screening for cholesterol abnormalities for men and women (starting at age 20 years); use to identify increased risk for lipid disorders
Parental history of fracture	To inform (in combination with other risk factors) earlier start to screening for osteoporosis in women
Family history, especially siblings, with hereditary hemochromatosis	Counseling for genetic testing for hereditary hemochromatosis among a symptomatic people
Family history of breast or ovarian cancer that includes a relative with a known deleterious BRCA mutation	Referral to counseling for BRCA genetic testing for women

BRCA = breast cancer; HLA = human leukocyte antigen;
HIV = human immunodeficiency virus; HER2 = human epidermal growth receptor 2;
EGFR = epidermal growth factor receptor; KRAS = Kirsten rat sarcoma viral oncogene homolog; mCRC = metastic colorectal cancer.
Note: Tier 1 genomic and family health history applications are recommended for clinical use by evidence-based panels based on a systematic review of analytic validty, clinical validity and utility for specific clinical scenarios.

SOURCE: Adapted from "Tier 1 Genomic and Family Health History Applications Are Recommended for Clinical Use by Evidence-Based Panels Based on a Systematic Review of Analytic Validity, Clinical Validity and Utility for Specific Clinical Scenarios," in *Genomic Tests by Levels of Evidence*, Centers for Disease Control and Prevention, Center for Surveillance, Epidemiology, and Laboratory Services, Public Health Genomics, April 15, 2013, http://www.cdc.gov/genomics/gtesting/file/print/tier.pdf (accessed December 19, 2015)

Genetic screening aims to identify disorders that require early detection and benefit from timely treatment to prevent serious illness, disability, or death. The determination of which disorders to include in screening programs is made by each state; as such, the tests that are conducted vary from state to state. To determine which disorders to screen for, states generally consider criteria such as how often the disorder occurs in the population, whether screening is effective, and whether the disease or disorder is treatable. Figure 4.2 shows a method developed by the Health Resources and Services Administration's Maternal and Child Health Bureau that may be used to score and evaluate conditions to determine whether they should be included in routine newborn screening.

In 2008 the Newborn Screening Saves Lives Act was signed into law. Coleen A. Boyle, Joseph A. Bocchini Jr., and James Kelly report in "Reflections on 50 Years of Newborn Screening" (*Pediatrics*, vol. 133, no. 6, June 2014) that by 2009 most states were screening for a recommended panel of 29 disorders. They describe newborn screening as "an unqualified public health success; it saves lives, prevents severe disability, and is a good use of limited health care dollars," explaining that it leads to early diagnosis and treatment of more than 12,500 newborns annually.

In January 2016 Michele A. Gatheridge et al. suggested that DMD should be added to the recommended panel of newborn screening tests. In "Identifying Non-Duchenne Muscular Dystrophy-Positive and False Negative Results in Prior Duchenne Muscular Dystrophy Newborn Screening Programs: A Review" (*JAMA Neurology*, vol. 73, no. 1), the researchers explain that screening for DMD is important because early treatment improves how patients fare and because new genetic therapies require early diagnosis to be optimally effective. Gatheridge et al. also note that screening for DMD will result in identification of other muscle diseases.

GENETIC TESTING AND HUMAN REPRODUCTION

By March 2016 thousands of genetic diseases, both frequently occurring disorders and extremely rare ones, had been identified that may be conveyed from one generation to the next. As genetic research advances, many more genetic diseases will be uncovered and additional tests will be developed to screen parents who are at risk of passing on genetic disease to their children and to identify embryos, fetuses, and newborns that suffer from genetic diseases.

FIGURE 4.2

Decision-making process to determine which conditions to include in newborn screening programs

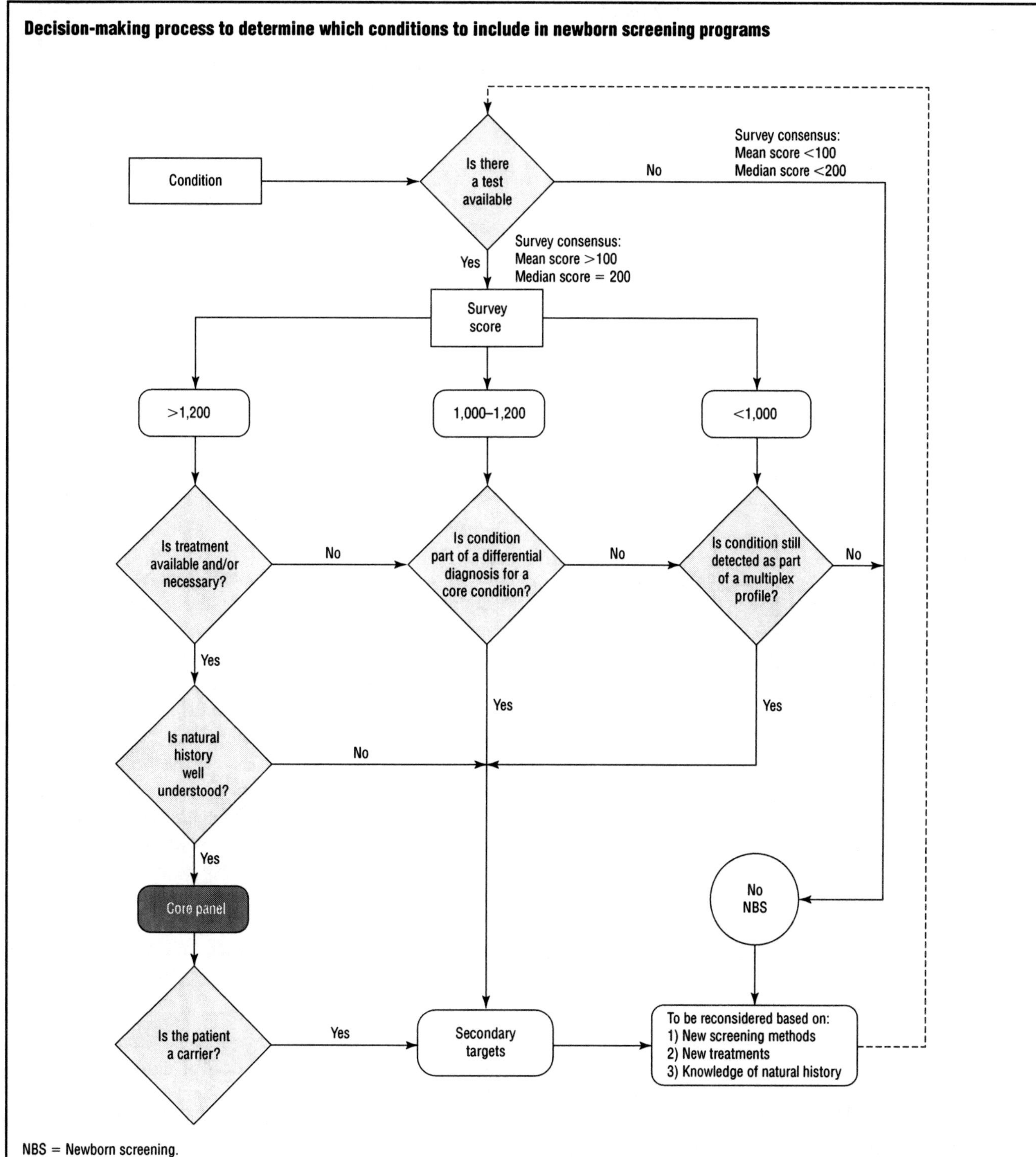

NBS = Newborn screening.

SOURCE: "Figure 9. Survey Scores Sorted by Testing Platforms," in *Newborn Screening: Toward a Uniform Screening Panel and System*, Health Resources and Services Administration, Maternal and Child Health Bureau, September 23, 2011, http://www.hrsa.gov/advisorycommittees/mchbadvisory/heritabledisorders/uniformscreening.pdf (accessed December 19, 2015)

Carrier Identification

Carrier identification is used to determine whether a healthy individual has a gene that may cause disease if passed on to his or her offspring. It is nearly always performed on populations that are deemed to be at a higher-than-average risk, such as those of Ashkenazi Jewish descent. Carrier testing is important because many people have just one copy of a gene for an autosomal recessive trait and because they are unaffected by the trait or disorder and are unaware that they may pass it on to their children. Only an individual with two copies of the gene will actually have the disorder. So although it is generally assumed that everyone is an unaffected carrier of at least one autosomal recessive gene, it only becomes a problem in terms of genetic inheritance when both parents are carriers—meaning that the mother and the father both have the same recessive disorder gene. When both parents are carriers, the offspring each have a one in four chance of receiving a defective copy of the gene from each parent and developing the disorder. (See Figure 4.3.)

An example of carrier identification is the test for a deletion in the dystrophin gene, which results in DMD, the most common form of muscular dystrophy in children. Carriers may avoid having an affected child by preventing pregnancy or by undergoing prenatal testing for DMD, with the option of ending the pregnancy if the fetus is found to be affected. Carrier identification is also important for CF and TSD.

Using genetic testing to detect carriers poses some challenges. Typically, a carrier has inherited a mutant gene from one parent and a normal gene from another parent. If, however, the carrier harbors a mutation that is only found in germ cells (the sperm or eggs), and only in some of these germ cells, then conventional genetic testing, which is performed on white blood cells, will miss the mutation.

FIGURE 4.3

Chances of inheriting a recessive disorder when both parents carry the gene for the disorder

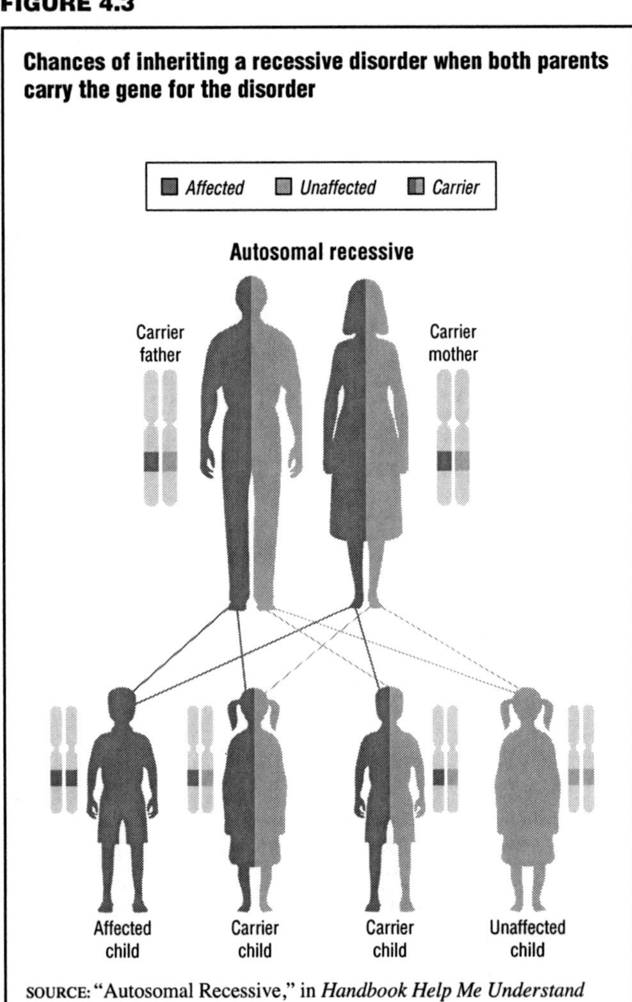

SOURCE: "Autosomal Recessive," in *Handbook Help Me Understand Genetics: Inheriting Genetic Conditions*, Lister Hill National Center for Biomedical Communications, U.S. National Library of Medicine, National Institutes of Health, Department of Health & Human Services, December 15, 2015, http://ghr.nlm.nih.gov/handbook/inheritance.pdf (accessed December 19, 2015)

Preimplantation Genetic Diagnosis

Preimplantation genetic diagnosis (PGD) permits prospective parents using in vitro fertilization (fertilization that takes place outside the body) to screen an embryo for specific genetic mutations before it is implanted in the uterus—when it is no larger than six or eight cells. One advantage of PGD is that it can screen for any congenital disorder for which the causative gene is known and may be used by couples who wish to avoid traditional prenatal diagnosis and the possibility of termination of pregnancy.

Prenatal Genetic Testing

Most prenatal genetic tests examine blood or other tissue from the mother to detect abnormalities in the fetus. The most common prenatal genetic blood test is the quad screen, which measures the levels of four substances in the blood (alpha fetoprotein, human chorionic gonadotropin, inhibin A [a hormone made by the placenta], and unconjugated estriol) and can identify selected birth defects such as Down syndrome and neural tube defects. (Two common neural tube defects are anencephaly [absence of the majority of the brain] and spina bifida [incomplete development of the back and spine].) The results of the quad screen are available within several days, and women with abnormal results are often advised to undergo further diagnostic testing such as chorionic villus sampling (CVS), amniocentesis, or percutaneous umbilical blood sampling. Table 4.2 describes six prenatal diagnostic procedures and when they are performed in terms of the weeks or trimesters of pregnancy.

CVS permits physicians to monitor the progress of pregnancy during the first trimester (the first three months). Laboratory examination of cells obtained via CVS can detect chromosomal abnormalities that produce genetic disorders such as Down syndrome, TSD, CF, and thalassemia (an inherited disorder of the hemoglobin in red blood cells). Some test results are available within a few days and others take one to two weeks, depending on the complexity of the laboratory analysis. CVS provides comparable diagnostic information as amniocentesis; however, the risks (miscarriage, infection, vaginal bleeding, and birth defects) that are associated with CVS are slightly higher. CVS may also be performed earlier in pregnancy, at 10 to 12 weeks, than amniocentesis, which is generally performed at 15 to 20 weeks. Approximately one out of 100 pregnancies is miscarried as a result of CVS.

TABLE 4.2

Prenatal tests

Amniocentesis	This test takes a small sample of the amniotic fluid surrounding the baby.	This test can be given after 14 weeks or during the third trimester. The former checks for genetic defects like Down Syndrome; the latter checks for abnormal lung development.
Chorionic villus sampling (CVS)	This test withdraws a small sample of tissue from just outside the amniotic sac in which the baby grows.	Taken between 10 and 12 weeks, this test checks for the possibility of such genetic diseases as Huntington's Disease and Duchenne muscular dystrophy.
Quad-screen test	This is a blood test taken from the mother that checks several different components.	This test is usually performed in the second trimester (15–20 weeks). The screening looks for several things, particularly the risk of Down Syndrome.
Rh incompatibility	This test determines whether the mother and baby have incompatible blood types.	This test can be done before pregnancy or at the first prenatal visit. If there is Rh incompatibility, treatments can help prevent later complications.
Ultrasound	This test uses high frequency sound waves to show internal organs and the growing baby within the womb.	Ultrasound can be used during the first, second, and third trimesters to show the gender, status, position, health, and growth of the baby.
Cell free fetal DNA	This new test uses the mother's blood to look for increased amounts of material from chromosomes 21, 18, and 13.	This test may be given as early as 10 weeks to women whose age, family history, or standard screening results place them at higher risk for having a child with a chromosome disorder.

SOURCE: Adapted from "Understanding Prenatal Tests," in "What Makes a Healthy Pregnancy?" *Medline Plus*, vol. 3, no. 1, Winter 2008, http://www.nlm.nih.gov/medlineplus/magazine/issues/winter08/articles/winter08pg22.html (accessed December 19, 2015)

Amniocentesis involves taking a sample of the fluid that surrounds the fetus in the uterus for chromosome analysis. Like CVS, amniocentesis samples and analyzes cells that are derived from the fetus to enable parents to learn of chromosomal abnormalities and the gender of the unborn child. The results are available in about two weeks after the test is performed. The risk of miscarriage (about one out of 200 pregnancies) resulting from amniocentesis is lower than the risk that is associated with CVS.

Down syndrome is the genetic disease most often identified by amniocentesis or CVS. Down syndrome is rarely inherited; most cases arise from an error in the formation of the egg or sperm, which results in the addition of an extra chromosome 21 at conception. Like most prenatal diagnoses for inherited genetic diseases, this use of genetic testing is intended to help prospective parents make informed decisions about the viability of a pregnancy. In "Data and Statistics" (October 21, 2014, http://www.cdc.gov/ncbddd/birthdefects/downsyndrome/data.html), the CDC indicates that there are approximately 6,000 diagnoses of Down syndrome each year in the United States—one out of every 700 babies is born with Down syndrome.

Periumbilical blood sampling (PUBS) is the most invasive prenatal genetic test. Using a high-resolution ultrasound, a physician inserts a needle through the expectant mother's abdominal wall to extract a sample of fetal blood from the umbilical cord. PUBS may be performed from approximately 16 weeks' gestation to term. PUBS poses a high risk to the fetus—one out of 50 procedures results in miscarriage. Because it is an invasive, relatively high-risk procedure, it is primarily used when a diagnosis must be made quickly. For example, if an expectant mother is exposed to an infectious agent with the potential to produce birth defects, PUBS may be used to detect an infection in the blood of the fetus.

GENETIC TESTING IN CHILDREN AND ADULTS

Genetic testing may also be performed to find out which children and adults are at an increased risk for developing specific diseases. Predictive genetic testing can identify which individuals are at risk for many heritable diseases including CF, TSD, HD, and amyotrophic lateral sclerosis (a degenerative neurologic condition commonly known as Lou Gehrig's disease), as well as some cancers (including some cases of breast, colon, and ovarian cancer).

The presence of a defective or altered gene is considered a "positive" result from predictive genetic testing. Nevertheless, a positive result does not guarantee that the person will develop the disease; it simply indicates genetic susceptibility and increased risk of developing the disease. Also, like other types of diagnostic medical testing, genetic tests are not 100% predictive—the results rely on the quality of laboratory procedures and the accuracy of interpretations—and there is always the chance of obtaining false-positive and false-negative test results.

Health professionals are optimistic that positive test results will motivate people at higher-than-average risk of developing a disease to be particularly attentive to disease prevention activities and to seek regular and periodic screening to detect the disease early, when it is most successfully treated. There is an expectation that genetic information will increasingly be used in routine population screening to determine individual susceptibility to common disorders such as heart disease, diabetes, and cancer. This type of screening will identify groups at risk so that primary prevention efforts such as diet and exercise or secondary prevention efforts such as early detection can be directed to them.

Symptomatic Genetic Testing

Although the majority of genetic testing is performed on people who are healthy and symptom-free to determine if they are carriers or to assess their risk of developing a specific disease or disorder, some testing is performed on people with symptoms of a disease to establish the diagnosis and calculate the risk of developing the disease for other family members. This type of testing is known as symptomatic genetic testing (it is also called diagnostic genetic testing or predictive genetic testing).

Symptomatic genetic testing is used to predict the likelihood that a healthy person with a family history of a disorder will develop the disease. Testing positive for a specific genetic mutation indicates an increased susceptibility to the disorder but does not confirm the diagnosis. For example, a woman may opt to undergo testing to learn whether she has a genetic mutation (BRCA1 or BRCA2, respectively) that would indicate the likelihood of developing hereditary breast or ovarian cancer. If she tests positive for the genetic mutation, she may then choose to undergo some form of preventive treatment. Preventive measures may include increased surveillance, such as more frequent mammography and breast ultrasound examinations; chemoprevention (prescription drug therapy that is intended to reduce risk); or surgical prophylaxis, such as mastectomy (surgical removal of one or both breasts) and/or oophorectomy (surgical removal of one or both ovaries).

Interestingly, researchers have discovered that these preventive measures are not as widely used as might be expected. For example, Richard G. Roetzheim et al. report in "Acceptance and Adherence to Chemoprevention among Women at Increased Risk of Breast Cancer" (*Breast*, vol. 24, no. 1, February 2015) that in their study 54.4% of women offered chemoprevention began it and of that group just 60% completed the five years of recommended therapy. The researchers observe that barriers to completing the course of chemoprevention include its negative side effects, such as worsening of menopausal symptoms, sexual dysfunction, weight gain, and joint symptoms.

It also seems likely that some people might forgo genetic testing and the opportunity to take preventive action because they fear discrimination. Until 2008, when the Genetic Information Nondiscrimination Act (GINA) became law, these fears were justified. GINA prevents health insurers from denying coverage, adjusting premiums on the basis of genetic test results, or requesting that an individual undergo genetic testing.

Symptomatic genetic testing may also assist in directing the treatment for symptomatic patients in whom a mutation in a single gene (or in a gene pair) accounts for a disorder. CF and myotonic dystrophy (the most common adult form of muscular dystrophy) are examples of disorders that may be confirmed or ruled out by symptomatic genetic testing and other methods (the sweat test for CF and a neurologic evaluation for myotonic dystrophy).

One issue involved in symptomatic genetic testing is the appropriate frequency of testing in view of rapidly expanding genetic knowledge and identification of genes that are linked to disease. Physicians frequently see symptomatic patients for whom there is neither a definitive diagnosis nor a genetic test. The as yet unanswered question is: Should such people be recalled for genetic testing each time a new test becomes available? Although clinics that perform genetic testing counsel patients to maintain regular contact to learn about the availability of new tests, there is no uniform guideline about the frequency of testing.

Testing Children for Adult-Onset Disorders

In 2000 the American Academy of Pediatrics Committee on Genetics recommended genetic testing for people under the age of 18 years only when testing offers immediate medical benefits or when there is a benefit to another family member and there is no anticipated harm to the person being tested.

The American Academy of Pediatrics Committee on Bioethics and Newborn Screening Task Force advocates informed consent for newborn screening. (As of March 2016, most states did not require informed consent.) The committee does not endorse carrier screening in people under the age of 18 years, except in the case of a pregnant teenager. It also recommends against predictive testing for adult-onset disorders in people under the age of 18 years.

The American College of Medical Genetics, the American Society of Human Genetics, and the World Health Organization have also weighed in about genetic testing of asymptomatic (exhibiting no symptoms of illness or disease) children, asserting that decision making should emphasize the children's well-being. One issue involves the value of testing asymptomatic children for genetic mutations that are associated with adult-onset conditions such as HD. Because treatment can only begin with the onset of the disease and because there is no treatment to alter the course of the disease, it may be ill advised to test for it. Another concern is testing for the carrier status of autosomal-recessive or X-linked conditions such as CF. Experts caution that children might confuse carrier status with actually having the condition, which in turn might provoke needless anxiety.

There are, however, circumstances in which genetic testing of children may be appropriate and useful. Examples are children with symptoms of suspected hereditary disorders or those who are at risk for cancers in which inheritance plays a primary role.

In "Points to Consider: Ethical, Legal, and Psychosocial Implications of Genetic Testing in Children and Adolescents" (*American Journal of Human Genetics*, vol. 97, no. 1, July 2, 2015), Jeffrey R. Botkin et al. present the

American Society of Human Genetics's (ASHG) updated recommendations about genetic testing of children. The ASHG continues to advise, "Unless there is a clinical intervention appropriate in childhood, parents should be encouraged to defer predictive or pre-dispositional testing for adult-onset conditions until adulthood or at least until the child is an older adolescent who can participate in decision making in a relatively mature manner." The ASHG also explains that although genomic sequencing may be appropriate for children with genetic disorders for whom genetic testing has failed to identify a causative mutation, "genome-scale sequencing is not indicated for screening in healthy children."

ETHICAL CONSIDERATIONS AND GENETIC TESTING

Since the 1990s rapid advances in genetic research have challenged scientists, health care professionals, ethicists, government regulators, legislators, and consumers to stay abreast of new developments. Understanding the scientific advances and their implications is critical for everyone involved in making informed decisions about the ways in which genetic research and information will affect the lives of current and future generations. As of March 2016, consideration of these ethical issues had not produced simple or universally applicable answers to the many questions that are posed by the increasing availability of genetic information. Ongoing public discussion and debate are intended to inform, educate, and assist people in every walk of life to make personal decisions about their health and participate in decisions that concern others.

Some of the as yet unresolved issues include whether to disclose incidental or secondary discoveries such as carrier status, whether an effective treatment must exist as a rationale for screening, when to screen, and determining whether specific tests should be universal or target selected populations. For example, the ASHG recommends that parents should be able to decline receiving secondary findings before genetic testing is performed but favors disclosing secondary findings to the child's parents regardless of their stated preference only when the information will help prevent serious illness.

As researchers learn more about the genes that are responsible for a variety of illnesses, they can design more tests with ever-increasing accuracy and reliability to predict whether an individual is at risk of developing specific diseases. However, the ethical issues involved in genetic testing have turned out to be far more complicated than originally anticipated. Physicians and researchers initially believed that at-risk families would welcome a test to determine in advance who would develop or escape a disease. They would be able to plan more realistically about having children, choosing jobs, obtaining insurance, and living their life. Nevertheless, many people with family histories of a genetic disease have decided that not knowing is better than anticipating a grim future and an agonizing, slow death. They prefer to live with the hope that they will not develop the disease rather than having the certain knowledge that they will.

The discovery of genetic links and the development of tests that predict the likelihood or certainty of developing a disease raise ethical questions for people who carry a defective gene. Should women who are carriers of HD or CF have children? Should a fetus with a defective gene be carried to term or aborted?

Concerns persist about privacy and the confidentiality of medical records, as well as the possibility that the results of genetic testing can lead to stigmatization despite GINA, the legislation passed in 2008 that prevents such discrimination. Some people remain reluctant to be tested because they still fear they may lose their health, life, and disability insurance, or even their jobs, if they are found to have an increased risk of developing a chronic disease that is costly to treat or that may produce significant disability.

Predictive and Personalized DNA Testing Is Popular but Controversial

Direct-to-consumer genomic testing to assess disease risk offers information about a person's genetic risk of common polygenic diseases. The tests are sold via the Internet and can be relatively inexpensive. Consumers purchase the tests and receive their results without any contact with a health care professional. Advocates of direct-to-consumer genomic testing contend that providing this type of information may motivate consumers to obtain timely health screening and pursue healthful lifestyle choices. Detractors allege that this type of testing may cause undue harm, including anxiety about the results and their interpretation, and increase the use of unnecessary and expensive screening and medical procedures.

In October 2015, 23andMe became the first direct-to-consumer genetic testing company to obtain approval from the U.S. Food and Drug Administration (FDA). In 2013 the company was ordered to stop selling its DNA analysis because the FDA was concerned that users might make health care decisions based on inaccurate results. Prior to the ban, 23andMe analyzed users' saliva for dozens of diseases and conditions; however, the FDA-approved test offers users information about their carrier status for 36 diseases and conditions such as CF and TSD. Andrew Pollack notes in "23andMe Will Resume Giving Users Health Data" (NYTimes.com, October 21, 2015) that Anne Wojcicki, the cofounder and chief executive officer of 23andMe, still aims to gain FDA approval to provide data about health risks, as it did before the FDA ban.

Botkin et al. observe that "in the absence of professional counseling and interpretation, there are concerns that consumers might make misguided changes in their health care or lifestyle," but note that to date, studies have found that users of direct-to-consumer genetic tests generally do not make inappropriate changes in lifestyle or health-related behaviors.

Stacie D. Adams, James P. Evans, and Arthur S. Aylsworth express in "Direct-to-Consumer Genomic Testing Offers Little Clinical Utility but Appears to Cause Minimal Harm" (*North Carolina Medical Journal*, vol. 74, no. 6, November 19, 2013) concern about the analytic validity of the tests and state that "risk estimates from different companies for the same individual vary significantly, and the companies sometimes provide contradictory recommendations—which highlights the fact that no one yet understands how to validly interpret genomic data." They are also concerned about the clinical validity and utility of the tests because the risks identified by the tests are often insignificant compared with those a physician might identify while obtaining a medical history.

COMMON GENETICALLY INHERITED DISEASES

Although many diseases, disorders, and conditions are called genetic, classifying a disease as genetic simply means that there is an identified genetic component to either its origin or expression. Many medical geneticists contend that most diseases cannot be classified as strictly genetic or environmental. Environmental factors can greatly influence the way disease-causing genes express themselves. They can even prevent the genes from being expressed at all. Similarly, environmental (infectious) diseases may not be expressed because of some genetic predisposition to immunity. Each disease, in each individual, exists along a continuum between a genetic disease and an environmental disease.

A multitude of diseases are believed to have strong genetic contributions, including:

- Heart disease—coronary atherosclerosis (a disease in which cholesterol and other deposits build up on the inner walls of the arteries and limit the flow of blood), hypertension (high blood pressure), and hyperlipidemia (elevated blood levels of cholesterol and other lipids)
- Diabetes
- Cancer—retinoblastomas (cancer of the eye), colon, stomach, ovarian, uterine, lung, bladder, breast, skin (melanoma), pancreatic, and prostate
- Neurological disorders—Alzheimer's disease, amyotrophic lateral sclerosis, Gaucher's disease (a disease of fat processing that is linked to the lack of an enzyme), HD, multiple sclerosis, narcolepsy (a neurological disorder that is marked by a sudden recurrent uncontrollable compulsion to sleep), neurofibromatosis (a hereditary disorder that is characterized by widespread abnormalities in the nervous system, skin, and bones), Parkinson's disease, TSD, and Tourette syndrome (a neurological disorder that is characterized by repeated, involuntary movements and uncontrollable vocal sounds)
- Mental illnesses, mental retardation, and behavioral conditions—alcoholism, anxiety disorders, attention-deficit/hyperactivity disorder, eating disorders, Lesch-Nyhan's syndrome (a rare disorder that disrupts the ability to build and break down purines and can produce self-destructive behavior), manic depression, and schizophrenia
- Other disorders—cleft lip and cleft palate, clubfoot, CF, DMD, hemophilia (a genetic blood disorder in which blood does not clot properly), Hurler's syndrome (a rare disorder in which the enzyme that breaks down long chains of sugar molecules is absent), Marfan's syndrome (a disease that is characterized by elongated bones, especially in limbs and digits, and by abnormalities of the eyes and circulatory system), phenylketonuria, SCD, and thalassemia
- Medical and physical conditions with genetic links—alpha-1-antitrypsin deficiency (the lack of this liver protein may result in emphysema and liver and skin disease), arthritis, asthma, baldness, congenital adrenal hyperplasia (lack of an enzyme that is necessary to make the hormones cortisol and aldosterone), migraine headaches, obesity, periodontal disease, porphyria (a genetic abnormality of metabolism that causes abdominal pains and mental confusion), and selected speech disorders

Cystic Fibrosis

CF is the most common inherited fatal disease of children and young adults in the United States. The National Library of Medicine's Genetics Home Reference reports in "Conditions: Cystic Fibrosis" (March 14, 2016, http://ghr.nlm.nih.gov/condition/cystic-fibrosis) that CF occurs in about one out of 2,500 to 3,500 whites, one out of 17,000 African Americans, and one out of 31,000 Asian Americans. In "Learning about Cystic Fibrosis" (December 27, 2013, http://www.genome.gov/10001213), the National Institutes of Health's National Human Genome Research Institute observes that one out of 31 Americans—over 10 million people—are symptom-free carriers of the CF gene. Because it is a recessive genetic disorder, a child must receive the CF gene from both parents to inherit CF.

The CF gene was identified in 1989 and was cloned and sequenced in 1991. The gene was originally called cystic fibrosis transmembrane conductance regulator (CFTR) because it encodes a cell membrane protein that controls the movement of chloride ions across the plasma membrane of cells. Chloride transport is crucial because chloride is a component of salt, which is involved in fluid absorption and volume regulation. Mutations of this gene prevent the chloride ions from operating properly, which can cause disease that affects organs and tissues throughout the body, provoking abnormal, thick secretions from glands and epithelial cells. Over time, a thick, viscous mucus fills the lungs and pancreas, which produces difficulty in breathing and interference with digestion. Eventually, affected children die of respiratory failure.

CF is usually diagnosed by the time an affected child is three years old. Often, the only signs are a persistent cough, a large appetite but poor weight gain, an extremely salty taste to the skin, and large, foul-smelling bowel movements. A simple sweat test is the standard diagnostic test for CF. The test measures the amount of salt in the sweat; abnormally high levels are the hallmark of CF.

Harriet Corvol et al. report in "Translating the Genetics of Cystic Fibrosis to Personalized Medicine" (*Translational Research*, vol. 168, February 2016) that genetic research and technologies such as next gene sequencing and novel genomic editing tools promise to provide new ways to identify CFTR variants and modifier genes and to correct them. Approximately 2,000 mutations have been identified and are classified according to their damaging effects on the cell membrane protein. Personalized medicine, also called P4 medicine (personalized medicine, which considers how each individual's genetics influence his or her care; predictive medicine, which enables physicians to assess the risks that an individual will develop the disease or that the disease will progress; preventive medicine, which focuses on promoting overall health and well-being rather than on a disease cure; and participative medicine, which encourages the patient to make informed decisions and be responsible for his or her own health), is used to guide the development of specific, personalized therapies for CF that target the dysfunctional gene or protein.

Huntington Disease

HD is one of the more common hereditary diseases. It is an inherited, progressive brain disorder that causes the degeneration of cells in a pair of nerve clusters deep in the brain that affect both the body and the mind. HD is caused by a single dominant gene and affects men and women of all races and ethnic groups.

According to Genetics Home Reference, in "Conditions: Huntington Disease" (March 14, 2016, http://ghr.nlm.nih.gov/condition/huntington-disease), HD affects three to seven per 100,000 people of European ancestry. It seems to be less common in other populations, including people of Japanese, Chinese, and African descent. In "Learning about Huntington's Disease" (November 17, 2011, http://www.genome.gov/10001215), the National Human Genome Research Institute reports that 30,000 people in the United States have HD, an additional 35,000 display some symptoms, and 75,000 carry the gene mutation that will cause them to develop the disease.

The gene mutation responsible for HD was mapped to chromosome 4 in 1983 and was cloned in 1993. The mutation occurs in the DNA that codes for the protein called huntingtin. The number of repeated triplets of nucleotides—cytosine (C), adenine (A), and guanine (G), known as CAG (nucleotides are nitrogen-containing molecules that link together to form strands of DNA and RNA)—is inversely related to the age when the individual first experiences symptoms: the more repeated triplets, the younger the age at which the disease first appears.

HD generally begins during the third and fourth decades of life; however, there is a form of the disease that can affect children and adolescents. It is easy to overlook early symptoms, such as forgetfulness, a lack of muscle coordination, or a loss of balance, and as a result the diagnosis is often delayed. The disease progresses gradually, usually over a 10- to 25-year period.

As HD progresses, patients develop involuntary movement (chorea) of the body, limbs, and facial muscles; speech becomes slurred; and swallowing becomes increasingly difficult. HD patients' cognitive abilities decline and there are distinct personality changes—depression and withdrawal, sometimes countered with euphoria. By the late stages of the illness, nearly all patients must be institutionalized, and they usually die as a result of choking or infections.

PREDICTION TEST. In 1983 researchers identified a DNA marker that made it possible to offer a test to determine, before symptoms appear, whether an individual has inherited the HD gene. It is even possible to make a prenatal diagnosis by testing DNA from fetal cells that are removed via CVS or amniocentesis. Some people, however, prefer not to know whether or not they carry the defective gene.

TREATMENT AND PROMISING RESEARCH. According to Praveen Dayalu and Roger L. Albin of the University of Michigan, in "Huntington Disease: Pathogenesis and Treatment" (*Neurologic Clinics*, vol. 33, no. 1, February 2015), although there is not yet any direct treatment of HD to slow the progression of the disease, its symptoms, both the chorea and psychiatric symptoms, may be treated with tetrabenazine, which was approved by the FDA in 2008 for the treatment of chorea. However, drug treatment that effectively suppresses HD-related involuntary movements may produce some undesirable side effects, such as sleep disturbances, depression, and anxiety.

In "Huntington Disease" (*Nature Reviews Disease Primers*, April 23, 2015), Gillian P. Bates et al. report that in 2015 clinical trials focusing on gene silencing (regulation of gene expression, specifically the ability of a cell to prevent the expression of a certain gene) and on huntingtin-lowering agents aimed at diminishing production of the mutant protein were under way.

Muscular Dystrophy

Muscular dystrophy (MD) is a term that describes a group of hereditary muscle-destroying disorders. The CDC estimates in "Muscular Dystrophy: Data & Statistics" (August 7, 2015, http://www.cdc.gov/ncbddd/musculardystrophy/data.html) that Duchenne/Becker muscular dystrophy (DBMD) is diagnosed in one out of 5,600 to 7,700 males aged five to 24 years, which translates to a prevalence rate of 1.3 to 1.8 per 10,000 males aged five to 24 years. All forms of the disease are caused by defects in genes that play key roles in the growth and development of muscles. The gene is passed from the mother to her children. Females who inherit the defective gene generally do not display symptoms—instead they become carriers, and their children have a 50% chance of inheriting the disease.

Because the proteins that are produced by the defective genes are abnormal, the muscles begin to atrophy (waste away). As the muscle cells die, they are replaced by fat and connective tissue. The symptoms of MD often progress slowly, so they may not be noticed until as much as 50% of the muscle tissue has been affected.

Although all the various forms of MD cause progressive weakening and wasting of muscle tissues, they vary in terms of the usual age when symptoms appear, the rate of progression, and the initial group of muscles affected. The most common childhood type, DMD, affects young boys, who exhibit symptoms in early childhood and generally die from respiratory weakness or damage to the heart before adulthood. Other forms of MD develop later in life and are usually not fatal.

In 1992 scientists discovered the defect in the gene that causes myotonic dystrophy, the most common adult form of MD. In people with this disorder, a segment of the gene is enlarged and unstable. This finding helps physicians to diagnose myotonic dystrophy. Researchers have since identified genes that are linked to other types of MD, including DMD, DBMD, limb-girdle MD, and Emery-Dreifuss MD.

TREATMENT AND HOPE. Although there is no cure for MD, treatment modalities such as physical therapy, exercise programs, and orthopedic devices (special shoes, braces, or powered wheelchairs) can help patients maintain mobility and independence as long as possible.

Many researchers believe that genetic research holds the key to development of effective treatments, and even cures, for these diseases. Because defective or absent proteins cause MD, researchers hope that experimental treatments to transplant normal muscle cells into wasting muscles will replace the diseased cells. Muscle cells, unlike other cells in the body, fuse together to become giant cells. It is hoped that by introducing cells with healthy genes the muscle cells will start to produce the deficient or entirely absent proteins.

The challenge is to get the body to accept the new muscle cells without mounting an immune attack against them. Researchers are experimenting with new delivery methods called vectors to help the healthy genes gain access to the body. One such vector implants a healthy gene into a virus that has been stripped of all its harmful properties. The modified virus containing the gene is then injected into a patient. Researchers hope this will sharply reduce the patient's immune system response, which will enable the healthy gene to restore the missing muscle protein.

In "A New Therapeutic Effect of Simvastatin Revealed by Functional Improvement in Muscular Dystrophy" (*Proceedings of the National Academy of Sciences*, vol. 112, no. 41, October 13, 2015), Nicholas P. Whitehead et al. report the promising results of animal research using simvastatin, a statin drug, to treat dystrophic muscles. Statin drugs lower cholesterol and have historically been used to improve cardiovascular health; however, they also reduce inflammation and fibrosis (thickening and scarring of connective tissue). Whitehead et al. find that "simvastatin dramatically improves muscle strength and fatigue resistance" in mice with DMD.

Sickle-Cell Disease

SCD is a group of inherited blood disorders (including sickle-cell anemia, sickle-hemoglobin C disease, sickle beta-plus thalassemia, and sickle beta-zero thalassemia) that affects red blood cells. In SCD the red blood cells contain an abnormal type of hemoglobin, called hemoglobin S, which is responsible for hemolysis (the premature destruction of red blood cells). It also causes the red blood cells to stiffen and change shape; they become sickle, or crescent shaped, particularly in parts of the body where the amount of oxygen is relatively low. These abnormally shaped cells have shorter life spans than normal red blood cells and they have difficulty passing through the smaller blood vessels and capillaries. Unlike normal red blood cells, they tend to clog the vessels, which prevent blood and oxygen from reaching vital tissues. The lack of oxygen damages the tissue, which in turn causes more sickling and more damage.

Figure 4.4 shows how a mutation in an amino acid produces the abnormal hemoglobin, which in turn can produce the sickled cells that cause illness.

SYMPTOMS OF SCD. SCD produces symptoms that are comparable to those of anemia, including fatigue, weakness, fainting, and palpitations or an increased awareness of the heartbeat. The palpitations result from the heart's attempts to compensate for the anemia by pumping blood faster than normal.

Sickle-cell patients experience periodic sickle-cell crises—attacks of pain in the bones and stomach. Blood clots may also develop in the lungs, kidneys, brain, and other organs. A severe crisis or several acute crises can damage the organs of the body by impeding blood flow. The frequency of these crises varies from patient to patient. However, sickle-cell crises are more likely to occur during times of stress, such as when the body is combating an infection or after an accident or injury. Cumulative damage can lead to death from heart failure, kidney failure, or stroke.

FIGURE 4.4

Sickle-cell anemia

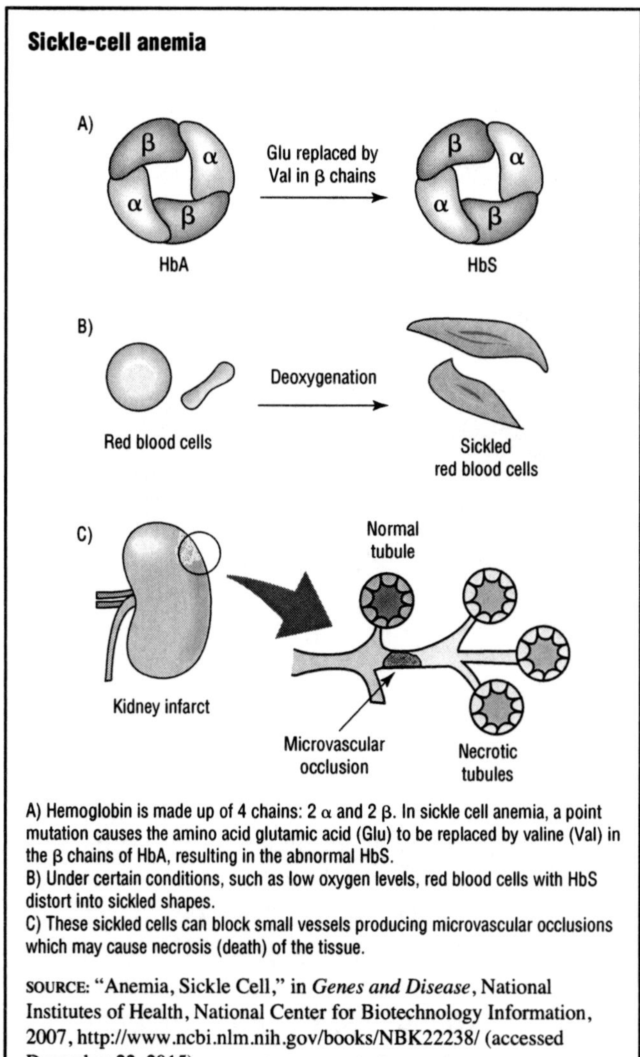

A) Hemoglobin is made up of 4 chains: 2 α and 2 β. In sickle cell anemia, a point mutation causes the amino acid glutamic acid (Glu) to be replaced by valine (Val) in the β chains of HbA, resulting in the abnormal HbS.
B) Under certain conditions, such as low oxygen levels, red blood cells with HbS distort into sickled shapes.
C) These sickled cells can block small vessels producing microvascular occlusions which may cause necrosis (death) of the tissue.

SOURCE: "Anemia, Sickle Cell," in *Genes and Disease*, National Institutes of Health, National Center for Biotechnology Information, 2007, http://www.ncbi.nlm.nih.gov/books/NBK22238/ (accessed December 22, 2015)

WHO CONTRACTS SCD? SCD occurs most frequently in people of African, Native American, and Hispanic descent. However, it also occurs in Portuguese, Spanish, French Corsicans, Sardinians, Sicilians, mainland Italians, Greeks, Turks, and Cypriots. There are also occurrences of SCD in the Middle East and Asia. According to the World Health Organization, in "Genes and Human Disease: Monogenic Diseases" (2016, http://www.who.int/genomics/public/geneticdiseases/en/index2.html), SCD is the most common inherited blood disorder in the United States, affecting an estimated 72,000 Americans, most of whom have African ancestry. SCD occurs in approximately one out of 500 African American births and in one out of 1,000 to 1,400 Hispanic American births.

When one parent has the sickle-cell gene, the offspring will carry the trait, but only when both the mother and the father have the trait can they produce a child with SCD. Figure 4.5 shows the inheritance pattern for the sickle-cell trait. The sickle-cell trait is present in one out of 12 African Americans, or about 2 million people.

Examining amniotic fluid or tissue that is taken from the placenta as early as the first trimester of pregnancy enables detection of the likelihood the unborn child will have the sickle-cell trait or SCD. A genetic counselor evaluates the results and can inform the expectant parents of the chances that their child will have the sickle-cell trait or SCD.

BENEFITS OF UNIVERSAL SCREENING. The National Heart, Lung, and Blood Institute notes in "What Is Sickle Cell Anemia?" (June 12, 2015, http://www.nhlbi.nih.gov/health/dci/Diseases/Sca/SCA_WhatIs.html) that SCD screening of all newborns is important because early diagnosis and treatment significantly improves future health. Early diagnosis and timely treatments, such as with antibiotics to fight infections, reduce the number of deaths that are attributable to SCD and enable most children who are born with SCD to live well into adulthood.

THE CURE FOR SCD. According to the CDC, in "Facts about Sickle Cell Disease" (September 14, 2015, http://www.cdc.gov/ncbddd/sicklecell/facts.html), bone marrow transplant and stem cell treatment can cure SCD. Bone marrow is the spongy tissue in the cavities of bones that creates and contains blood cells. A bone marrow/stem cell transplant procedure extracts blood stem cells (the cells that form blood) from a healthy donor and places them into a person whose bone marrow is not functioning properly. Bone marrow/stem cell transplants carry significant risks, which even include death of the recipient. To be optimally effective, the bone marrow must be a close match and the ideal donor is most often a sibling. Because of the associated risks, bone marrow/stem cell transplants are reserved for children with severe cases of SCD.

FIGURE 4.5

Inheritance of sickle-cell trait

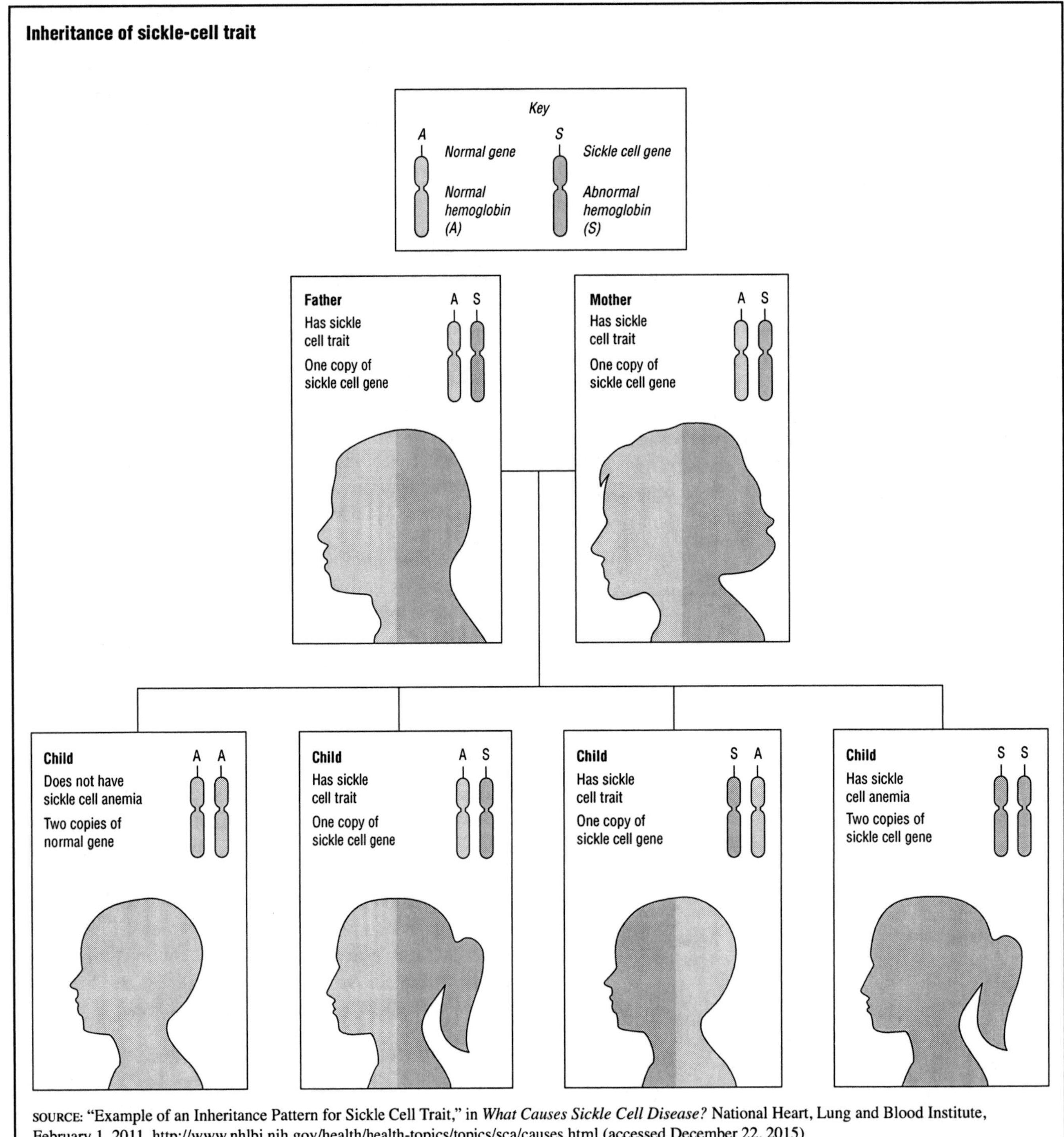

SOURCE: "Example of an Inheritance Pattern for Sickle Cell Trait," in *What Causes Sickle Cell Disease?* National Heart, Lung and Blood Institute, February 1, 2011, http://www.nhlbi.nih.gov/health/health-topics/topics/sca/causes.html (accessed December 22, 2015)

Tay-Sachs Disease

TSD is a fatal genetic disorder in children that causes the progressive destruction of the central nervous system. It is named for Warren Tay (1843–1927), a British ophthalmologist, and Bernard Sachs (1858–1944), an American neurologist, the physicians who first identified and described the disease. It is caused by insufficient activity of, or the complete absence of, an important enzyme called hexosaminidase A (hex-A). Without hex-A, a fatty substance called ganglioside GM2 builds up abnormally in the cells, particularly the brain's nerve cells. Ultimately, this buildup causes these cells to degenerate and die. This destructive process begins well before birth, but the disease is usually not diagnosed until the baby is several months old.

SYMPTOMS OF TSD. A baby with TSD appears healthy at birth and usually develops normally during the first months of life, but then development slows. The child begins to regress and loses skills one by one—the ability to crawl, to sit, to reach out, and to turn over. Gradually, the child becomes blind, deaf, and unable to swallow. Muscles atrophy, and paralysis sets in. Mental retardation occurs, and the child is unable to interact with the outside world. There is no cure for this disease. Even with optimal medical care and treatment, death from infection usually occurs by age four.

HOW IS TSD INHERITED? TSD is transmitted from parent to child the same way eye or hair color is inherited. It is an autosomal recessive genetic disorder caused by mutations in both alleles of the HEXA gene on chromosome 15. Both parents must be carriers of the TSD gene to give birth to a child with the disease.

People who carry the TSD gene have no signs of the disease and are generally unaware that they have the potential to pass this disease on to their offspring. When just one parent is a carrier, the offspring will not have TSD, but there is a 50% chance of having a child who is a carrier. When both parents carry the recessive TSD gene, there is a 25% chance of having a child with the disease and a 50% chance of bearing a child who is a carrier. Prenatal diagnosis early in pregnancy, using CVS or amniocentesis, can accurately predict if the fetus is affected by TSD.

WHO IS AT RISK? Like SCD, TSD occurs most frequently in specific populations. People of Ashkenazi Jewish descent have the highest risk of being carriers of TSD. According to the National Tay-Sachs and Allied Diseases Association of Delaware Valley, in "Tay-Sachs Disease" (2016, http://www.tay-sachs.org/taysachs_disease.php), approximately one out of 27 Jewish people in the United States is a carrier of the TSD gene. French Canadians and Cajuns also have the same carrier rate as people of Ashkenazi Jewish descent, and one out of 50 Irish Americans is a carrier.

CHAPTER 5
CHRONIC DISEASES: CAUSES, TREATMENT, AND PREVENTION

The Centers for Disease Control and Prevention (CDC) defines chronic diseases as prolonged illnesses that do not resolve spontaneously and are rarely cured completely. According to the CDC, in "Chronic Disease Overview" (February 23, 2016, http://www.cdc.gov/nccdphp/overview.htm), chronic illnesses such as cardiovascular disease, cancer, respiratory disease, cerebrovascular disease, and diabetes are the leading causes of death and disability in the United States and are among the most preventable of all health problems.

CARDIOVASCULAR DISEASES

Cardiovascular disease, which includes coronary heart diseases, arrhythmias, diseases of the arteries, congestive heart failure, rheumatic heart disease, high blood pressure, cerebrovascular disease (stroke), and congenital heart defects, continued to be the leading cause of death in the United States in 2014. According to Dariush Mozaffarian et al., in "Heart Disease and Stroke Statistics—2016 Update" (*Circulation*, vol. 133, no. 4, January 26, 2016), an estimated 85.6 million American adults have some form of cardiovascular disease; of these, approximately 44% are over the age of 60 years.

Mozaffarian et al. indicate that based on 2013 data about 2,200 Americans die from cardiovascular disease each day. In 2013 one out of every three (800,937) deaths was attributable to cardiovascular disease. An estimated 15.5 million people suffer from coronary heart disease, and in 2013 it claimed 370,213 lives in the United States, or about one out of every seven deaths. Each year approximately 660,000 Americans will have a new coronary attack, and roughly 305,000 will have a recurrent (second or third) attack. An additional 160,000 silent first myocardial infarctions (heart attacks that produce no symptoms or such mild symptoms that they go unnoticed) occur each year.

Heart Attack and Angina Pectoris

A heart attack, or myocardial infarction, occurs when the blood supply from a coronary artery to the heart muscle (the myocardium) is cut off abruptly. This happens when one of the coronary arteries that supply blood to the heart is obstructed (blocked). When the blood supply is eliminated, the heart's muscle cells are deprived of oxygen and die. Disability or death can result, depending on how much of the heart muscle has been damaged.

Angina pectoris is not a disease; it is a symptom and the name for chest pain or pressure that occurs when poor blood flow through a partially occluded (blocked) artery to the heart quickly and temporarily reduces its supply of oxygen. When the blood flow is restored, the pain subsides. A common condition, angina is often a warning sign of the risk of heart attack. Its dull, constricting pain typically occurs when an individual is physically active or excited but subsides when activity ceases. In men, angina usually occurs after the age of 50 years, whereas women tend to develop angina later in life.

WARNING SIGNALS OF A HEART ATTACK. In "Warning Signs of Heart Attack, Stroke & Cardiac Arrest" (2016, http://www.heart.org/HEARTORG/Conditions/Conditions_UCM_305346_SubHomePage.jsp), the American Heart Association (AHA) describes several warning signs of a heart attack:

- An uncomfortable pressure, squeezing, fullness, or pain in the center of the chest behind the breastbone
- Pain that spreads to the shoulders, neck, arms, back, jaw, or stomach
- Chest discomfort that is accompanied by sweating, nausea, shortness of breath, or a feeling of weakness

IMMEDIATE CARE IS CRUCIAL. Immediate medical care dramatically improves the odds of surviving a heart attack. Treatments are most effective if given within an hour of when the attack begins. According to the AHA, intensive emergency care during the first 12 hours after a heart attack improves the patient's chance of survival and recovery. Researchers believe that patients who suffer heart attacks benefit from early intensive treatment—such as improved monitoring of their conditions and aggressive use of pharmacologic (drug) therapy, including appropriate reperfusion (the action of restoring the flow of blood to the heart) therapies and "clot-busting" medications—that is initiated with as little delay as possible.

Treatments for Heart Disease

Drug treatment for heart disease focuses on improving blood flow to the heart, controlling abnormal heart rhythms, reducing the heart's workload, and preventing blood clots. Frequently prescribed heart disease medications include:

- Angiotensin converting enzyme (ACE) inhibitors, which widen blood vessels to ease the heart's workload and reduce blood pressure
- Angiotensin II receptor blockers, which exert the same effects as ACE inhibitors but act using a different mechanism
- Antiarrhythmia drugs, which help regulate abnormal heart rhythms that are caused by erratic electrical activity of the heart
- Antiplatelet drugs, which help prevent blood clots from forming
- Aspirin, which reduces inflammation and pain and inhibits blood clots
- Beta-blockers, which ease the heart's workload by slowing the heart rate and improving the heart's ability to pump blood through the body
- Digoxin, which slows the heart rate, strengthens contractions, and boosts blood circulation
- Diuretics, which remove excess water and salt from the body to reduce the heart's workload and help lower blood pressure
- Nitrates, which widen and relax the coronary arteries, thereby easing blood flow to the heart
- Warfarin, which prevents blood clots from forming

Once it is clear that a person is having a heart attack, immediate treatment usually includes administering drugs to help open the blocked artery, which restores blood flow to the heart and prevents clots from forming again. If the patient gets to an emergency department quickly, reperfusion might be done. Drugs may be administered to decrease the workload of the heart, relieve chest pain, reduce blood pressure, and thin the blood to prevent clot formation in the arteries and promote reperfusion. Patients with heart disease may also undergo other procedures, including:

- Balloon angioplasty or percutaneous transluminal coronary angioplasty to widen narrowed arteries with an inflated balloon
- Placement of wire mesh tubes, called stents, into arteries after angioplasty to prevent later collapse or restenosis (renarrowing)
- Coronary artery bypass graft surgery to improve blood supply to parts of the heart muscle that have decreased blood flow

Once emergency care and immediate treatment is completed, most communities have cardiac rehabilitation programs that help people recover from a heart attack and reduce the chances of having another one.

New Stents Debut

Traditional metal stents effectively open occluded blood vessels, but permanent stents pose some long-term risks. Specifically, there is increasing risk for thrombosis (formation of a blood clot in the artery). Even newer polymer-coated drug-eluting stents (scaffolding that slowly releases a drug that prevents any further blockage or obstruction occurring in the artery) carry the risk of thrombosis and restenosis.

In 2011 a new kind of stent that gradually disappears over the course of five years was approved for use in Europe. The bioresorbable vascular scaffold (BVS) leaves two tiny markers that enable physicians to see where the stent was placed. In "Everolimus-Eluting Bioresorbable Vascular Scaffolds versus Everolimus-Eluting Metallic Stents: A Meta-analysis of Randomised Controlled Trials" (*Lancet*, vol. 387, no. 10018, February 2016), Salvatore Cassese et al. review the results of six studies comparing BVS to metal drug-eluting stents. Although the BVS was generally comparable to the metal stent, patients with the BVS had increased risk of thrombosis. The researchers assert that studies involving larger numbers of patients with longer periods of follow-up are needed to evaluate the risks and benefits of BVS, which, as of 2016, was not yet approved for use in the United States.

Bypass Surgery

Coronary artery bypass graft (CABG) surgery, commonly known as bypass surgery, can improve blood flow to the heart, relieve chest pains, and help the heart pump more efficiently. Generally, a segment of a large healthy vein, usually taken from the patient's leg, is spliced between the aorta (the main vessel carrying blood from the left side of the heart to all the arteries of the body and limbs) and the blocked coronary arteries. The coronary bypass operation thus supplies blood to the area of the heart that has a deficient blood supply. During the operation the patient is placed on a heart-lung machine that takes over the function of the heart and lungs while the surgery is proceeding. Usually, patients recovering from CABG surgery spend two or three days in the intensive care unit and several additional days in the hospital following the surgery.

An alternative to CABG surgery is minimally invasive direct coronary bypass surgery. In this procedure, the surgeon makes one or more small incisions (about 3 inches [7.6 cm] long) in the chest wall and works directly on the clogged artery while the heart is beating. Some surgeons use fiber-optic techniques similar to those used in gallbladder and other procedures. Another technique actually stops the heartbeat and uses a modified heart-lung machine that is connected to a large artery in the groin while the surgeon operates through small incisions using a video camera and long-handled instruments.

Catheter-Based Interventions

Simpler procedures called catheter-based interventions are performed via a thin tube that is inserted into an artery, rather than operating on the coronary artery by cutting through the chest wall. One such catheter-based intervention is percutaneous coronary intervention (PCI; this procedure is also called percutaneous transluminal coronary angioplasty). A physician punctures an artery in the patient's groin and threads a balloon-tipped catheter into the artery. The tip of the catheter is slowly advanced up through the arterial system and positioned in the coronary artery at the point of the blockage or stenosis (narrowing). The small, sausage-shaped balloon on the end of the catheter is then inflated, flattening the fatty plaque and widening the artery. The balloon is sometimes inflated and deflated several times to clear the artery.

PCI has several obvious advantages over bypass surgery. It is performed under a local rather than a general anesthetic and does not involve opening the chest or using a heart-lung machine. It is less expensive, and the patient is usually out of the hospital and recovering in a few days. Still, PCI is not always completely effective, and nearly one-third of patients who receive PCI eventually require bypass surgery or another PCI because the initial procedure is unsuccessful or the blockage recurs.

As technology advances, catheter-based interventions using fiber optics and laser methods may replace angioplasty as the treatments of choice. For example, some physicians use a tiny cutting blade that is attached to the end of a fiber-optic tube to remove accumulated plaque; however, this method has not yet been proven to be more effective than balloon angioplasty.

Cardiovascular therapies such as the use of statins (drugs that reduce cholesterol) and beta-blockers (drugs that decrease the force and rate of the heart's contractions, which lowers blood pressure and reduces the heart's demand for oxygen) and decreasing rates of myocardial infarction have resulted in decreasing numbers of bypass surgeries and other revascularization procedures. Robert W. Yeh et al. report in "Population Trends in Rates of Coronary Revascularization" (*JAMA Internal Medicine*, vol. 175, no. 3, March 2015) that revascularizations decreased between 2003 and 2012. Over the course of the study period, the rate of revascularizations fell from 423 to 258 per 100,000 residents.

HEART TRANSPLANTS. In 1967 the South African heart surgeon Christiaan Barnard (1922–2001) performed the first successful heart transplant. This feat was repeated one month later in the United States by Norman E. Shumway (1923–2006) at Stanford University Hospital in California. Early heart transplant patients did not live long, largely because of the body's tendency to reject new tissue. The use of immunosuppressant drugs helped overcome this obstacle and transplant patients' life expectancies increased. However, immunosuppressant drugs may also accelerate atherosclerosis (commonly known as "hardening of the arteries") in the transplanted heart because they suppress the body's normal immune responses. In 2016 research focused on the development of more specific immunosuppressants and ways to prevent atherosclerosis in transplanted hearts.

According to the Health Resources and Services Administration's (HRSA) Organ Procurement and Transplantation Network (March 21, 2016, https://optn.transplant.hrsa.gov/data/view-data-reports/national-data/), in the United States in 2014, 2,655 heart transplants were performed, and in 2015, 2,804 heart transplants were performed.

Risk Factors for Heart Disease

Various risk factors exist for heart disease. Although some cannot be changed, others can be modified.

UNCHANGEABLE RISK FACTORS. Four risk factors for heart disease that cannot be altered are heredity, race, sex, and increasing age. People whose parents had or have cardiovascular diseases are more likely to develop them. Race is also a significant factor. For example, Mozaffarian et al. note that African American adults have the highest rates of high blood pressure in the world (greater than 45%), which increases the risk for heart disease. Men have a greater risk of heart attack than do women. Heart attacks are the leading cause of death among men older than the age of 40 years, but heart disease is not a major cause of death among women until they reach the age of 60 years. Heart attacks are also more likely to occur as a person ages. More than half of the Americans who experience heart attacks are aged 65 years and older. Of those who die from their attacks, the vast majority are older than the age of 65 years.

CHANGEABLE RISK FACTORS. Cigarette smoking doubles the risk of heart attack. A smoker who suffers a heart attack is more likely to die from it and more likely to die suddenly than a nonsmoker. However, once people stop smoking, regardless of the length of time or the amount they smoked, the risk of heart disease decreases significantly. Between 2000 and 2013 the prevalence of cigarette smoking among adults aged 18 years and older decreased from 23.1% to 17.9%. (See Table 5.1.) In contrast, the percentage of smokers remained relatively

TABLE 5.1

Smoking among adults by sex, race, and age, selected years 1965–2013

[Data are based on household interviews of a sample of the civilian noninstitutionalized population]

Sex, race, and age	1965[a]	1974[a]	1979[a]	1985[a]	1990[a]	2000	2005	2010	2011	2012	2013
18 years and over, age-adjusted[b]	Percent of adults who were current cigarette smokers[c]										
All persons	41.9	37.0	33.3	29.9	25.3	23.1	20.8	19.3	19.0	18.2	17.9
Male	51.2	42.8	37.0	32.2	28.0	25.2	23.4	21.2	21.2	20.6	20.5
Female	33.7	32.2	30.1	27.9	22.9	21.1	18.3	17.5	16.8	15.9	15.5
White male[d]	50.4	41.7	36.4	31.3	27.6	25.4	23.3	21.4	21.4	20.7	20.5
Black or African American male[d]	58.8	53.6	43.9	40.2	32.8	25.7	25.9	23.3	23.2	22.0	21.8
White female[d]	33.9	32.0	30.3	27.9	23.5	22.0	19.1	18.3	17.7	16.9	16.3
Black or African American female[d]	31.8	35.6	30.5	30.9	20.8	20.7	17.1	16.6	15.2	14.2	14.9
18 years and over, crude											
All persons	42.4	37.1	33.5	30.1	25.5	23.2	20.9	19.3	19.0	18.1	17.8
Male	51.9	43.1	37.5	32.6	28.4	25.6	23.9	21.5	21.6	20.5	20.5
Female	33.9	32.1	29.9	27.9	22.8	20.9	18.1	17.3	16.5	15.8	15.3
White male[d]	51.1	41.9	36.8	31.7	28.0	25.7	23.6	21.4	21.6	20.3	20.3
Black or African American male[d]	60.4	54.3	44.1	39.9	32.5	26.2	26.5	24.3	23.8	22.0	21.9
White female[d]	34.0	31.7	30.1	27.7	23.4	21.4	18.7	17.9	17.2	16.6	15.9
Black or African American female[d]	33.7	36.4	31.1	31.0	21.2	20.8	17.3	17.0	15.3	14.7	15.1
All males											
18–44 years	57.9	47.9	40.4	35.2	31.4	29.2	27.1	23.9	23.6	24.0	22.9
18–24 years	54.1	42.1	35.0	28.0	26.6	28.1	28.0	22.8	21.3	20.1	21.9
25–34 years	60.7	50.5	43.9	38.2	31.6	28.9	27.7	26.1	27.5	28.0	24.4
35–44 years	58.2	51.0	41.8	37.6	34.5	30.2	26.0	22.5	21.2	22.8	22.1
45–64 years	51.9	42.6	39.3	33.4	29.3	26.4	25.2	23.2	24.4	20.2	21.9
45–54 years	55.9	46.8	42.0	34.9	32.1	28.8	28.1	25.2	27.0	21.4	21.4
55–64 years	46.6	37.7	36.4	31.9	25.9	22.6	21.1	20.7	21.4	18.8	22.6
65 years and over	28.5	24.8	20.9	19.6	14.6	10.2	8.9	9.7	8.9	10.6	10.6
White male[d]											
18–44 years	57.1	46.8	40.0	34.6	31.3	30.2	27.7	24.6	24.3	24.8	23.4
18–24 years	53.0	40.8	34.3	28.4	27.4	30.4	29.7	23.8	22.1	21.9	23.5
25–34 years	60.1	49.5	43.6	37.3	31.6	29.7	27.7	26.6	28.6	28.4	24.6
35–44 years	57.3	50.1	41.3	36.6	33.5	30.6	26.3	23.1	21.4	23.3	21.9
45–64 years	51.3	41.2	38.3	32.1	28.7	25.8	24.5	22.5	24.0	19.4	21.7
45–54 years	55.3	45.0	40.9	33.7	31.3	28.0	27.4	24.5	26.6	20.7	21.2
55–64 years	46.1	36.6	35.3	30.5	25.6	22.5	20.4	20.1	20.8	17.9	22.2
65 years and over	27.7	24.3	20.5	18.9	13.7	9.8	7.9	9.6	8.6	10.3	10.0
Black or African American male[d]											
18–44 years	66.3	58.1	45.2	39.6	32.9	25.5	25.1	22.6	22.7	21.3	20.9
18–24 years	62.8	54.9	40.2	27.2	21.3	20.9	21.6	18.8	18.4	13.2	*13.2
25–34 years	68.4	58.5	47.5	45.6	33.8	23.2	29.8	25.7	25.0	24.9	24.8
35–44 years	67.3	61.5	48.6	45.0	42.0	30.7	23.3	22.6	24.3	24.7	24.0
45–64 years	57.9	57.8	50.0	46.1	36.7	32.2	32.4	31.8	28.9	24.6	25.7
45–54 years	62.4	63.6	51.5	47.7	42.0	35.6	33.9	33.2	29.2	23.3	25.7
55–64 years	51.8	50.1	47.9	44.4	30.2	26.3	29.8	29.6	28.4	26.4	25.6
65 years and over	36.4	29.7	26.2	27.7	21.5	14.2	16.8	10.0	13.7	17.4	15.5
All females											
18–44 years	42.1	37.5	34.7	31.4	25.6	24.5	21.2	19.1	18.8	16.9	16.6
18–24 years	38.1	34.1	33.8	30.4	22.5	24.9	20.7	17.4	16.4	14.5	15.4
25–34 years	43.7	38.8	33.7	32.0	28.2	22.3	21.5	20.6	19.5	19.4	17.9
35–44 years	43.7	39.8	37.0	31.5	24.8	26.2	21.3	19.0	19.9	16.1	16.3
45–64 years	32.0	33.4	30.7	29.9	24.8	21.7	18.8	19.1	18.5	18.9	18.1
45–54 years	37.5	36.0	32.6	32.4	28.5	22.2	20.9	21.3	21.6	21.3	20.6
55–64 years	25.0	30.4	28.6	27.4	20.5	20.9	16.1	16.5	15.0	16.2	15.2
65 years and over	9.6	12.0	13.2	13.5	11.5	9.3	8.3	9.3	7.1	7.5	7.5
White female[d]											
18–44 years	42.2	37.3	35.1	31.6	26.5	26.5	22.6	20.5	20.3	18.6	17.8
18–24 years	38.4	34.0	34.5	31.8	25.4	28.5	22.6	18.4	18.4	16.9	17.0
25–34 years	43.4	38.6	34.1	32.0	28.5	24.9	23.1	22.0	20.6	20.7	19.2
35–44 years	43.9	39.3	37.2	31.0	25.0	26.6	22.2	20.5	21.5	17.6	17.0
45–64 years	32.7	33.0	30.6	29.7	25.4	21.4	18.9	19.5	19.0	19.4	18.4
45–54 years	38.2	34.9	32.5	32.4	29.1	21.9	21.0	22.4	22.5	22.7	21.2
55–64 years	25.7	30.6	28.5	27.2	21.2	20.6	16.2	15.9	15.1	15.8	15.5
65 years and over	9.8	12.3	13.8	13.3	11.5	9.1	8.4	9.4	7.0	7.5	7.9

TABLE 5.1

Smoking among adults by sex, race, and age, selected years 1965–2013 [CONTINUED]

[Data are based on household interviews of a sample of the civilian noninstitutionalized population]

Sex, race, and age	1965[a]	1974[a]	1979[a]	1985[a]	1990[a]	2000	2005	2010	2011	2012	2013
Black or African American female[d]	Percent of adults who were current cigarette smokers[c]										
18–44 years	42.9	41.1	34.7	33.5	22.8	20.8	16.9	17.1	15.0	12.3	15.1
18–24 years	37.1	35.6	31.8	23.7	10.0	14.2	14.2	14.2	9.1	*7.4	11.8
25–34 years	47.8	42.2	35.2	36.2	29.1	15.5	16.9	19.3	17.5	17.3	16.4
35–44 years	42.8	46.4	37.7	40.2	25.5	30.2	19.0	17.2	17.4	11.2	16.4
45–64 years	25.7	38.9	34.2	33.4	22.6	25.6	21.0	19.8	18.3	20.4	18.8
45–54 years	32.3	46.2	36.2	36.4	26.5	26.5	22.2	20.4	20.1	20.1	22.2
55–64 years	16.5	29.3	31.9	29.8	17.6	24.2	19.1	18.9	16.0	20.8	14.8
65 years and over	7.1	*8.9	*8.5	14.5	11.1	10.2	10.0	9.4	9.1	9.1	6.5

*Estimates are considered unreliable. Data preceded by an asterisk have a relative standard error of 20%–30%.
[a]Data prior to 1997 are not strictly comparable with data for later years due to the 1997 questionnaire redesign.
[b]Estimates are age-adjusted to the year 2000 standard population using five age groups: 18–24 years, 25–34 years, 35–44 years, 45–64 years, and 65 years and over. Age-adjusted estimates in this table may differ from other age-adjusted estimates based on the same data and presented elsewhere if different age groups are used in the adjustment procedure.
[c]Starting with 1993 data, current cigarette smokers were defined as ever smoking 100 cigarettes in their lifetime and smoking now every day or some days.
[d]The race groups, white and black, include persons of Hispanic and non-Hispanic origin. Starting with 1999 data, race-specific estimates are tabulated according to the 1997 *Revisions to the Standards for the Classification of Federal Data on Race and Ethnicity* and are not strictly comparable with estimates for earlier years. The single-race categories shown in the table conform to the 1997 Standards. Starting with 1999 data, race-specific estimates are for persons who reported only one racial group. Prior to 1999, data were tabulated according to the 1977 Standards. Estimates for single-race categories prior to 1999 included persons who reported one race or, if they reported more than one race, identified one race as best representing their race. Starting with 2003 data, race responses of other race and unspecified multiple race were treated as missing, and then race was imputed if these were the only race responses. Almost all persons with a race response of other race were of Hispanic origin.

SOURCE: "Table 52. Current Cigarette Smoking among Adults Aged 18 and over, by Sex, Race, and Age: United States, Selected Years 1965–2013," in *Health, United States, 2014: With Special Feature on Adults Aged 55–64*, Centers for Disease Control and Prevention, National Center for Health Statistics, 2015, http://www.cdc.gov/nchs/data/hus/hus14.pdf (accessed December 15, 2015)

constant among male and female adults aged 55 to 64 years and 65 years and older.

High blood pressure (often referred to as hypertension), which usually has no symptoms or warning signs, is called the "silent killer." High blood pressure means that it is more difficult for blood to pump through the arteries, which increases the heart's workload, causing it to weaken and enlarge over time. Generally, blood pressure increases with age. Men have a higher incidence of high blood pressure than women until 45 to 54 years of age, when the risks become equal for both sexes. According to the National Center for Health Statistics (NCHS), in *Health, United States, 2014* (2015, http:// www.cdc.gov/nchs/data/hus/hus14.pdf), the prevalence of uncontrolled high blood pressure for men and women of all age groups decreased from 77.2% in 1988–94 to 54.6% in 2011–12. (See Table 5.2.)

High serum cholesterol levels increase the risk of coronary heart disease. High serum cholesterol is defined as greater than or equal to 240 milligrams per deciliter (mg/dL). Borderline high serum cholesterol is defined as greater than or equal to 200 mg/dL and less than 240 mg/dL. The NCHS indicates that 12.7% of adults aged 20 years and older had high serum cholesterol levels in 2011–12, down from 20.8% in 1988–94. (See Table 5.2.) This decline is likely the result of heightened awareness of the importance of reducing cholesterol levels and increased use of cholesterol-lowering drugs—statins are the most commonly prescribed class of cholesterol-lowering drugs. Maintaining a healthy weight, eating a healthful diet, and exercising can also enhance the effectiveness of cholesterol-lowering drugs.

A lack of physical exercise is also a risk factor for heart disease. According to the NCHS, between 1998 and 2013 the percentage of adults aged 18 years and older who met the 2008 federal aerobic activity and muscle-strengthening guidelines increased from 14.3 % to 21%. (See Table 5.3.) In 2013, however, the percentage of Americans who were engaged in regular leisure-time physical activity declined with increasing age, decreasing from 30.3% of people aged 18 to 24 years to just 11.7% of those aged 65 years and older.

For adults aged 18 to 64 years, the U.S. Department of Health and Human Services recommends in "Physical Activity Guidelines: Adults" (2016, http://health.gov/paguidelines/guidelines/adults.aspx) 2 hours and 30 minutes (150 minutes) per week of moderate-intensity, 1 hour and 15 minutes (75 minutes) per week of vigorous-intensity aerobic physical activity, or an equivalent combination of moderate- and vigorous-intensity aerobic physical activity. Aerobic activity should be performed in episodes of at least 10 minutes, preferably spread throughout the week. Adults should also engage in muscle-strengthening activities that involve all the major muscle groups on two or more days per week. The Department of Health and Human Services asserts that additional health benefits are provided by increasing to 5 hours (300 minutes) per week of moderate-intensity aerobic physical activity, 2 hours and 30 minutes (150 minutes) per week of vigorous-intensity physical activity, or an equivalent combination of both.

TABLE 5.2

Selected health conditions and risk factors, selected years 1988–2012

[Data are based on interviews and physical examinations of a sample of the civilian noninstitutionalized population]

Health condition	1988–1994	1999–2000	2001–2002	2003–2004	2005–2006	2007–2008	2009–2010	2011–2012
Diabetes[a]	Percent of adults aged 20 and over							
Total, age-adjusted[b]	8.8	9.0	10.6	10.9	10.4	11.4	11.5	11.9
Total, crude	8.3	8.6	10.3	10.9	10.9	11.9	12.1	12.5
Hypercholesterolemia[c]								
Total, age-adjusted[d]	22.8	25.5	24.6	27.9	27.4	27.6	27.2	28.2
Total, crude	21.5	24.5	24.2	27.9	28.1	28.8	28.6	30.4
High cholesterol[e]								
Total, age-adjusted[d]	20.8	18.3	16.5	16.9	15.6	14.2	13.2	12.7
Total, crude	19.6	17.7	16.4	17.0	15.9	14.6	13.6	13.1
Hypertension[f]								
Total, age-adjusted[d]	25.5	30.0	29.7	32.1	30.5	31.2	30.0	30.0
Total, crude	24.1	28.9	28.9	32.5	31.7	32.6	31.9	32.5
Uncontrolled high blood pressure among persons with hypertension[g]								
Total, age-adjusted[d]	77.2	71.9	68.3	63.8	63.0	56.2	55.7	54.6
Total, crude	73.9	69.1	65.4	60.8	56.6	51.8	46.7	48.0
Overweight (includes obesity)[h]								
Total, age-adjusted[d]	56.0	64.5	65.6	66.4	66.9	68.1	68.8	68.6
Total, crude	54.9	64.1	65.6	66.5	67.3	68.3	69.2	69.0
Obesity[i]								
Total, age-adjusted[d]	22.9	30.5	30.5	32.3	34.4	33.7	35.7	34.9
Total, crude	22.3	30.3	30.6	32.3	34.7	33.9	35.9	35.1
Untreated dental caries[j]								
Total, age-adjusted[d]	27.7	24.4	21.3	29.8	24.4	21.7	—	25.5
Total, crude	28.2	25.0	21.7	30.2	24.5	21.8	—	25.5
Obesity[k]	Percent of persons under age 20							
2–5 years	7.2	10.3	10.6	14.0	11.0	10.1	12.1	8.4
6–11 years	11.3	15.1	16.3	18.8	15.1	19.6	18.0	17.7
12–19 years	10.5	14.8	16.7	17.4	17.8	18.1	18.4	20.5
Untreated dental caries[j]								
5–19 years	24.3	23.6	21.2	25.6	16.2	16.9	14.6	17.5

—Data not available.
[a]Includes physician-diagnosed and undiagnosed diabetes. Estimates were obtained using fasting weights. Physician-diagnosed diabetes was obtained by self-report and excludes women who reported having diabetes only during pregnancy. Undiagnosed diabetes is defined as a fasting plasma glucose (FPG) of at least 126 mg/dL or a hemoglobin A1c of at least 6.5% and no reported physician diagnosis. Pregnant women were excluded. Adjustments to FPG recommended by NHANES for trend analysis were incorporated into the data presented here. The revised definition of undiagnosed diabetes was based on recommendations from the American Diabetes Association.
[b]Estimates are age-adjusted to the year 2000 standard population using three age groups: 20–44 years, 45–64 years, and 65 years and over. Age-adjusted estimates in this table may differ from other age-adjusted estimates based on the same data presented elsewhere if different age groups are used in the adjustment procedure.
[c]Hypercholesterolemia is defined as measured serum total cholesterol greater than or equal to 240 mg/dL or reporting taking cholesterol-lowering medication. Respondents were asked, "Are you now following this advice [from a doctor or health professional] to take prescribed medicine [to lower your cholesterol]?" Risk levels for serum total cholesterol have been defined by the Third Report of the National Cholesterol Education Program Expert Panel on Detection, Evaluation, and Treatment of High Blood Cholesterol in Adults. National Heart, Lung, and Blood Institute, National Institutes of Health. September 2002.
[d]Estimates are age-adjusted to the year 2000 standard population using five age groups: 20–34 years, 35–44 years, 45–54 years, 55–64 years, and 65 years and over. Age-adjusted estimates in this table may differ from other age-adjusted estimates based on the same data and presented elsewhere if different age groups are used in the adjustment procedure.
[e]High cholesterol is defined as greater than or equal to 240 mg/dL (6.20 mmol/L). This second measure of cholesterol presented in Health, United States is based solely on measured high serum total cholesterol.
[f]Hypertension is defined as having measured high blood pressure and/or taking antihypertensive medication. High blood pressure is defined as having measured systolic pressure of at least 140 mm Hg or diastolic pressure of at least 90 mm Hg. Those with high blood pressure also may be taking prescribed medicine for high blood pressure. For antihypertensive medication use, respondents were asked, "Are you now taking prescribed medicine for your high blood pressure?"
[g]Uncontrolled high blood pressure among persons with hypertension is defined as measured systolic pressure of at least 140 mm Hg or diastolic pressure of at least 90 mm Hg, among those with measured high blood pressure or reporting taking antihypertensive medication.
[h]Overweight is defined as body mass index (BMI) greater than or equal to 25, based on the NHANES variable, Body Mass Index. Excludes pregnant women.
[i]Obesity is defined as body mass index (BMI) greater than or equal to 30, based on the NHANES variable, Body Mass Index. Excludes pregnant women.
[j]Untreated dental caries refers to decay on the crown or enamel surface of a tooth (i.e., coronal caries) that has not been treated or filled. The presence of caries was evaluated in primary and permanent teeth for persons aged 5 and older. The third molars were not included. Persons without at least one natural tooth (primary or permanent) were excluded. Over time, there have been changes in the NHANES oral health examination process, ages examined, and methodology.
[k]Obesity is defined as body mass index (BMI) at or above the sex- and age-specific 95th percentile BMI (based on the variable BMXBMI) using cutoff points from the 2000 CDC growth charts for the United States. Starting with Health, United States, 2010, the terminology describing height for weight among children changed from previous editions. The term obesity now refers to children who were formerly labeled as overweight. This is a change in terminology only and not measurement; the previous definition of overweight is now the definition of obesity. Excludes pregnant girls.

SOURCE: "Table 59. Selected Health Conditions and Risk Factors, by Age: United States, Selected Years 1988–1994 through 2011–2012," in *Health, United States, 2014: With Special Feature on Adults Aged 55–64*, Centers for Disease Control and Prevention, National Center for Health Statistics, 2015, http://www.cdc.gov/nchs/data/hus/hus14.pdf (accessed December 15, 2015)

TABLE 5.3

Participation in activities that meet the 2008 federal physical activity guidelines for adults aged 18 and older, by selected characteristics, selected years 1998–2013

[Data are based on household interviews of a sample of the civilian noninstitutionalized population]

	2008 Physical Activity Guidelines for Americans[a]									
	Met both aerobic activity and muscle-strengthening guidelines					Met neither aerobic activity nor muscle-strengthening guideline				
Characteristic	**1998**	**2000**	**2010**	**2012**	**2013**	**1998**	**2000**	**2010**	**2012**	**2013**
	Percent									
18 years and over, age-adjusted[b,c]	14.3	15.0	20.7	20.8	21.0	56.6	54.7	49.1	46.6	46.5
18 years and over, crude[c]	14.5	15.1	20.4	20.3	20.4	56.3	54.6	49.5	47.1	47.2
Age										
18–44 years	18.9	18.9	25.7	25.7	25.7	50.7	49.1	43.1	41.0	40.3
18–24 years	23.8	23.8	29.6	29.7	30.3	46.5	44.5	39.4	37.9	35.5
25–44 years	17.4	17.3	24.3	24.2	24.0	51.9	50.6	44.4	42.2	42.0
45–64 years	11.4	12.8	17.7	17.2	17.8	58.8	57.6	51.0	49.6	50.2
45–54 years	13.2	14.5	19.2	18.2	20.1	56.9	55.4	48.9	48.3	48.4
55–64 years	8.6	10.1	15.9	16.0	15.3	61.8	61.0	53.7	51.2	52.1
65 years and over	5.5	6.8	10.4	11.9	11.7	71.0	67.0	64.6	58.4	59.4
65–74 years	7.0	8.4	13.6	14.8	14.7	65.6	60.3	59.9	51.7	54.0
75 years and over	3.5	4.9	6.4	7.9	7.6	77.8	75.0	70.3	67.2	66.8
Sex[b]										
Male	17.5	17.9	25.1	24.6	25.0	50.8	49.6	43.8	42.2	42.0
Female	11.4	12.3	16.5	17.1	17.2	61.9	59.4	54.0	50.7	50.7
Sex and age										
Male:										
18–44 years	23.0	23.0	31.8	31.8	31.7	44.3	43.0	37.1	35.9	34.7
45–54 years	16.1	16.0	20.9	18.7	22.3	52.9	52.7	45.2	45.9	46.3
55–64 years	9.4	11.3	19.1	16.8	17.6	58.2	58.7	50.1	49.1	49.6
65–74 years	9.5	9.4	16.6	17.1	15.9	58.9	55.3	55.6	45.9	49.7
75 years and over	4.9	7.1	9.1	10.5	7.8	69.5	66.7	62.8	61.3	60.6
Female:										
18–44 years	14.9	15.0	19.6	19.8	19.8	56.9	55.0	49.0	46.0	45.7
45–54 years	10.5	13.1	17.5	17.7	18.0	60.8	57.9	52.4	50.5	50.5
55–64 years	7.8	9.0	13.1	15.3	13.2	65.0	63.1	57.0	53.2	54.4
65–74 years	5.1	7.7	11.0	12.8	13.6	70.9	64.3	63.6	56.7	57.7
75 years and over	2.6	3.6	4.6	6.2	7.5	83.0	80.0	75.3	71.2	71.0
Race[b,d]										
White only	14.8	15.7	21.4	21.5	21.7	55.2	53.1	47.6	45.4	45.2
Black or African American only	11.7	12.2	17.2	16.8	17.7	65.7	64.6	58.5	55.0	54.7
American Indian or Alaska Native only	16.0	10.6*	12.7*	18.7	16.8	57.6	67.1	54.0	50.8	50.8
Asian only	13.5	14.1	17.8	17.1	18.3	59.1	55.0	51.7	47.8	47.6
Native Hawaiian or other Pacific Islander only	—	*	*	*	*	—	*	*	*	*
2 or more races	—	19.0	25.9	28.7	22.4	—	52.8	45.0	40.5	44.4
Hispanic origin and race[b,d]										
Hispanic or Latino	9.4	9.2	14.4	15.7	16.6	67.7	66.5	60.2	54.5	53.8
Mexican	8.7	8.1	13.2	14.9	15.0	69.5	67.0	60.7	53.8	53.4
Not Hispanic or Latino	14.9	15.8	21.9	21.7	21.9	55.3	53.2	47.2	45.1	45.2
White only	15.5	16.5	22.9	23.0	22.9	53.6	51.4	45.0	43.2	43.1
Black or African American only	11.7	12.2	17.4	16.7	17.8	65.8	64.6	58.4	55.1	54.7
Education[e,f]										
No high school diploma or GED	4.6	4.3	7.7	7.6	8.0	76.3	74.0	69.8	66.3	66.6
High school diploma or GED	8.6	9.5	12.7	12.4	13.8	64.6	61.7	59.0	57.4	57.0
Some college or more	18.2	18.9	25.0	24.9	24.4	48.0	47.1	42.1	39.7	40.6

CONTRIBUTING FACTORS. Diabetes, or elevated blood glucose, affects cholesterol and triglyceride levels. The disease can sharply increase the risk of heart attack, especially when blood glucose is uncontrolled or poorly controlled. According to the National Institute of Diabetes and Digestive and Kidney Diseases, in *National Diabetes Statistics Report, 2014* (2014, http://www.cdc.gov/diabetes/pubs/statsreport14/national-diabetes-report-web.pdf), in 2010 hospitalization rates for heart attack were 1.8 times higher among adults aged 20 years and older with diabetes than among adults without diabetes. The CDC reports that 11.9% of adults had diabetes in 2011–12. (See Table 5.2.)

Obesity is also a factor that contributes to heart disease. Men with a waistline measurement that exceeds their hip measurement and women whose waistline measurement is more than 80% of their hip measurement are at greater risk. Although obesity is directly associated with an increased risk for cardiovascular disease, being overweight to any degree strains the heart.

TABLE 5.3

Participation in activities that meet the 2008 federal physical activity guidelines for adults aged 18 and older, by selected characteristics, selected years 1998–2013 [CONTINUED]

[Data are based on household interviews of a sample of the civilian noninstitutionalized population]

*Estimates are considered unreliable.
—Data not available.
[a]Starting with *Health, United States, 2010,* measures of physical activity shown in this table changed to reflect the federal *2008 Physical Activity Guidelines for Americans.* This table presents four measures of physical activity that are of interest to the public health community: the percentage of adults who met the federal 2008 guidelines for both aerobic activity and muscle strengthening; the percentage who met neither the aerobic activity guideline nor the muscle-strengthening guideline; the percentage who met the aerobic activity guideline; and the percentage who met the muscle-strengthening guideline. Persons who met neither the aerobic activity nor the muscle-strengthening guideline were unable to be active, were completely inactive, or had some aerobic or muscle-strengthening activities but amounts were insufficient to meet the guidelines. The percentage of persons who met the aerobic activity guideline includes those who may or may not have also met the muscle-strengthening guideline. Similarly, the percentage of persons who met the muscle-strengthening guideline includes those who may or may not have also met the aerobic activity guideline. The federal 2008 guidelines recommend that for substantial health benefits adults perform at least 150 minutes (2 hours and 30 minutes) a week of moderate-intensity, or 75 minutes (1 hour and 15 minutes) a week of vigorous-intensity aerobic physical activity, or an equivalent combination of moderate- and vigorous-intensity aerobic activity. Aerobic activity should be performed in episodes of at least 10 minutes, and preferably should be spread throughout the week. The 2008 guidelines also recommend that adults perform muscle-strengthening activities that are moderate or high intensity and involve all major muscle groups on 2 or more days a week, because these activities provide additional health benefits.
[b]Estimates are age-adjusted to the year 2000 standard population using five age groups: 18–44 years, 45–54 years, 55–64 years, 65–74 years, and 75 years and over. Age-adjusted estimates in this table may differ from other age-adjusted estimates based on the same data and presented elsewhere if different age groups are used in the adjustment procedure.
[c]Includes all other races not shown separately, unknown education level, and unknown disability status.
[d]The race groups, white, black, American Indian or Alaska Native, Asian, Native Hawaiian or Other Pacific Islander, and 2 or more races, include persons of Hispanic and non-Hispanic origin. Persons of Hispanic origin may be of any race. Starting with 1999 data, race-specific estimates are tabulated according to the 1997 *Revisions to the Standards for the Classification of Federal Data on Race and Ethnicity* and are not strictly comparable with estimates for earlier years. The five single-race categories plus multiple-race categories shown in the table conform to the 1997 Standards. Starting with 1999 data, race-specific estimates are for persons who reported only one racial group; the category 2 or more races includes persons who reported more than one racial group. Prior to 1999, data were tabulated according to the 1977 Standards with four racial groups, and the Asian only category included Native Hawaiian or Other Pacific Islander. Estimates for single-race categories prior to 1999 included persons who reported one race or, if they reported more than one race, identified one race as best representing their race. Starting with 2003 data, race responses of other race and unspecified multiple race were treated as missing, and then race was imputed if these were the only race responses. Almost all persons with a race response of other race were of Hispanic origin.
[e]Estimates are for persons aged 25 and over and are age-adjusted to the year 2000 standard population using five age groups: 25–44 years, 45–54 years, 55–64 years, 65–74 years, and 75 years and over.
[f]GED is General Educational Development high school equivalency diploma.

SOURCE: "Table 63. Participation in Leisure-Time Aerobic and Muscle-Strengthening Activities That Meet the Federal *2008 Physical Activity Guidelines for Americans* among Adults Aged 18 and over, by Selected Characteristics: United States, Selected Years 1998–2013," in *Health, United States, 2014: With Special Feature on Adults Aged 55–64*, Centers for Disease Control and Prevention, National Center for Health Statistics, 2015, http://www.cdc.gov/nchs/data/hus/hus14.pdf (accessed December 15, 2015)

The prevalence of obesity among adults over the age of 20 years has increased from 22.9% in 1988–94 to 34.9% in 2011–12. (See Table 5.2.) During the same period the prevalence of overweight rose from 56% to 68.6%. The NCHS notes in *Early Release of Selected Estimates Based on Data from the January–June 2015 National Health Interview Survey* (November 2015, http://www.cdc.gov/nchs/data/nhis/earlyrelease/earlyrelease201511_06.pdf) that although the prevalence of overweight and obesity increased in both males and females in all racial and ethnic groups between 1997 and 2015, non-Hispanic whites were less likely to be obese than Hispanics and non-Hispanic African Americans. (See Figure 5.1.) Obesity was highest among non-Hispanic African American women (45.4%).

Women and Heart Disease

Until the early 1990s almost all research on heart disease was carried out on middle-aged men. Nevertheless, heart disease affects women, too. At menopause, women begin to lose the protection provided by the hormones that appear to reduce the risk of heart disease. As a result, the rates of coronary heart disease are two to three times higher among postmenopausal women than among premenopausal women. In fact, starting at age 75 the prevalence of cardiovascular disease is higher among women than among men of the same age group.

Women are more seriously affected by heart disease than men are because women have smaller arteries, they frequently wait longer to get care, and they are generally older (typically by 10 years) when heart disease strikes. Another reason is that women's early symptoms of heart disease often differ from those of the "classic" heart attack. Before a heart attack women may experience unusual fatigue, sleep disturbance, shortness of breath, indigestion, and anxiety. Although many symptoms that may occur during a heart attack are comparable to the symptoms men experience (shortness of breath, weakness, unusual fatigue, cold sweat, and dizziness), women may also experience nausea. According to Nancy Brown, in "How the American Heart Association Helped Change Women's Heart Health" (*Circulation Cardiovascular Quality Outcomes*, vol. 8, no. 2, March 2015), in 2004 the AHA launched Go Red for Women, a program to increase awareness efforts about the effect of heart disease in women. Brown notes that since 2004, awareness of heart disease as the number-one killer of women has increased to 54% and fewer women have died from cardiovascular disease.

Stroke

Stroke (cerebrovascular disease) is a cardiovascular disease that affects the blood vessels of the central nervous system. When an artery supplying oxygen and nutrients to

FIGURE 5.1

Prevalence of obesity among adults, by sex and race/ethnicity, January–June 2015

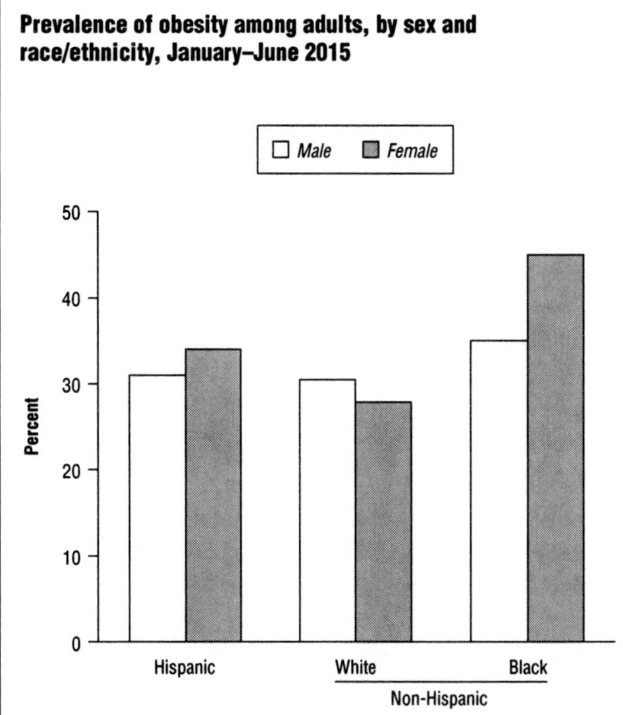

Notes: Data are based on household interviews of a sample of the civilian noninstitutionalized population. Obesity is defined as a body mass index (BMI) of 30 kg/m² or more. The measure is based on self-reported height (m) and weight (kg). Estimates of obesity are restricted to adults aged 20 and over for consistency with the Healthy People 2020 (3) initiative. The analyses excluded the 4.0% of persons with unknown height or weight. Estimates are age-adjusted using the projected 2000 U.S. population as the standard population and using five age groups: 20–24, 25–34, 35–44, 45–64, and 65 and over.

SOURCE: "Figure 6.3. Age-Adjusted Prevalence of Obesity among Adults Aged 20 Years and over, by Sex and Race/Ethnicity: United States, January–June 2015," in *Early Release of Selected Estimates Based on Data from the January–June 2015 National Health Interview Survey*, Centers for Disease Control and Prevention, National Center for Health Statistics, November 2015, http://www.cdc.gov/nchs/data/nhis/earlyrelease/earlyrelease201511_06.pdf (accessed December 26, 2015)

the brain bursts or becomes clogged with a blood clot, a part of the brain does not receive the oxygen it needs. Without the necessary oxygen, the affected nerve cells die within moments. The parts of the body that are controlled by these nerve cells also become dysfunctional. Because dead brain cells cannot be replaced, the damage done by a stroke is often permanent.

Stroke affects people in different ways. The extent of the resulting damage or loss depends on the type of stroke and the area of the brain that has been damaged. Physicians can often identify the location of a stroke in the brain from the symptoms and deficits that are observed during a neurologic examination, even before an imaging study (computed tomography [CT] or magnetic resonance imaging) confirms the region of the brain affected. The senses, speech, the ability to understand speech, behavioral patterns, thought, and memory are affected most frequently. The most common effect is for one side of the body to become paralyzed or severely weakened. A loss of sensation or vision as the result of the stroke can result in a loss of awareness of the affected parts, so many stroke victims may forget or "neglect" the parts of the body that are weakened or paralyzed. Falls, bumping into objects, or dressing only one side of the body tend to result from this sudden lack of awareness.

INCIDENCE OF STROKE DEATHS IS DECLINING. In *Health, United States, 2014*, the NCHS notes that stroke (cerebrovascular diseases) was the fifth-leading cause of death in the United States in 2013, following heart disease, cancer, chronic lower respiratory diseases, and unintentional injuries, and that 128,978 Americans died of stroke. (See Table 1.5 in Chapter 1.) Mozaffarian et al. indicate that each year about 795,000 people suffer a new stroke and 185,000 experience recurrent strokes. The AHA explains in the fact sheet "Older Americans & Cardiovascular Diseases" (2015, https://www.heart.org/idc/groups/heart-public/@wcm/@sop/@smd/documents/downloadable/ucm_472923.pdf) that among people aged 60 to 79 years, 6.1% of men and 5.2% of women have had a stroke. Among those aged 80 years and older, 15.8% of men and 14% of women have had a stroke.

The death rate for stroke declined between 2000 and 2013. Mozaffarian et al. attribute this decline in stroke mortality to improved control of high blood pressure, diabetes, and high cholesterol and reduced prevalence of smoking.

Two blood thinners, heparin and warfarin, are often used to reduce the chance of blood clots and recurrent strokes, although these drugs pose some risk of bleeding problems. Clinical trials show that the drugs are safe if their use is closely monitored. Another drug, tissue plasminogen activator (tPA), is a "clot-busting drug" approved specifically for fighting strokes. tPA must be administered within three hours after the onset of a stroke. The drug works to stop the swift advance of damage that is caused by clots shutting off blood flow to the brain, which accounts for four-fifths of strokes. Early detection and immediate treatment are vital for tPA treatment to be optimally effective. The use of statin drugs and regular, low doses of aspirin have also proved effective in preventing stroke.

Aspirin not only helps prevent ischemic stroke (the most common type of stroke; it is usually caused by a clot occluding a blood vessel that supplies the brain) but also helps when given to a person immediately after an ischemic stroke to reduce the risk of suffering another stroke. Aspirin confers protection against stroke by preventing the formation of the clots that can block blood vessels. Nevertheless, aspirin does not help prevent hemorrhagic stroke (another common type of stroke) because this type of stroke is caused by the rupture of a blood vessel in the brain and results in an accumulation of blood.

REHABILITATION FOR STROKE SURVIVORS. Stroke is a leading cause of serious long-term disability. The AHA asserts that stroke accounts for more than half of all patients who are hospitalized for acute brain diseases. According to the National Stroke Association, in the fact sheet "Recovery after Stroke: Recurrent Stroke" (March 2014, https://www.stroke.org/sites/default/files/resources/NSAFactSheet_RecurrentStroke_2014.pdf), 3% to 10% of stroke victims will suffer a second stroke within 30 days of the first one, and between 5% and 14% will have a second stroke within one year of the first.

Many survivors lose mental and physical abilities and need expensive, long, and intensive rehabilitation to regain their independence. In some cases independence is not achievable. Stroke can affect most senses and perception, and patients who have had a stroke may find even familiar surroundings incomprehensible. They may be unable to recognize or understand well-known objects or people. The simplest activities become difficult, and depression is a common problem because patients who have had a stroke may feel overwhelmed and develop a sense of despair.

Alexander W. Dromerick et al. note in "Critical Periods after Stroke Study: Translating Animal Stroke Recovery Experiments into a Clinical Trial" (*Frontiers in Neuroscience*, vol. 9, no. 231, April 29, 2015) that the duration of recovery depends on the severity of the stroke. Rehabilitation consists of compensation and learning. Patients relearn ways to accomplish everyday tasks such as washing dishes and when necessary learn new ways to accomplish tasks through a combination of newly acquired compensatory strategies and restoration of motor, sensory, and cognitive function in uninjured tissues.

Spontaneous recovery during the initial 30 days after a stroke probably accounts for the highest levels of regained functional ability. However, rehabilitation to reduce dependency and improve physical ability is also vital. The patient's attitude, the skills of the rehabilitation team, and the support and understanding from the patient's family all affect the quality of recovery.

Dromerick et al suggest that the timing of stroke rehabilitation may be critical in terms of its effectiveness. For example, some studies indicate that very intense motor training early after stroke lead to worse outcomes. Animal studies find that the best response to rehabilitation training occurred when it began at five days post-stroke. Rehabilitation was somewhat less effective when training was initiated at 14 days. When it was started 30 days post-stroke, results were comparable to animals that received no rehabilitation training at all.

In "Advances in Stroke: Recovery and Rehabilitation" (*Stroke*, vol. 44, no. 2, February 2013), Michael Brainin and Richard D. Zorowitz review studies of the effectiveness of different types of stroke therapy. They find that for patients with moderate to severe motor function problems, early prescription of the drug fluoxetine in conjunction with physiotherapy enhanced motor recovery after three months. The researchers note that electromechanical and robot-assisted arm training helped patients regain arm function and arm muscle strength and improved their ability to perform the activities of daily living. Brainin and Zorowitz also report that repetitive transcranial magnetic stimulation (which uses magnetic pulses to stimulate brain nerve cells) improved upper limb motor function in patients with stroke.

High Blood Pressure

Blood pressure is a combination of two forces: the heart pumping blood into the arteries and the resistance of small arteries called arterioles to the flow of blood. The greater the resistance, the greater the pressure that is needed by the heart to keep the blood moving. The walls of the arterioles are elastic enough to allow for the expansion and contraction that is caused by the constantly changing rate of blood flow, thus allowing for a steady blood pressure in normal bodies. If the arterioles stay contracted or lose their elasticity as a result of atherosclerosis, the resistance to blood flow increases and blood pressure rises.

Blood pressure is measured in millimeters of mercury (mm Hg) by an instrument known as a sphygmomanometer. The sphygmomanometer produces two values: the systolic pressure (a measurement of the maximum pressure of the blood flow when the heart contracts or beats) and the diastolic pressure (the minimum pressure of the blood flow between beats). A typical normal range of values may vary, but the more resistance there is to blood flow, the higher the reading. High blood pressure (hypertension) for adults is defined as a systolic pressure equal to or greater than 140 mm Hg and/or a diastolic pressure equal to or greater than 90 mm Hg.

Prehypertension is defined as systolic pressure of 120 mm Hg to 139 mm Hg and diastolic pressure of 80 mm Hg to 89 mm Hg. According to the CDC, in "High Blood Pressure Facts" (February 19, 2015, http://www.cdc.gov/bloodpressure/facts.htm), in 2011–12 nearly one out of three adults in the United States had prehypertension.

Elevated blood pressure causes the heart to work harder than normal and places the arteries under a strain that might contribute to a heart attack, stroke, or atherosclerosis. When the heart works too hard, it can become enlarged and will eventually be unable to function at maximum pumping capacity.

Figure 5.2 shows the prevalence of hypertension, the risks and costs associated with it, and the importance of

FIGURE 5.2

High blood pressure prevalence, risks, costs, and ways to control blood pressure, 2014

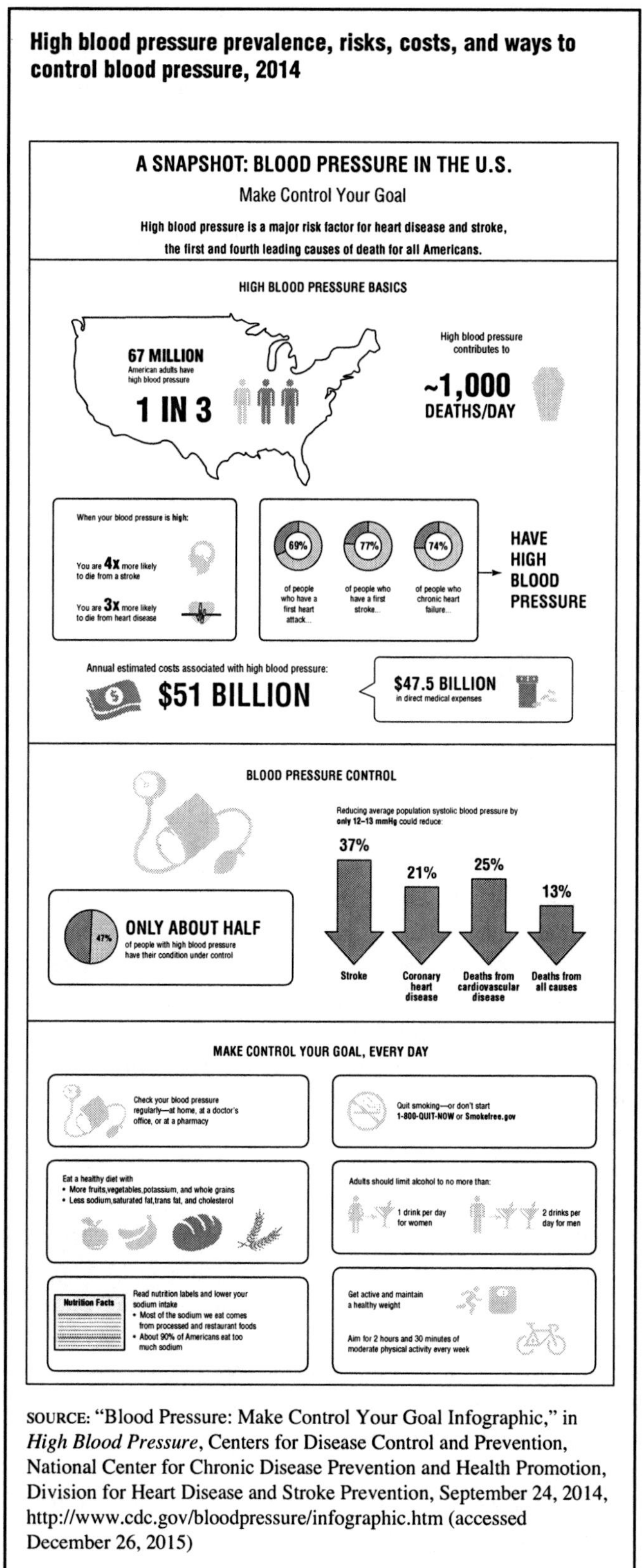

SOURCE: "Blood Pressure: Make Control Your Goal Infographic," in *High Blood Pressure*, Centers for Disease Control and Prevention, National Center for Chronic Disease Prevention and Health Promotion, Division for Heart Disease and Stroke Prevention, September 24, 2014, http://www.cdc.gov/bloodpressure/infographic.htm (accessed December 26, 2015)

blood pressure control. It also presents the health and lifestyle choices that help control blood pressure.

TREATMENT. In almost all cases, hypertension is treatable. A variety of medications, including diuretics, which rid the body of excess fluid and salt, can lower blood pressure.

Diet and lifestyle changes are also essential to control hypertension. (See Figure 5.2.) Some people with only mildly elevated blood pressure need only to reduce or eliminate salt in their diet. Blood pressure in overweight or obese people often declines when they lose weight. Heavy drinkers often see improved blood pressure when they abstain from alcohol or drink less. Similarly, smokers and people who use chewing tobacco are advised to quit because tobacco use causes an immediate spike in blood pressure and can also cause arterial narrowing, which increases blood pressure. Some people find exercise, stress management techniques, and relaxation therapy helpful. When people are aware of the problem and follow prescribed treatments, hypertension can be controlled and need not be fatal. However, patients often stop taking high blood pressure medication once their hypertension is controlled. This poses a serious danger; it is essential that patients continue to take the medication even though they feel perfectly well.

CANCER

Cancer (also called malignant neoplasms) is a large group of diseases that are characterized by the uncontrolled growth and spread of abnormal cells. These cells may grow into masses of tissue called tumors. Tumors made up of cells that are not cancerous are called benign tumors. Tumors consisting of cancer cells are called malignant tumors. The dangerous aspect of cancer is that cancer cells invade and destroy normal tissue.

The spread of cancer cells occurs either by a local growth of the tumor or by some of the cells becoming detached and traveling through the blood and lymph systems to start additional tumors in other parts of the body. Metastasis (the spread of cancer cells) may be confined to a region of the body, but if left untreated (and often despite treatment), the cancer cells can spread throughout the entire body, causing death. The rapid, invasive, and destructive nature of cancer makes it, arguably, the most feared of all diseases, even though it was second to heart disease as the leading cause of death in the United States in 2013. (See Table 1.5 in Chapter 1.)

What Causes Cancer, Who Gets Cancer, and Who Survives?

Cancer may be caused by both external factors (chemicals, radiation, and viruses) and internal factors (hormones, immune conditions, and inherited mutations). These factors act together or in sequence to begin or promote cancer.

No one is immune to cancer. Because the incidence increases with age, most cases are found among adults in midlife or older. However, in *Health, United States, 2014*, the NCHS reports that in 2013 cancer was the second-leading cause of death in the United States among children aged five to 14 years. (See Table 1.7 in Chapter 1.) The American Cancer Society (ACS) estimates in *Cancer Facts and Figures, 2015* (2015, http://www.cancer.org/acs/groups/content/@editorial/documents/document/acspc-044552.pdf) that about one out of two men and one out of three women in the United States will have some type of cancer at some point during their lifetime.

The ACS indicates that in 2015, 1.7 million new cancer cases were diagnosed and 589,430 people died of cancer. In the United States cancer causes one out of every four deaths. Although the five-year survival rate for all cancers diagnosed between 2004 and 2010 was 68%, up from 49% between 1975 and 1977, the death rates for many forms of cancer have remained fairly steady since the 1930s. Three exceptions are stomach, uterine, and lung cancer. During the 1930s stomach cancer and uterine cancer had some of the highest death rates, but they have since declined to some of the lowest death rates. Meanwhile, the lung cancer death rate increased dramatically from 1930 until about 1990, especially for men, and then began to decline.

The improved rates of survival are largely attributable to earlier diagnosis and improved treatment. Just 50 years ago fewer than one out of four patients treated for cancer were still living after five years. Nearly 14.5 million Americans have a history of cancer. Many of these individuals are considered "cured," meaning that there is no evidence of the disease, and survivors have a life expectancy that is comparable to people who have never had cancer.

Research reveals that long-term survivors of childhood cancers are at an increased risk for subsequent health problems. For example, many childhood cancer survivors have endocrine conditions (disorders of the glands that secrete hormones into the bloodstream). Mark A. Applebaum and Susan L. Cohn of the University of Chicago explain in "Surveillance of Childhood Cancer Survivors: A Lifelong Affair" (*Journal of Clinical Oncology*, vol. 33, no. 31, November 1, 2015) that one of the most serious consequences of treatment is the development of subsequent malignant neoplasms. These subsequent cancers are a major cause of premature death, and patients who survive their first subsequent malignant neoplasm remain at risk for additional cancers.

BEHAVIORAL AND ENVIRONMENTAL RISK FACTORS CONTRIBUTE TO CANCER DEATHS. In the landmark study "Causes of Cancer in the World: Comparative Risk Assessment of Nine Behavioural and Environmental Risk Factors" (*Lancet*, vol. 366, no. 9499, November 19, 2005), Goodarz Danaei et al. collaborated with more than 100 scientists around the world in 2001 to estimate mortality for 12 types of cancer that are linked to certain risk factors. They find that of the 7 million cancer deaths worldwide, 35% were attributable to nine potentially modifiable behavioral and environmental risk factors: overweight and obesity, low fruit and vegetable intake, physical inactivity, smoking, alcohol consumption, unsafe sex, urban air pollution, indoor smoke from household use of coal, and contaminated injections in health care settings.

Worldwide, the nine risk factors caused 1.6 million cancer deaths among men and 830,000 cancer deaths among women. Smoking alone was estimated to have caused 21% of deaths from cancer worldwide. Smoking, which is linked to lung, mouth, stomach, pancreatic, and bladder cancers, was the biggest avoidable risk factor, followed by alcohol consumption and low fruit and vegetable intake. In high-income countries the nine risk factors caused 760,000 cancer deaths; smoking, alcohol consumption, and overweight and obesity were the most important causes of cancer in these nations.

In low- and middle-income regions the nine risk factors caused nearly 1.7 million cancer deaths; smoking, alcohol consumption, and low fruit and vegetable intake were the leading risk factors for these deaths. The sexual transmission of the human papillomavirus (HPV) was the leading risk factor for uterine cancer in women in low- and middle-income countries, particularly in sub-Saharan Africa and South Asia, mainly because access to cervical cancer screening is limited.

Danaei et al. conclude that "these results clearly show that many globally important types of cancer are preventable by changes in lifestyle behaviors and environmental interventions. To win the war against cancer we must focus not just on advances in biomedical technologies, but also on technologies and policies that change the behaviors and environments that cause those cancers."

Signs and Symptoms of Cancer

In "Signs and Symptoms of Cancer" (August 11, 2014, http://www.cancer.org/Cancer/CancerBasics/signs-and-symptoms-of-cancer), the ACS identifies the general signs and symptoms that may be associated with cancer, such as fever, unexplained weight loss, fatigue, pain, and skin changes such as hyperpigmentation (darker looking skin), jaundice (yellow-tinged eyes and skin), erythema (reddened skin), itching, and excessive hair growth. The ACS also lists the following symptoms or changes as possible signs of cancer and indications to see a physician:

- Change in bowel or bladder habits
- Sores that do not heal
- White patches inside the mouth or white spots on the tongue
- Unusual bleeding or discharge
- Thickening or lump in breast or elsewhere

- Indigestion or difficulty swallowing
- Obvious change in wart or mole
- Persistent cough or hoarseness

Preventing Cancer and Improving Survival

The ACS estimates in *Cancer Facts and Figures, 2015* that many more lives could be saved with early detection and treatment. For example, in 2015 nearly 171,000 of the estimated 589,430 U.S. cancer deaths were caused by tobacco smoking. Regular screening can detect cancers of the breast, oral cavity, colon, rectum, cervix, and skin at early stages, when treatment is more likely to be successful. For example, 91% of female breast cancer patients currently survive five years or more, up from 75% during the mid-1970s. With early detection, the ACS points out that for women who are diagnosed with localized breast cancer (cancer that has not spread to lymph nodes or other locations outside the breast), the five-year survival rate is 98%. Table 5.4 shows how the use of mammography has increased from 29% in 1987 to 65.7% in 2013.

Protecting skin from sunlight would prevent many of the more than 3 million skin cancers found annually. Besides limiting excess sun exposure, avoiding sunbeds and tanning salons can help prevent many cases of melanoma, the deadliest form of skin cancer. In "Preventing Skin Cancer through Reduction of Indoor Tanning: Current Evidence" (*American Journal of Preventive Medicine*, vol. 44, no. 6, June 2013), Meg Watson et al. explain that melanoma is one of the most commonly diagnosed cancers among teens and young adults. It is responsible for more than 9,000 deaths each year, and its prevalence has been increasing in recent years, particularly among non-Hispanic whites. Indoor tanning before age 35 increases the risk of melanoma by 60% to 80%.

Watson et al. note that the U.S. Food and Drug Administration (FDA) and the Federal Trade Commission regulate indoor tanning devices and advertising at the national level. State regulation and enforcement of indoor tanning devices, including restrictions on youth access to indoor tanning, varies throughout the United States. According to the National Conference of State Legislatures, in "Indoor Tanning Restrictions for Minors—A State-by-State Comparison" (http://www.ncsl.org/research/health/indoor-tanning-restrictions.aspx), in 2016, 12 states (California, Delaware, Hawaii, Illinois, Louisiana, Minnesota, Nevada, New Hampshire, North Carolina, Oregon, Texas, and Vermont) and the District of Columbia prohibited indoor tanning for people under the age of 18 years.

Christopher P. Wild et al. observe in "Translational Cancer Research: Balancing Prevention and Treatment to Combat Cancer Globally" (*Journal of the National Cancer Institute*, vol. 107, no. 1, 2015) that more than 50% of all cancers could be prevented "if the specific risk factors were identified and exposures controlled effectively." Primary prevention is effective as evidenced by declining lung cancer rates following reductions in smoking. However, primary prevention requires the identification of risk factors, and for some common cancers such as prostate, kidney, pancreas, and brain malignancies the identity of major risk factors is as yet unknown. Secondary prevention is frequently impeded by the inability to detect many types of cancer early enough to permit successful treatment or the inability to distinguish between findings identified at screening that would or would not progress to malignancy. Breast and prostate cancers are examples of the latter circumstance, and there is concern that some patients may be subjected to overtreatment.

Cancer among African Americans

African Americans are more likely to be diagnosed with cancer and to die from the disease than any other racial or ethnic population. In 2013 the rate of cancer deaths among African American males was 238.7 per 100,000 population, compared with 195.5 per 100,000 population among white men. (See Table 5.5.) According to the ACS, in *Cancer Facts and Figures, 2015*, most of these differences are not likely due to genetics; they are more likely due to social, economic, cultural, behavioral, and environmental factors. Examples of social and economic inequities include a lack of health insurance, transportation, or access to quality, affordable health care, which prevents or delays testing and timely treatment.

Sex and Cancer

Men and women are each more prone to certain types of cancer—most obviously, the cancers of the reproductive system, such as ovarian and cervical cancer in women and prostate and testicular cancer in men. Breast cancer also occurs mainly in women, although some men do die from this disease. For men, the lifetime risk of getting breast cancer is very small—about one in 1,000. The ACS estimates in *Cancer Facts and Figures, 2015* that 2,350 new cases of breast cancer were diagnosed in men in 2015 and 440 men died as a result of breast cancer.

Similarly, cancer rates are different for men and women, and the disease claims more men than women. In 2013 there were 196 cancer deaths per 100,000 males, compared with 139.5 cancer deaths per 100,000 females. (See Table 5.5.)

Lung Cancer

The ACS estimates in *Cancer Facts and Figures, 2015* that 221,200 new cases of lung cancer were diagnosed in 2015. The incidence of lung cancer increased until 1991, but has been declining in men since then. The incidence rate began to decline in women in 2003.

TABLE 5.4

Use of mammography by selected age groups, selected years 1987–2013

[Data are based on household interviews of a sample of the civilian noninstitutionalized population]

Characteristic	1987	1993	1994	2000	2003	2005	2008	2010	2013
	Percent of women having a mammogram within the past 2 years[a]								
40 years and over, age-adjusted[b,c]	29.0	59.7	61.0	70.4	69.5	66.6	67.1	66.5	65.7
40 years and over, crude[b]	28.7	59.7	60.9	70.4	69.7	66.8	67.6	67.1	66.8
50 years and over, age-adjusted[b,c]	27.3	59.7	60.9	73.7	72.4	68.2	70.3	68.8	69.1
50 years and over, crude[b]	27.4	59.7	60.6	73.6	72.4	68.4	70.5	69.2	69.5
Age									
40–49 years	31.9	59.9	61.3	64.3	64.4	63.5	61.5	62.3	59.6
50–64 years	31.7	65.1	66.5	78.7	76.2	71.8	74.2	72.6	71.4
65 years and over	22.8	54.2	55.0	67.9	67.7	63.8	65.5	64.4	66.9
65–74 years	26.6	64.2	63.0	74.0	74.6	72.5	72.6	71.9	75.3
75 years and over	17.3	41.0	44.6	61.3	60.6	54.7	57.9	55.7	56.5
Race[d]									
40 years and over, crude:									
White only	29.6	60.0	60.6	71.4	70.1	67.4	67.9	67.4	66.8
Black or African American only	24.0	59.1	64.3	67.8	70.4	64.9	68.0	67.9	67.1
American Indian or Alaska Native only	*	49.8	65.8	47.4	63.1	72.8	62.7	71.2	62.6
Asian only	*	55.1	55.8	53.5	57.6	54.6	66.1	62.4	66.6
Native Hawaiian or Other Pacific Islander only	—	—	—	*	*	*	*	*	*
2 or more races	—	—	—	69.2	65.3	63.7	55.2	51.4	65.4
Hispanic origin and race[d]									
40 years and over, crude:									
Hispanic or Latina	18.3	50.9	51.9	61.2	65.0	58.8	61.2	64.2	61.4
Not Hispanic or Latina	29.4	60.3	61.5	71.1	70.1	67.5	68.3	67.4	67.5
White only	30.3	60.6	61.3	72.2	70.5	68.3	68.7	67.8	67.6
Black or African American only	23.8	59.2	64.4	67.9	70.5	65.2	68.3	67.4	67.2
Age, Hispanic origin, and race[d]									
40–49 years:									
Hispanic or Latina	*15.3	52.6	47.5	54.1	59.4	54.2	54.1	59.8	56.4
Not Hispanic or Latina:									
White only	34.3	61.6	62.0	67.2	65.2	65.5	64.1	62.6	60.3
Black or African American only	27.8	55.6	67.2	60.9	68.2	62.1	59.5	63.5	59.4
50–64 years:									
Hispanic or Latina	23.0	59.2	60.1	66.5	69.4	61.5	71.3	68.6	65.6
Not Hispanic or Latina:									
White only	33.6	66.2	67.5	80.6	77.2	73.5	74.1	73.5	72.1
Black or African American only	26.4	65.5	63.6	77.7	76.2	71.6	76.7	74.0	71.7
65 years and over:									
Hispanic or Latina	*	*35.7	48.0	68.3	69.5	63.8	59.0	65.2	63.2
Not Hispanic or Latina:									
White only	24.0	54.7	54.9	68.3	68.1	64.7	66.1	65.0	67.3
Black or African American only	14.1	56.3	61.0	65.5	65.4	60.5	66.4	60.9	68.8
Age and percent of poverty level[e]									
40 years and over, crude:									
Below 100%	14.6	41.1	44.2	54.8	55.4	48.5	51.4	51.4	49.9
100%–199%	20.9	47.5	48.6	58.1	60.8	55.3	55.8	53.8	56.7
200%–399%	29.7	63.2	65.0	68.8	69.9	67.2	64.4	66.2	66.0
400% or more	42.9	74.1	74.1	81.5	77.7	76.6	79.0	78.1	77.2
40–49 years:									
Below 100%	18.6	36.1	43.0	47.4	50.6	42.5	46.6	48.1	43.3
100%–199%	18.4	47.8	47.6	43.6	54.0	49.8	46.5	46.2	52.0
200%–399%	31.2	63.0	64.5	60.2	63.0	61.8	56.8	59.2	58.5
400% or more	44.1	69.6	69.9	75.8	71.6	73.6	72.5	73.6	69.0
50–64 years:									
Below 100%	14.6	47.3	46.2	61.7	58.3	50.4	57.5	54.7	55.0
100%–199%	24.2	47.0	49.0	68.3	64.0	58.8	58.9	57.3	57.2
200%–399%	29.7	66.1	69.6	75.1	74.1	70.7	69.8	70.7	69.5
400% or more	44.7	78.7	78.0	86.9	84.9	80.6	84.3	82.8	80.9

Lung cancer was estimated to claim 158,040 lives in 2015, accounting for 27% of all cancer deaths. Each year since 1987 more women have died of lung cancer than breast cancer, which had been the leading cause of cancer deaths for women for more than 40 years. Lung cancer is also the leading cause of cancer-related deaths for men.

TABLE 5.4

Use of mammography by selected age groups, selected years 1987–2013 [CONTINUED]

[Data are based on household interviews of a sample of the civilian noninstitutionalized population]

Characteristic	1987	1993	1994	2000	2003	2005	2008	2010	2013
65 years and over:				Percent of women having a mammogram within the past 2 years[a]					
Below 100%	13.1	40.4	43.9	54.8	57.0	52.3	49.1	50.6	49.8
100%–199%	19.9	47.6	48.8	60.3	62.8	56.1	59.4	55.5	59.3
200%–399%	27.7	60.3	61.0	71.1	72.3	68.6	65.0	67.2	68.1
400% or more	34.7	71.3	73.0	81.9	73.0	72.6	78.3	74.5	79.0

*Estimates are considered unreliable. Data preceded by an asterisk have a relative standard error (RSE) of 20%–30%. Data not shown have an RSE greater than 30%.
—Data not available.
[a]Questions concerning use of mammography differed slightly on the National Health Interview Survey across the years for which data are shown.
[b]Includes all other races not shown separately, unknown poverty level in 1987, unknown health insurance status, unknown education level, and unknown disability status.
[c]Estimates for women aged 40 and over are age-adjusted to the year 2000 standard population using four age groups: 40–49 years, 50–64 years, 65–74 years, and 75 years and over. Estimates for women 50 years of age and over are age-adjusted using three age groups.
[d]The race groups, white, black, American Indian or Alaska Native, Asian, Native Hawaiian or Other Pacific Islander, and 2 or more races, include persons of Hispanic and non-Hispanic origin. Persons of Hispanic origin may be of any race. Starting with 1999 data, race-specific estimates are tabulated according to the 1997 *Revisions to the Standards for the Classification of Federal Data on Race and Ethnicity* and are not strictly comparable with estimates for earlier years. The five single-race categories plus multiple-race categories shown in the table conform to the 1997 Standards. Starting with 1999 data, race-specific estimates are for persons who reported only one racial group; the category 2 or more races includes persons who reported more than one racial group. Prior to 1999, data were tabulated according to the 1977 Standards with four racial groups, and the Asian only category included Native Hawaiian or Other Pacific Islander. Estimates for single-race categories prior to 1999 included persons who reported one race or, if they reported more than one race, identified one race as best representing their race. Starting with 2003 data, race responses of other race and unspecified multiple race were treated as missing, and then race was imputed if these were the only race responses. Almost all persons with a race response of other race were of Hispanic origin.
[e]Percent of poverty level is based on family income and family size and composition using U.S. Census Bureau poverty thresholds. Poverty level was unknown for 11% of women aged 40 and over in 1987. Missing family income data were imputed for 1997 and beyond.

SOURCE: Adapted from "Table 732. Use of Mammography among Women 40 Years of Age and over, by Selected Characteristics: United States, Selected Years 1987–2013," in *Health, United States, 2014: With Special Feature on Adults Aged 55–64*, Centers for Disease Control and Prevention, National Center for Health Statistics, 2015, http://www.cdc.gov/nchs/data/hus/hus14.pdf (accessed December 15, 2015)

The main risk factor for lung cancer is cigarette smoking, especially a long history of smoking (20 years or more). In addition, exposure to certain industrial substances, such as asbestos, organic chemicals, and radon, can increase the risk of developing the disease.

Passive, or involuntary or secondhand smoking (inhaling other people's smoke), also increases the risk for nonsmokers. Research shows that the risk to a nonsmoking woman who is married to a smoker is 30% greater than for a woman with a nonsmoking spouse. In "Secondhand Tobacco Smoke and Smoke-Free Homes" (November 16, 2015, http://www.epa.gov/indoor-air-quality-iaq/secondhand-tobacco-smoke-and-smoke-free-homes), the U.S. Environmental Protection Agency claims that an estimated 3,000 nonsmokers die each year from secondhand-smoke-induced lung cancer. The agency added secondhand smoke to its list of known carcinogens in 1993.

Lowell Dale explains in "What Is Thirdhand Smoke, and Why Is It a Concern?" (July 10, 2014, http://www.mayoclinic.com/health/third-hand-smoke/AN01985) that thirdhand smoke, the residue of nicotine and other toxic chemicals in tobacco that coats indoor surfaces such as walls, carpets, drapes, furniture, and bedding, has been identified as a health hazard. Thirdhand smoke, which can interact with other indoor pollutants to form cancer-causing compounds, poses a risk to both the skin and lungs.

The ACS explains that early diagnosis of lung cancer is difficult. By the time a tumor is visible on x-rays, it is often in the advanced stages. However, if an individual stops smoking before cellular changes occur, damaged tissues often return to normal. Diagnostic tests such as low-dose spiral CT scans, which provide detailed three-dimensional images of the lungs, and laboratory procedures that can detect molecular markers for cancer in sputum have demonstrated an ability to diagnose lung cancer earlier than conventional tests, and research to evaluate their effects on survival rates is under way. The National Lung Screening Trial (http://www.cancer.gov/clinicaltrials/noteworthy-trials/nlst), a clinical trial to determine the effectiveness of lung cancer screening in high-risk people (people who smoked at least a pack of cigarettes per day for 30 years), reports 20% fewer lung cancer deaths among current and former heavy smokers who were screened with spiral CT, compared with standard chest x-ray. However, this detection method may not be useful in the general population because this study considered only subjects with a history of heavy smoking. Furthermore, the risks that are associated with screening, including radiation exposure from multiple CT scans and unnecessary lung biopsy and surgery, may outweigh the benefits in the general population. The treatment options for lung cancer include surgery, radiation therapy, and chemotherapy (anticancer drugs).

The U.S. Preventive Services Task Force (USPSTF; December 2013, http://www.uspreventiveservicestaskforce.org/Page/Document/UpdateSummaryFinal/lung-cancer-screening?ds=1&s=lung%20cancer%20screening) recommends annual screening for lung cancer with an imaging study called low-dose CT in adults aged 55 to

TABLE 5.5

Death rates for cancer by sex, age, race, and Hispanic origin, selected years 1950–2013

[Data are based on death certificates]

Sex, race, Hispanic origin, and age	1950[a]	1960[a]	1970	1980	1990	2000	2012	2013
All persons				Deaths per 100,000 resident population				
All ages, age-adjusted[b]	193.9	193.9	198.6	207.9	216.0	199.6	166.5	163.2
All ages, crude	139.8	149.2	162.8	183.9	203.2	196.5	185.6	185.0
Under 1 year	8.7	7.2	4.7	3.2	2.3	2.4	1.6	1.6
1–4 years	11.7	10.9	7.5	4.5	3.5	2.7	2.4	2.1
5–14 years	6.7	6.8	6.0	4.3	3.1	2.5	2.2	2.2
15–24 years	8.6	8.3	8.3	6.3	4.9	4.4	3.6	3.4
25–34 years	20.0	19.5	16.5	13.7	12.6	9.8	8.7	8.6
35–44 years	62.7	59.7	59.5	48.6	43.3	36.6	28.0	28.1
45–54 years	175.1	177.0	182.5	180.0	158.9	127.5	108.5	105.5
55–64 years	390.7	396.8	423.0	436.1	449.6	366.7	293.2	288.2
65–74 years	698.8	713.9	754.2	817.9	872.3	816.3	632.2	616.9
75–84 years	1,153.3	1,127.4	1,169.2	1,232.3	1,348.5	1,335.6	1,161.7	1,139.4
85 years and over	1,451.0	1,450.0	1,320.7	1,594.6	1,752.9	1,819.4	1,658.9	1,635.4
Male								
All ages, age-adjusted[b]	208.1	225.1	247.6	271.2	280.4	248.9	200.3	196.0
All ages, crude	142.9	162.5	182.1	205.3	221.3	207.2	197.9	197.6
Under 1 year	9.7	7.7	4.4	3.7	2.4	2.6	1.7	1.5
1–4 years	12.5	12.4	8.3	5.2	3.7	3.0	2.7	2.2
5–14 years	7.4	7.6	6.7	4.9	3.5	2.7	2.4	2.2
15–24 years	9.7	10.2	10.4	7.8	5.7	5.1	4.1	3.8
25–34 years	17.7	18.8	16.3	13.4	12.6	9.2	8.4	8.6
35–44 years	45.6	48.9	53.0	44.0	38.5	32.7	24.0	24.0
45–54 years	156.2	170.8	183.5	188.7	162.5	130.9	110.1	106.5
55–64 years	413.1	459.9	511.8	520.8	532.9	415.8	336.9	331.3
65–74 years	791.5	890.5	1,006.8	1,093.2	1,122.2	1,001.9	746.7	726.2
75–84 years	1,332.6	1,389.4	1,588.3	1,790.5	1,914.4	1,760.6	1,447.6	1,414.5
85 years and over	1,668.3	1,741.2	1,720.8	2,369.5	2,739.9	2,710.7	2,303.1	2,272.6
Female								
All ages, age-adjusted[b]	182.3	168.7	163.2	166.7	175.7	167.6	142.1	139.5
All ages, crude	136.8	136.4	144.4	163.6	186.0	186.2	173.7	172.8
Under 1 year	7.6	6.8	5.0	2.7	2.2	2.3	1.5	1.8
1–4 years	10.8	9.3	6.7	3.7	3.2	2.5	2.2	1.9
5–14 years	6.0	6.0	5.2	3.6	2.8	2.2	2.0	2.1
15–24 years	7.6	6.5	6.2	4.8	4.1	3.6	3.0	3.0
25–34 years	22.2	20.1	16.7	14.0	12.6	10.4	8.9	8.6
35–44 years	79.3	70.0	65.6	53.1	48.1	40.4	31.9	32.1
45–54 years	194.0	183.0	181.5	171.8	155.5	124.2	107.0	104.6
55–64 years	368.2	337.7	343.2	361.7	375.2	321.3	252.5	248.1
65–74 years	612.3	560.2	557.9	607.1	677.4	663.6	531.9	520.8
75–84 years	1,000.7	924.1	891.9	903.1	1,010.3	1,058.5	950.0	933.3
85 years and over	1,299.7	1,263.9	1,096.7	1,255.7	1,372.1	1,456.4	1,336.4	1,310.1
White male[c]								
All ages, age-adjusted[b]	210.0	224.7	244.8	265.1	272.2	243.9	199.7	195.5
All ages, crude	147.2	166.1	185.1	208.7	227.7	218.1	213.1	213.0
25–34 years	17.7	18.8	16.2	13.6	12.3	9.2	8.5	8.5
35–44 years	44.5	46.3	50.1	41.1	35.8	30.9	24.2	23.9
45–54 years	150.8	164.1	172.0	175.4	149.9	123.5	108.2	105.7
55–64 years	409.4	450.9	498.1	497.4	508.2	401.9	329.4	323.1
65–74 years	798.7	887.3	997.0	1,070.7	1,090.7	984.3	742.8	723.3
75–84 years	1,367.6	1,413.7	1,592.7	1,779.7	1,883.2	1,736.0	1,453.0	1,421.7
85 years and over	1,732.7	1,791.4	1,772.2	2,375.6	2,715.1	2,693.7	2,318.7	2,290.7
Black or African American male[c]								
All ages, age-adjusted[b]	178.9	227.6	291.9	353.4	397.9	340.3	246.1	238.7
All ages, crude	106.6	136.7	171.6	205.5	221.9	188.5	166.4	165.6
25–34 years	18.0	18.4	18.8	14.1	15.7	10.1	9.1	10.2
35–44 years	55.7	72.9	81.3	73.8	64.3	48.4	26.6	27.3
45–54 years	211.7	244.7	311.2	333.0	302.6	214.2	145.0	132.4
55–64 years	490.8	579.7	689.2	812.5	859.2	626.4	468.8	464.0
65–74 years	636.5	938.5	1,168.9	1,417.2	1,613.9	1,363.8	970.2	941.5
75–84 years[d]	853.5	1,053.3	1,624.8	2,029.6	2,478.3	2,351.8	1,685.7	1,633.2
85 years and over	—	1,155.2	1,387.0	2,393.9	3,238.3	3,264.8	2,540.2	2,465.6

80 years who have a 30 pack-year smoking history and currently smoke or have quit within the past 15 years. The rationale for annual screening is that non-small cell lung cancer, the most common type of lung cancer, can sometimes be cured by removing part of the affected lung, if it is detected early enough.

TABLE 5.5

Death rates for cancer by sex, age, race, and Hispanic origin, selected years 1950–2013 [CONTINUED]

[Data are based on death certificates]

—Data not available.
*Rates based on fewer than 20 deaths are considered unreliable and are not shown.
[a]Includes deaths of persons who were not residents of the 50 states and the District of Columbia (D.C.).
[b]Age-adjusted rates are calculated using the year 2000 standard population. Prior to 2001, age-adjusted rates were calculated using standard million proportions based on rounded population numbers. Starting with 2001 data, unrounded population numbers are used to calculate age-adjusted rates.
[c]The race groups, white, black, Asian or Pacific Islander, and American Indian or Alaska Native, include persons of Hispanic and non-Hispanic origin. Persons of Hispanic origin may be of any race. Death rates for Hispanic, American Indian or Alaska Native, and Asian or Pacific Islander persons should be interpreted with caution because of inconsistencies in reporting Hispanic origin or race on the death certificate (death rate numerators) compared with population figures (death rate denominators). The net effect of misclassification is an underestimation of deaths and death rates for races other than white and black.
[d]In 1950, rate is for the age group 75 years and over.
Notes: Starting with *Health, United States, 2003,* rates for 1991–1999 were revised using intercensal population estimates based on the 1990 and 2000 censuses. For 2000, population estimates are bridged-race April 1 census counts. Starting with *Health, United States, 2012,* rates for 2001–2009 were revised using intercensal population estimates based on the 2000 and 2010 censuses. For 2010, population estimates are bridged-race April 1 census counts. Rates for 2011 and beyond were computed using 2010-based postcensal estimates. Age groups were selected to minimize the presentation of unstable age-specific death rates based on small numbers of deaths and for consistency among comparison groups. Starting with 2003 data, some states allowed the reporting of more than one race on the death certificate. The multiple-race data for these states were bridged to the single-race categories of the 1977 Office of Management and Budget standards, for comparability with other states.

SOURCE: "Table 26. Death Rates for Malignant Neoplasms, by Sex, Race, Hispanic Origin, and Age: United States, Selected Years 1950–2013," in *Health, United States, 2014: With Special Feature on Adults Aged 55–64,* Centers for Disease Control and Prevention, National Center for Health Statistics, 2015, http://www.cdc.gov/nchs/data/hus/hus14.pdf (accessed December 15, 2015)

Colon and Rectal Cancer

The ACS reports in *Cancer Facts and Figures, 2015* that in 2015 an estimated 93,090 cases of colon cancer and 39,610 cases of rectal cancer were diagnosed and that an estimated 49,700 people died of the diseases. The incidence of colorectal cancer has been decreasing since the mid-1980s, and among adults aged 50 years and older it declined 4.3% per year between 2007 and 2011.

When colorectal cancer is detected early, the ACS indicates that the five-year survival rate is 90%. However, only 40% of this type of cancer is found at this stage. If the malignancy has spread regionally, the five-year survival rate drops to 71%.

Colon cancer occurs most often in people without any known risk factors. However, people with a family history of polyps in the colon or rectum and people who have suffered from ulcerative colitis and other diseases of the bowel are considered to be at a greater risk for developing the disease. Other significant risk factors may be physical inactivity, obesity, diabetes, smoking, heavy alcohol consumption, and a diet high in fat and low in fiber.

The ACS recommends a variety of screening tests to detect bowel cancer in its early stages. For people over the age of 50 years, an annual stool test for fecal occult blood (hidden blood) is recommended, along with flexible sigmoidoscopy (examination of the lower colon and rectum using a hollow, lighted tube) every five years or as often as recommended by the physician. The ACS also recommends an imaging procedure called a double-contrast barium enema, which provides a complete radiologic examination of the colon, every five years for people over the age of 50 years and a screening colonoscopy (examination of the entire colon) every 10 years or as often as recommended by their physician. Although it is a costlier screening test, some people prefer a virtual colonoscopy, which uses x-rays and computers to produce images of the entire length of the colon.

Despite overwhelming evidence that screening and early detection save lives, many adults do not receive even the simplest of the colon cancer screening tests. The CDC asserts in "Screening for Colorectal Cancer: It's the Right Choice" (September 22, 2015, http://www.cdc.gov/cancer/colorectal/basic_info/screening/infographic.htm) that if everyone aged 50 years and older had regular screening tests and all precancerous polyps were removed, as many as 60% of deaths from colorectal cancer could be prevented.

The most common treatment for cancer of the bowel is surgery to remove the diseased area, in combination with radiation. Chemotherapy alone, or along with radiation, is given before or after surgery to most patients whose cancer has penetrated the bowel wall deeply or spread to the lymph nodes. A colostomy (an opening in the abdomen to allow for waste elimination) is seldom necessary for patients with colon cancer but may be required for patients with rectal cancer. The ACS reports that few patients with rectal cancer require a permanent colostomy if the cancer is detected in the early stages. Of those who do require a permanent colostomy, most go on to lead normal, active lives. Chemotherapeutic agents that are used to treat metastatic (spreading) colon and rectal cancer include the drugs oxaliplatin with 5-fluorouracil followed by leucovorin and bevacizumab, which block the growth of blood vessels to the tumor, and cetuximab and panitumumab, both of which block the effects of hormone-like factors that promote cancer cell growth.

Breast Cancer

Breast cancer is the most common form of cancer among women. According to the ACS, in *Cancer Facts and Figures, 2015*, an estimated 231,840 new cases of invasive breast cancer and 60,290 new cases of in situ breast cancer were diagnosed in women in 2015. (Invasive breast cancer spreads to the surrounding breast tissue, whereas in situ, or noninvasive, breast cancer is confined to the milk ducts or glands.) An estimated 40,290 women died from breast cancer in 2015. The disease ranks second in terms of cancer deaths in women, after lung cancer.

Both the incidence of breast cancer and deaths from the disease have been declining since 2000. According to the ACS, the declining incidence is due to earlier detection and improved treatment; however, the dramatic decrease of 7% between 2002 and 2003 has been attributed to the sharply decreased use of hormone replacement therapy, which was linked to increased breast cancer risk.

The five-year survival rates for breast cancer are encouraging. The ACS reports that if the cancer is localized, the survival rate is 99%. If the cancer is undetected and has spread regionally, however, the survival rate decreases to 85%, and for women whose cancer has spread to distant parts of the body, the survival rate is only 25%.

The precise causes of breast cancer are still unknown. The disease is most common in women older than the age of 50, and the risks are higher among women with a family history of breast cancer, women who have never had children, and women who gave birth to their first baby after the age of 30. Other factors that may contribute to increased risk for breast cancer include having a longer-than-average menstrual history (menstruation beginning at an early age and ending late in life), being obese after menopause, consuming alcohol, long-term smoking, and eating a high-fat diet.

CHOICES OF TREATMENT. Breast cancer treatment remains a subject of continuing medical debate. If a breast contains cancerous tissue, the patient and her physician have four standard treatment options: surgery, radiation therapy, chemotherapy, or hormone therapy. Treatment choices depend on the location and size of the tumor, the stage of the cancer (whether the cancer has spread within the breast or to other parts of the body affects staging), and the size of the breast. A small, contained tumor can be removed in a procedure commonly called a lumpectomy (removal of the tumor, or "lump") and a lymph node dissection (microscopic examination of lymph nodes to detect cancer cells), followed by radiation therapy to the whole breast. If the cancer is more advanced and invasive, removing the breast (mastectomy) and usually the adjoining lymph nodes, combined with chemotherapy or hormone therapy, may be the most effective treatment.

Favorable outcomes for women with early-stage breast cancer who undergo breast-conserving therapy (BCT; lumpectomy, usually with radiation therapy) have been confirmed in many studies. For example, in "Mastectomy and Breast-Conserving Therapy Confer Equivalent Outcomes in Young Women with Early-Stage Breast Cancer" (*CA: A Cancer Journal for Clinicians*, vol. 65, no. 5, September–October 2015), Mary Kay Barton reports that many rigorous studies have determined that BCT and mastectomy confer equivalent survival outcomes in women with early-stage breast cancer. Even women aged 40 years and younger who have a greater risk of an aggressive cancer and a higher rate of local recurrence have similar or better survival outcomes when treated with BCT versus mastectomy with no radiation therapy. In *Cancer Facts and Figures, 2015*, the ACS confirms that numerous studies show that the long-term survival rates after lumpectomy plus radiation therapy are similar to the survival rates after mastectomy for women whose cancer has not spread.

Sentinel lymph node (SLN; the first lymph node the cancer is likely to spread to from the tumor) biopsy is a form of treatment that was tested in two large clinical trials that compared SLN biopsy with conventional axillary lymph node dissection. The trials were conducted by the National Surgical Adjuvant Breast and Bowel Project and the American College of Surgeons Oncology Group—which are networks of institutions and physicians across the country that jointly conduct trials under the sponsorship of the National Cancer Institute. SLN biopsy is a surgical procedure involving the removal of the SLN. Either a radioactive substance or a blue dye (in some cases both) is injected near the tumor. This flows through the lymph ducts to the lymph nodes. The first lymph node to receive the substance or dye is removed for biopsy. If cancer cells are not found, no more lymph nodes may need to be removed. After the SLN biopsy, the surgeon performs a lumpectomy or mastectomy to remove the tumor.

Peer and professionally facilitated support groups are available to help patients deal with the emotional consequences and physical side effects of breast cancer treatment. Significant advances and techniques have made breast reconstruction possible—frequently during or immediately following surgery.

GENETIC RESEARCH. Physicians have known for some time that a predisposition to some forms of breast cancer is inherited. For this reason, physicians have been searching for the gene or genes responsible so that they can test patients and provide more careful monitoring for those who are at risk. In 1994 doctors identified the BRCA1 gene, and in 1995 they isolated the BRCA2 gene.

Kelly A. Metcalfe of the University of Toronto explains in "Oophorectomy for Breast Cancer Prevention in Women with BRCA1 or BRCA2 Mutations" (*Future Medicine*, vol. 5, no. 1, January 2009) that if a woman with a family history of breast cancer inherits a defective form of either BRCA1 or BRCA2, she has an estimated 80% to 90% risk of developing breast cancer. Researchers also think that the two genes are linked to ovarian, prostate, and colon cancer and that BRCA2 likely plays some role in breast cancer in men. Scientists suspect that the two genes may also participate in some way in the development of breast cancer in women with no family history of the disease. In *Cancer Facts and Figures, 2015*, the ACS reports that only 5% to 10% of all cases of female breast cancer are attributable to defects in BRCA1 and BRCA2. Variations of other genes are also associated with an increased risk for breast cancer.

In "Which Role for EGFR Therapy in Breast Cancer?" (*Frontiers in Bioscience*, no. 4, January 1, 2012), Vito Lorusso et al. indicate that other forms of breast cancer are driven by copies of the genes EGFR and HER2 and are expressed in up to 30% of the new cases of the disease in the United States each year. HER2/neu is an aggressive form of cancer with increased rates of recurrence and poor survival in node-positive breast cancer patients. The HER2 gene produces a protein on the surface of cells that serves as a receiving point for growth-stimulating hormones.

Trastuzumab, a genetically engineered antibody drug that became available in 1998, increases the benefits of chemotherapy by shrinking tumors and slowing the progression of HER2/neu. By 2016 promising therapies included treatment with the anti-HER2/neu antibody trastuzumab (for patients with high levels of the HER2 protein) and newer anti-HER2 antibody drugs such as pertuzumab and aromatase inhibitors. The results of clinical trials of trastuzumab and pertuzumab in combination with other chemotherapeutic agents were reported in 2012 and 2013. One such study was conducted by Luca Gianni et al. In "Efficacy and Safety of Neoadjuvant Pertuzumab and Trastuzumab in Women with Locally Advanced, Inflammatory, or Early HER2-Positive Breast Cancer (NeoSphere): A Randomised Multicentre, Open-Label, Phase 2 Trial" (*Lancet Oncology*, vol. 13, no. 1, January 2012), the researchers find the combination of pertuzumab or trastuzumab, or both, and docetaxel to be safe and effective therapy for HER2-positive locally advanced or metastatic breast cancer. Many breast tumors are "estrogen sensitive," meaning the hormone estrogen helps them to grow. Aromatase inhibitors help block the growth of these tumors by lowering the amount of estrogen in the body. In 2016 there were three aromatase inhibitors approved by the FDA: anastrozole, exemestane, and letrozole.

The ACA speculates in "Medicines to Reduce Breast Cancer Risk" (October 21, 2014, http://www.cancer.org/cancer/breastcancer/moreinformation/medicinestoreducebreastcancer/medicines-to-reduce-breast-cancer-risk-aromatase-inhibitors) that aromatase inhibitors may prove to be as effective as or more effective than tamoxifen or raloxifene in reducing breast cancer risk; however, their use for this purpose has not yet been fully evaluated.

Breast cancer genetic research is rapidly evolving. In "Large-Scale Genotyping Identifies 41 New Loci Associated with Breast Cancer Risk" (*Nature Genetics*, vol. 45, no. 4, April 2013), Kyriaki Michailidou et al. report that an analysis of nine genome-wide association studies and more than 45,000 breast cancer cases identified 41 new single nucleotide polymorphisms (genetic variations in a deoxyribonucleic acid sequence that occurs when a single nucleotide in a genome is altered) that are associated with breast cancer susceptibility. The researchers opine that more than 1,000 additional loci are involved in breast cancer susceptibility.

Jennifer J. Wheler et al. note in "Multiple Gene Aberrations and Breast Cancer: Lessons from Super-Responders" (*BMC Cancer*, vol. 15, no. 442, December 2015) that gene aberrations (mutations, amplifications, and rearrangements) promote tumor growth. The researchers observe that aberrations are common in breast cancer that involves genes such as HER2 (ERBB2), BRCA, PIK3CA, TP53, GATA3, and PTEN. They also indicate that patients with multiple gene abnormalities do not fare as well as those with no or a single identified abnormality and posit that the presence of multiple abnormalities may indicate genetic instability.

Skin Cancer

According to the ACS, in *Cancer Facts and Figures, 2015*, more than 3 million unreported cases of nonmelanoma (basal cell or squamous cell) cancers occur annually. The majority of these cancers are easily cured, especially if they are detected and treated early. The ACS estimates that 73,870 new cases of malignant melanoma, a far more serious form of skin cancer, were diagnosed in 2015.

The ACS reports that there were an estimated 13,340 deaths from skin cancer (9,940 from malignant melanoma) in 2015. Melanoma can spread to other parts of the body quickly, but if it is detected early and properly treated, it is highly curable. The five-year survival rate for localized malignant melanoma is 98%, and the five-year survival rates for regional- and distant-stage diseases are 63% and 16%, respectively.

Simple precautions can prevent most skin cancers. According to the ACS, avoiding the sun between 10 a.m. and 4 p.m. (when the ultraviolet rays are the strongest), using sunscreen with a sun protection factor of 30 or higher, avoiding tanning beds and sun lamps, and wearing protective clothing decrease the risk of skin cancer considerably.

Prostate Cancer

The ACS indicates in *Cancer Facts and Figures, 2015* that an estimated 220,800 American men were diagnosed with prostate cancer in 2015. Approximately 27,540 men died from the disease, making it the second-leading cause of cancer death in men, exceeded only by lung cancer. The probability of developing prostate cancer increases with advancing age.

During the late 1980s prostate-specific antigen (PSA) screening became available to test for the disease. This is a blood test that measures a protein that is made by prostate cells. PSA blood tests are reported in nanograms per milliliter (ng/mL). Results are considered to be normal if the reading is under 4 ng/mL; borderline results are between 4 and 10 ng/mL; and any reading of more than 10 ng/mL is high. The higher the reading, the more likely prostate cancer is present. However, normal levels increase with age, and older men with higher readings are frequently found to have no prostate cancer. For example, PSA levels greater than or equal to 2.5 ng/mL are considered to be abnormally high for men younger than the age of 49 years, whereas PSA levels greater than or equal to 4.5 ng/mL are considered to be abnormally high for men between the ages of 60 and 69 years.

In May 2012 the USPSTF (http://www.uspreventiveservicestaskforce.org/Page/Document/RecommendationStatementFinal/prostate-cancer-screening) recommended against routine PSA screening. The revised recommendation was based on a USPSTF review of the scientific evidence, which failed to support the premise that PSA-based early detection of prostate cancer prolongs lives. Furthermore, the USPSTF concluded that PSA-based screening may result in harm, specifically, overdiagnosis and overtreatment of prostate tumors that would not cause illness or death. In *Cancer Facts and Figures, 2015*, the ACS recommends that beginning at age 50 men at average risk for prostate cancer should discuss the benefits and limitations of PSA testing with their physician. African American men and men who have a first-degree relative who had prostate cancer should have this discussion at age 45 because they are at a higher risk of developing the disease. The ACS reports that two large clinical trials were conducted to help determine the efficacy (the ability of an intervention to produce the intended diagnostic or therapeutic effect in optimal circumstances) of PSA testing and they produced conflicting results. One study, which was conducted in Europe, reported a lower risk of death from prostate cancer among men receiving PSA screening, whereas the other study, which was conducted in the United States, did not.

In October 2015 the USPSTF (http://www.uspreventiveservicestaskforce.org/Page/Document/draft-research-plan/prostate-cancer-screening1) began a review of the evidence in the medical literature to update its prostate cancer screening guideline. Figure 5.3 shows the key questions the USPSTF will consider as it reviews the screening guidelines. These include:

- How effective is screening with the PSA test in reducing mortality (deaths) and morbidity (illnesses) from prostate cancer?

FIGURE 5.3

U.S. Preventive Services Task Force draft research plan for prostate cancer screening, October 2015

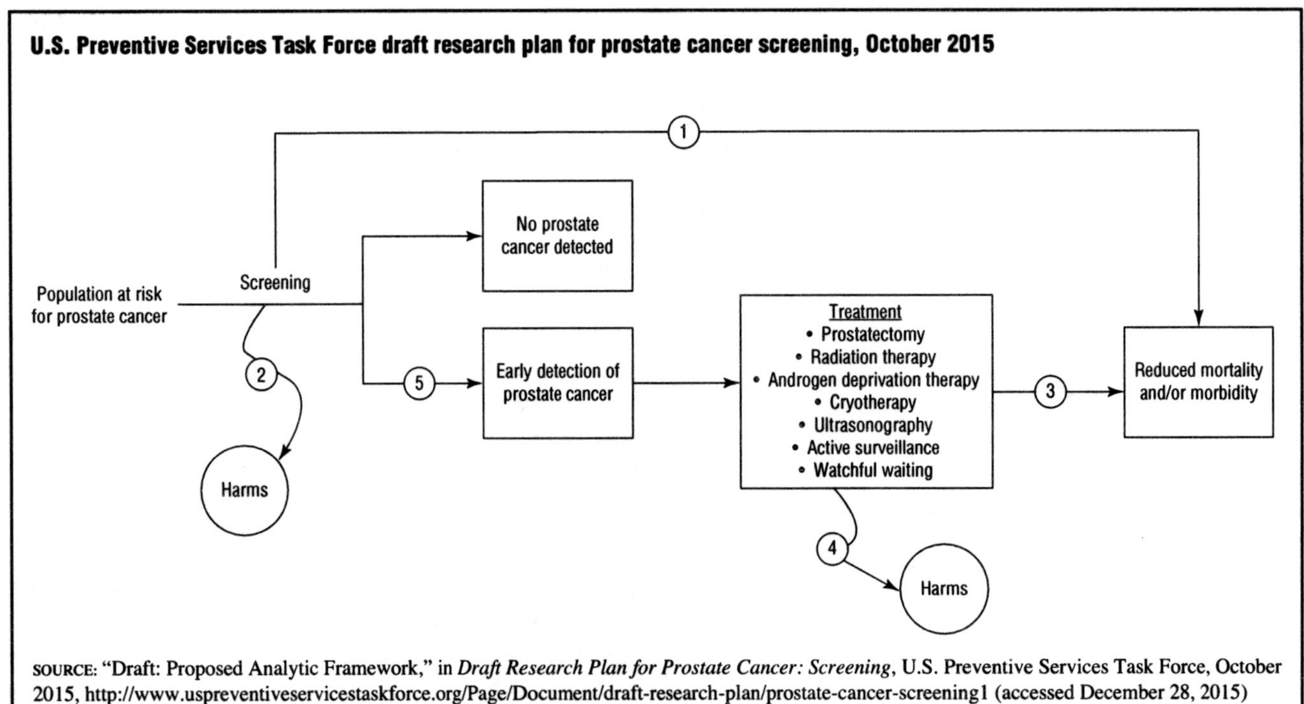

SOURCE: "Draft: Proposed Analytic Framework," in *Draft Research Plan for Prostate Cancer: Screening*, U.S. Preventive Services Task Force, October 2015, http://www.uspreventiveservicestaskforce.org/Page/Document/draft-research-plan/prostate-cancer-screening1 (accessed December 28, 2015)

- What are the harms of PSA-based screening?
- How effective is treatment of early-stage or screen-detected prostate cancer in reducing morbidity and mortality?
- What are the harms of treatment of early-stage or screen-detected prostate cancer?
- How effective are prostate cancer risk calculators combined with PSA testing to increase the detection of clinically significant prostate cancer (cancer that is more likely to cause symptoms or lead to advanced disease)?

The USPSTF will also consider how often U.S. men with prostate cancer detected by PSA testing receive treatment, the treatment preferences of U.S. men with prostate cancer detected by PSA testing, and which newer tests or testing strategies can help identify prostate cancer that is more or less likely to cause symptoms or lead to advanced disease. The answers to these questions will form the basis for the USPSTF's recommendation about prostate cancer screening.

PROSTATE CANCER TREATMENTS. In *Cancer Facts and Figures, 2015*, the ACS explains that prostate cancer may be treated in several ways, depending on the age of the patient, the severity of the cancer, and any other medical conditions the patient may have. Radiation and surgery may be used if the disease is in an early stage. Hormone therapy (which shrinks the tumor, thus relieving pain and other symptoms for a long period), chemotherapy, and radiation may be used alone or in combination if the cancer has spread, and these methods may be effective as supplements to treatments during early stages. "Watchful waiting" (close observation with no treatment) may also be appropriate in patients who are older or who have less aggressive tumors.

A radical prostatectomy is the removal of the prostate and some of the tissue surrounding the gland. This is done when the cancer has not spread outside the gland. Radiation therapy kills cancer cells, shrinks tumors, and may be used before or after prostate surgery. Impotence (erectile dysfunction) and urinary incontinence occur slightly more often when radiation is used following surgery. Radiation therapy can also cause damage to the rectum.

Therapy to reduce hormone (testosterone) levels may be prescribed to limit prostate cancer cell growth. Patients may be given drugs such as luteinizing hormone-releasing hormone agonists, which decrease the amount of testosterone in the body, or antiandrogens, which block the activity of testosterone. These cause cancer cells to shrink because testosterone promotes the growth of prostate cancer cells.

Transurethral resection relieves the blockage of urinary flow that is caused by cancer of the prostate gland. This procedure is often performed to relieve symptoms of urinary obstruction caused by the tumor. Chemotherapy is used to treat prostate cancer if it returns after being treated with other types of treatment. For men who have less aggressive tumors, are older than 70 years of age, or have coexisting illnesses, many physicians will use a watch-and-wait approach before suggesting active treatment.

Men with advanced prostate cancer that no longer responds to hormones may be candidates for immunization with a cancer vaccine known as sipuleucel-T. The vaccine entails removing immune cells from the man's body, exposing them to prostate proteins, and then reinfusing them to combat the prostate cancer cells. In 2010 cabazitaxel, a chemotherapy drug, was approved to treat metastatic prostate cancer that fails to respond to other treatments. New types of hormone therapy, such as abiraterone and enzalutamide, have been shown to be helpful for treatment of metastatic disease that does not respond to initial hormone therapy and/or chemotherapy. In 2013 radium-223 was approved to treat hormone-resistant prostate cancer that has spread to the bones.

Because 93% of all prostate cancers are detected in the local and regional stages, the five-year relative survival rate for patients whose tumors are diagnosed at these stages approaches 100%. The ACS reports that since the mid-1980s the five-year survival rate for all stages combined has increased from 68% to almost 100%.

RESPIRATORY DISEASES AND LUNG HEALTH

The lungs are especially vulnerable to airborne particles, such as viruses, bacteria, tobacco smoke, pollen, fungi, and air pollution. Workers who are exposed to certain airborne hazards—cotton fibers, asbestos, and coal, metal, and silica dust—can also develop serious lung diseases. Pneumoconiosis is the general term for occupationally induced lung diseases.

Asthma

According to the NCHS, in *Summary Health Statistics: National Health Interview Survey, 2014* (October 19, 2015, http://ftp.cdc.gov/pub/Health_Statistics/NCHS/NHIS/SHS/2014_SHS_Table_A-2.pdf), an estimated 17.7 million American adults had asthma in 2014. In *Summary Health Statistics for U.S. Children: National Health Interview Survey, 2014* (October 19, 2015, http://ftp.cdc.gov/pub/Health_Statistics/NCHS/NHIS/SHS/2014_SHS_Table_C-1.pdf), the NCHS indicates that asthma is the most common chronic illness among children. In 2014 an estimated 6.3 million children younger than 18 years of age had asthma.

People with asthma experience acute attacks of wheezing and shortness of breath. This difficulty in breathing is caused by a sudden narrowing of the bronchial tubes. Usually, it is not life threatening, but asthma often limits activities and can be extremely serious for the very young and the very old.

The incidence of asthma has increased dramatically since the 1980s in the United States and in other industrialized nations as a result of lifestyle changes and living conditions in modern society. Exposure to air pollutants including tobacco smoke, ozone, and diesel exhaust may be contributing to this increased incidence. Indoor exposures to allergens may also contribute to the increase in asthma because many indoor environments have been made more airtight to improve energy efficiency. Other factors implicated in the rise in asthma include the increased incidence of obesity, decreased physical activity, change in diet, decreased exposure to microbes during early life, and increased viral respiratory infections such as those that are contracted by children in day care settings. Although children appear to be at highest risk, new cases are also occurring in adults, particularly older adults.

RACIAL, AGE, AND SEX DISPARITIES. The prevalence of asthma varies by race, age, and sex. In 2015 the asthma prevalence rates continued to be highest among non-Hispanic African Americans under the age of 15 years. (See Figure 5.4.)

FIGURE 5.4

Prevalence of current asthma among persons of all ages, by age group, race, and ethnicity, 2015

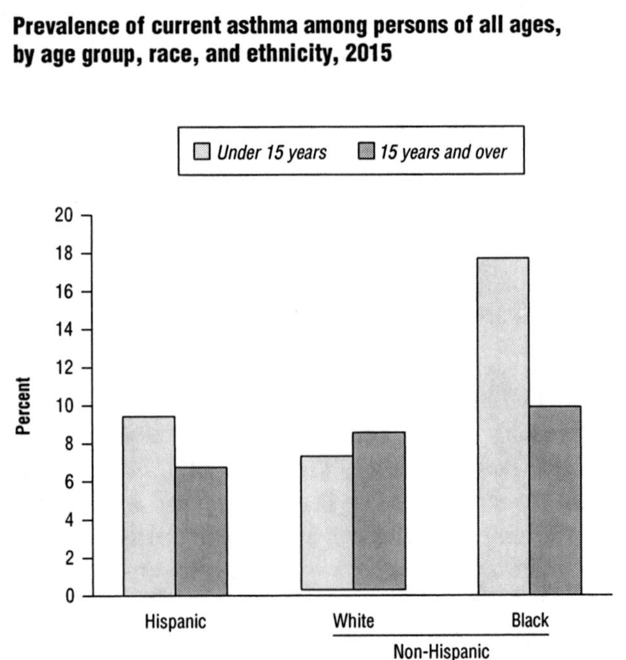

Notes: Data are based on household interviews of a sample of the civilian noninstitutionalized population. Information on current asthma is self-reported by adults aged 18 and over. For children under age 18, the information is collected from an adult family member, usually a parent, who is knowledgeable about the child's health. The analyses excluded the 0.2% of persons with unknown current asthma status.

SOURCE: "Figure 15.6. Sex-Adjusted Prevalence of Current Asthma among Persons of All Ages, by Age Group and Race/Ethnicity: United States, January–June 2015," in *Early Release of Selected Estimates Based on Data from the January–June 2015 National Health Interview Survey*, Centers for Disease Control and Prevention, National Center for Health Statistics, November 2015, http://www.cdc.gov/nchs/data/nhis/earlyrelease/earlyrelease201511_15.pdf (accessed December 28, 2015)

In 2015 asthma was more prevalent in children under the age of 15 years, and boys were more likely to have asthma than girls. (See Figure 5.5.) However, in all other age groups the prevalence was higher among females than among males.

CAUSES OF ASTHMA ATTACKS. Although the specific cause of asthma is not known, the disease appears to be associated with allergic reactions, heredity, and environment. Many environmental factors can trigger an asthma attack in susceptible individuals. Indoor and outdoor pollution do not cause the disease, but pollutants such as ozone, sulfur dioxide, nitrogen dioxide, and tobacco smoke can trigger an episode of asthma. Allergens such as pollen and dust mites can also provoke asthma attacks.

MANAGING ASTHMA SYMPTOMS. The National Heart, Lung, and Blood Institute (NHLBI) explains in *Asthma Care Quick Reference Guide: Diagnosing and Managing Asthma* (September 2012, https://www.nhlbi.nih.gov/files/docs/guidelines/asthma_qrg.pdf) that asthma control focuses on "reducing impairment—the frequency and intensity of symptoms and functional limitations currently or recently experienced by a patient; and... reducing risk—the likelihood of future asthma attacks, progressive decline in lung function (or, for children, reduced lung growth), or medication side effects." To achieve and maintain asthma control, environmental factors that trigger or worsen symptoms must be identified and addressed, prescription medication must be used appropriately, patients must learn self-care skills, and health professionals must monitor patients to ensure that control is maintained and, when needed, to change treatment.

Chronic Obstructive Pulmonary Disease

Chronic obstructive pulmonary disease (COPD), which includes emphysema and chronic bronchitis, is a progressive disease that causes the obstruction of airflow. The COPD Foundation indicates in "COPD Statistics across America" (2016, http://www.copdfoundation.org/What-is-COPD/COPD-Facts/Statistics.aspx) that COPD affects more than 24 million people in the United States. In *Health, United States, 2014*, the NCHS reports that deaths attributable to COPD have increased sharply. In 1980, 56,050 people died from COPD; by 2013 deaths attributable to chronic lower respiratory disease more than doubled to 149,205. (See Table 1.5 in Chapter 1.)

CHRONIC BRONCHITIS. Bronchitis is an inflammation of the lining of the bronchi (tubes that connect the trachea [windpipe] to the lungs). When the bronchi are inflamed and infected, less air is able to flow to and from the lungs,

FIGURE 5.5

Prevalence of current asthma among persons of all ages, by age group and sex, 2015

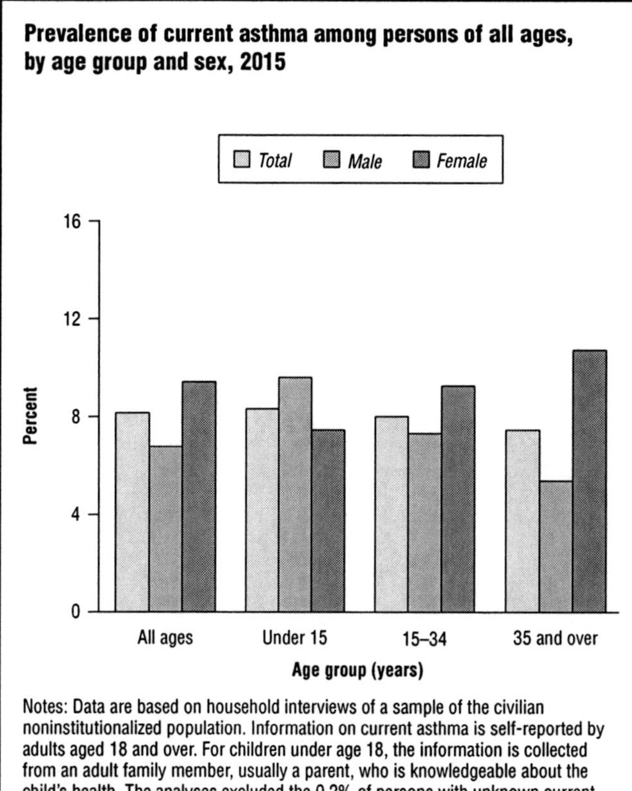

Notes: Data are based on household interviews of a sample of the civilian noninstitutionalized population. Information on current asthma is self-reported by adults aged 18 and over. For children under age 18, the information is collected from an adult family member, usually a parent, who is knowledgeable about the child's health. The analyses excluded the 0.2% of persons with unknown current asthma status.

SOURCE: "Figure 15.5. Prevalence of Current Asthma among Persons of All Ages, by Age Group and Sex: United States, January–June 2015," in *Early Release of Selected Estimates Based on Data from the January–June 2015 National Health Interview Survey*, Centers for Disease Control and Prevention, National Center for Health Statistics, November 2015, http://www.cdc.gov/nchs/data/nhis/earlyrelease/earlyrelease201511_15.pdf (accessed December 28, 2015)

and mucus forms and is coughed up. Acute bronchitis is usually brief in duration and follows the flu or a cold. Chronic bronchitis, however, lingers for months or even years and is characterized by a persistent mucus-producing cough. It is a long-term disease that is characterized by breathlessness and wheezing.

In 2014 nearly 8.7 million adults over the age of 18 years had chronic bronchitis. (See Table 5.6.) The NHLBI indicates in "What Causes Bronchitis?" (August 4, 2011, http://www.nhlbi.nih.gov/health/health-topics/topics/brnchi/causes) that people who smoke cigarettes are far more likely to develop chronic bronchitis than nonsmokers. Workers whose jobs involve inhaling large amounts of dust and irritating fumes are also more likely to get the disease. When air pollution becomes excessive, symptoms intensify.

Antibiotics and bronchodilator drugs are useful treatments, but even more important is the need to eliminate the sources of respiratory irritation. This could mean quitting smoking or avoiding polluted air, fumes, and dust. Chronic bronchitis is often the forerunner of emphysema.

EMPHYSEMA. Emphysema is a severe disease of the lungs that usually develops gradually. The air sacs on the walls of the lungs slowly lose their elasticity, and stale air becomes trapped in the lungs, which become overly inflated. This interferes with the normal exchange of oxygen and carbon dioxide. People with emphysema often feel as if they are drowning in a sea of air. In its late stage, emphysema also affects the heart, because the flow of blood from the lungs is disrupted by changes caused by the disease. The heart has to pump harder to compensate for the disease and may become enlarged. Death often results from heart failure. Approximately 3.4 million adults over the age of 18 years had emphysema in 2014. (See Table 5.6.)

DIABETES

Diabetes is a disease that affects the body's use of food, causing levels of blood glucose (sugar in the blood) to become too high. Normally, the body converts sugars, starches, and proteins into a form of sugar called glucose. The blood then carries glucose to all the cells throughout the body. In the cells, with the help of the hormone insulin, the glucose is either converted into energy for use immediately or stored for the future. Beta cells of the pancreas, a small organ located behind the stomach, manufacture insulin. The process of turning food into energy via glucose is important because the body depends on glucose for every function.

Because diabetes deprives body cells of the glucose that is needed to function properly, several complications can develop to threaten the lives of diabetics further. The healing process of the body is slowed or impaired, and the risk of infection increases. Complications of diabetes include higher risk and rates of heart disease; circulatory problems, especially in the legs, which often are severe enough to require surgery or even amputation; diabetic retinopathy, a condition that can cause blindness; kidney disease that may require dialysis; dental problems; and problems with pregnancy. Close attention to preventive health care such as regular eye, dental, and foot examinations and tight control of blood sugar levels have been shown to prevent some of the consequences of diabetes. The types of diabetes, the populations that are at risk of developing the disease, the complications of diabetes, and the measures to prevent the development of diabetes and its complications are described in Chapter 2.

Warning Signs of Prediabetes and Diabetes

To determine whether someone has prediabetes or diabetes, a fasting plasma glucose test or an oral glucose tolerance test is done in the doctor's office. A fasting blood glucose level between 100 and 125 mg/dL signals prediabetes, and a fasting blood glucose level of 126 mg/dL

TABLE 5.6

Frequency of selected respiratory diseases among persons aged 18 and older, by selected characteristics, 2014

Selected characteristic	All adults aged 18 and over	Emphysema[a]	Ever had asthma[a]	Still has asthma[a]	Hay fever[a]	Sinusitis[a]	Chronic bronchitis[a]
Total	**239,688**	**3,400**	**30,598**	**17,717**	**19,089**	**29,442**	**8,692**
Sex							
Male	115,541	1,623	12,387	5,889	7,824	10,139	2,993
Female	124,148	1,777	18,212	11,828	11,265	19,302	5,699
Age (years)							
18–44	112,149	98	15,651	8,404	6,315	9,997	2,835
45–64	82,605	1,511	10,032	6,230	8,986	12,653	3,600
65–74	26,362	1,052	3,103	1,945	2,392	4,372	1,285
75 and over	18,573	739	1,813	1,139	1,397	2,420	971
Race							
One race[b]	235,831	3,321	29,828	17,239	18,643	28,941	8,515
White	190,462	2,941	23,832	13,806	15,851	24,218	6,899
Black or African American	29,355	297	4,434	2,563	1,818	3,592	1,265
American Indian or Alaska Native	1,948	*43	292	218	165	213	*90
Asian	13,733	*35	1,226	621	785	893	218
Native Hawaiian or Other Pacific Islander	333	*	*43	*	*	*	*
Two or more races[c]	3,858	*79	771	478	447	501	176
Black or African American, white	760	—	109	*69	*30	*54	*
American Indian or Alaska Native, white	1,590	*71	382	267	255	275	127
Hispanic or Latino origin[d] and race							
Hispanic or Latino	36,571	237	3,823	2,135	1,957	3,073	645
Mexican or Mexican American	22,326	119	2,011	1,095	1,230	1,804	366
Not Hispanic or Latino	203,117	3,163	26,776	15,582	17,132	26,369	8,046
White, single race	157,364	2,716	20,496	11,942	14,075	21,427	6,332
Black or African American, single race	27,875	293	4,165	2,428	1,768	3,506	1,220
Education[e]							
Less than a high school diploma	27,612	1,023	3,206	2,159	1,665	3,004	1,443
High school diploma or GED[f]	52,697	1,135	5,807	3,695	3,943	7,005	2,361
Some college	59,919	898	8,152	4,744	5,685	8,895	2,698
Bachelor's degree or higher	67,940	288	8,081	4,462	6,429	8,733	1,523
Current employment status[g]							
Employed	146,624	642	17,187	9,336	11,223	16,452	3,628
Full-time	117,112	435	13,556	7,297	9,042	12,886	2,717
Part-time	27,205	162	3,483	1,919	2,070	3,284	811
Not employed but has worked previously	79,316	2,586	11,965	7,471	7,216	11,940	4,582
Not employed and has never worked	13,623	172	1,445	908	642	1,011	481
Family income[h]							
Less than $35,000	69,793	1,847	10,303	6,422	4,962	8,728	4,038
$35,000 or more	144,503	1,169	17,508	9,729	12,443	17,604	3,852
$35,000–$49,999	28,044	578	3,506	2,152	2,171	3,355	1,061
$50,000–$74,999	35,733	347	4,312	2,421	2,813	4,412	1,029
$75,000–$99,999	27,053	*63	3,086	1,732	2,071	3,228	717
$100,000 or more	53,673	181	6,604	3,424	5,388	6,610	1,045
Poverty status[i]							
Poor	31,383	719	5,054	3,271	2,046	3,631	1,684
Near poor	42,675	1,039	5,568	3,390	3,027	5,252	2,313
Not poor	152,199	1,412	18,393	10,130	13,219	18,959	4,219
Health insurance coverage[j]							
Under 65:							
Private	129,666	488	16,271	8,683	10,938	15,277	3,308
Medicaid	23,239	474	4,322	3,050	1,692	2,809	1,471
Other	9,095	421	1,546	890	893	1,693	702
Uninsured	31,587	213	3,380	1,929	1,740	2,805	933
65 and over:							
Private	22,525	747	2,471	1,567	1,859	3,546	1,128
Medicare and Medicaid	2,951	243	490	393	314	492	258
Medicare only	15,536	640	1,630	888	1,365	2,295	710
Other	3,513	154	285	200	232	448	142
Uninsured	313	*	*	*	*	*	*

or higher signals diabetes. With these tests, a patient fasts overnight, then drinks a solution that is rich in glucose. The patient's blood glucose level is then measured at one-hour intervals, commonly over two to five hours, to determine the rate at which the glucose is consumed. A diagnosis of prediabetes is made when the two-hour blood glucose level is between 140 and 199 mg/dL, and diabetes is diagnosed when the level is 200 mg/dL or higher.

TABLE 5.6

Frequency of selected respiratory diseases among persons aged 18 and older, by selected characteristics, 2014 [CONTINUED]

Selected characteristic	All adults aged 18 and over	Emphysema[a]	Ever had asthma[a]	Still has asthma[a]	Hay fever[a]	Sinusitis[a]	Chronic bronchitis[a]
Marital status							
Married	126,926	1,462	14,148	8,118	10,896	16,479	3,807
Widowed	14,312	703	1,754	1,153	1,156	2,265	955
Divorced or separated	26,802	799	3,953	2,639	2,606	4,336	1,895
Never married	53,788	274	7,953	4,275	3,302	4,732	1,558
Living with a partner	17,497	160	2,740	1,512	1,098	1,538	466
Place of residence[k]							
Large MSA	130,402	1,412	16,409	9,079	9,841	14,489	3,779
Small MSA	73,885	1,140	9,459	5,663	6,443	9,953	3,172
Not in MSA	35,402	848	4,731	2,975	2,806	5,000	1,741
Region							
Northeast	41,490	659	5,309	3,204	3,328	4,156	1,318
Midwest	55,095	772	7,129	4,209	3,894	6,786	2,162
South	89,270	1,452	11,065	6,346	6,674	13,181	3,656
West	53,834	517	7,095	3,958	5,193	5,320	1,556
Hispanic or Latino origin[d], race, and sex							
Hispanic or Latino, male	18,309	99	1,455	700	886	1,192	262
Hispanic or Latina, female	18,262	138	2,368	1,435	1,071	1,881	384
Not Hispanic or Latino:							
White, single race, male	76,277	1,297	8,351	4,098	5,798	7,400	2,232
White, single race, female	81,087	1,419	12,145	7,844	8,277	14,027	4,099
Black or African American, single race, male	12,626	133	1,636	671	664	1,097	332
Black or African American, single race, female	15,249	160	2,530	1,757	1,104	2,409	888

*Estimates are considered unreliable. Data preceded by an asterisk have a relative standard error (RSE) greater than 30% and less than or equal to 50% and should be used with caution. Data not shown have an RSE greater than 50%.
—Quantity zero.
[a]Respondents were asked in two separate questions if they had ever been told by a doctor or other health professional that they had emphysema or asthma. Respondents who had been told they had asthma were asked if they still had asthma. Respondents were asked in four separate questions if they had been told by a doctor or other health professional in the past 12 months that they had hay fever, sinusitis, or chronic bronchitis. A person may be represented in more than one column.
[b]Refers to persons who indicated only a single race group, including those of Hispanic or Latino origin.
[c]Refers to persons who indicated more than one race group, including those of Hispanic or Latino origin. Only two combinations of multiple race groups are shown due to small sample sizes for other combinations.
[d]Refers to persons who are of Hispanic or Latino origin and may be of any race or combination of races. "Not Hispanic or Latino" refers to persons who are not of Hispanic or Latino origin, regardless of race.
[e]Shown only for adults aged 25 and over.
[f]GED is General Educational Development high school equivalency diploma.
[g]"Full-time" employment is 35 or more hours per week. "Part-time" employment is 34 or fewer hours per week.
[h]Includes persons in families that reported either a dollar amount or would not provide a dollar amount but provided an income interval.
[i]"Poor" persons live in families defined as below the poverty threshold. "Near poor" persons live in families with incomes of 100% to less than 200% of the poverty threshold. "Not poor" persons live in families with incomes that are 200% of the poverty threshold or greater.
[j]Based on a hierarchy of mutually exclusive categories. Adults with more than one type of health insurance were assigned to the first appropriate category in the hierarchy. "Uninsured" includes adults who had no coverage as well as those who had only Indian Health Service coverage or had only a private plan that paid for one type of service such as accidents or dental care.
[k]MSA is metropolitan statistical area. Large MSAs have a population size of 1 million or more; small MSAs have a population size of less than 1 million. "Not in MSA" consists of persons not living in a metropolitan statistical area.
Notes: Estimates are based on household interviews of a sample of the civilian noninstitutionalized population. This table is based on data from the Sample Adult file and was weighted using the Sample Adult weight. Unknowns for the columns were not included in the frequencies, but they are included in the "All adults aged 18 and over" column. "Total" includes other races not shown separately and persons with unknown education, family income, poverty status, and health insurance characteristics.

SOURCE: "Table A-2b. Frequencies of Selected Respiratory Diseases among Adults Aged 18 and over, by Selected Characteristics: United States, 2014," in *Summary Health Statistics for U.S. Adults: National Health Interview Survey, 2014*, Centers for Disease Control and Prevention, National Center for Health Statistics, December 2015, http://ftp.cdc.gov/pub/Health_Statistics/NCHS/NHIS/SHS/2014_SHS_Table_A-2.pdf (accessed December 28, 2015)

The symptoms of type 1 diabetes usually occur suddenly. These include excessive thirst, frequent urination, weight loss, weakness and fatigue, nausea and vomiting, and irritability. The symptoms of type 2 diabetes generally appear gradually. These may include any of the symptoms seen in type 1 diabetes, plus recurring infections that are slow to heal, drowsiness, blurred vision, numbness in the hands or feet, and itching.

Prevalence of Diabetes

Between 1997 and 2015 there was an increase in diagnosed diabetes among U.S. adults aged 18 years and older. (See Figure 2.7 in Chapter 2.) By the first half of 2015, 9.6% of the U.S adult population aged 18 years and older had been diagnosed with diabetes. The prevalence of diabetes increases with age among men and women, with the highest rates among older adults—people aged 65 years and older. In all age categories except for ages 18 to 44 years, the prevalence of diagnosed diabetes in 2015 was higher in men than in women. (See Figure 5.6.) The prevalence of diagnosed diabetes was higher among Hispanics (13.3%) and non-Hispanic African Americans (12.8%) than among non-Hispanic whites (7.1%). (See Figure 5.7.)

FIGURE 5.6

Prevalence of diagnosed diabetes among adults aged 18 years and older, by age group and sex, 2013

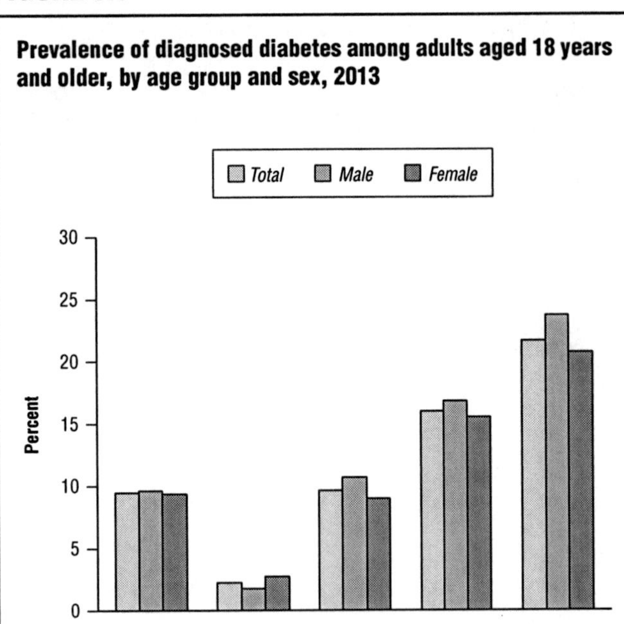

Notes: Data are based on household interviews of a sample of the civilian noninstitutionalized population. Prevalence of diagnosed diabetes is based on self-report of ever having been diagnosed with diabetes by a doctor or other health professional. Persons reporting "borderline" diabetes status and women reporting diabetes only during pregnancy were not coded as having diabetes in the analyses. The analyses excluded the 0.1% of persons with unknown diabetes status.

SOURCE: "Data Table for Figure 14.2. Prevalence of Diagnosed Diabetes among Adults Aged 18 Years and over, by Age Group and Sex: United States, January–June 2015," in *Early Release of Selected Estimates Based on Data from the January–June 2015 National Health Interview Survey*, Centers for Disease Control and Prevention, National Center for Health Statistics, November 2015, http://www.cdc.gov/nchs/data/nhis/earlyrelease/earlyrelease201511_14.pdf (accessed December 16, 2015)

FIGURE 5.7

Prevalence of diagnosed diabetes among adults aged 18 and older, by race/ethnicity, 2015

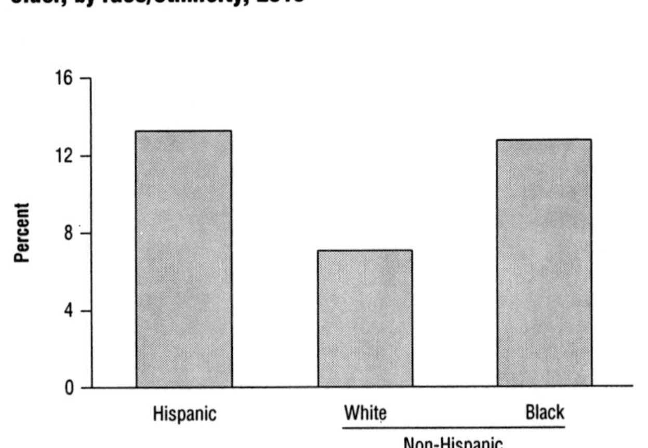

Notes: Data are based on household interviews of a sample of the civilian noninstitutionalized population. Prevalence of diagnosed diabetes is based on self-report of ever having been diagnosed with diabetes by a doctor or other health professional. Persons reporting "borderline" diabetes status and women reporting diabetes only during pregnancy were not coded as having diabetes in the analyses. The analyses excluded the 0.1% of persons with unknown diabetes status. Estimates are age-sex adjusted using the projected 2000 U.S. population as the standard population and using four age groups: 18–44, 45–54, 55–64, and 65 and over.

SOURCE: "Data Table for Figure 14.3. Age-Sex-Adjusted Prevalence of Diagnosed Diabetes among Adults Aged 18 Years and over, by Race/Ethnicity: United States, January–June 2015," in *Early Release of Selected Estimates Based on Data from the January–June 2015 National Health Interview Survey*, Centers for Disease Control and Prevention, National Center for Health Statistics, November 2015, http://www.cdc.gov/nchs/data/nhis/earlyrelease/earlyrelease201511_14.pdf (accessed December 16, 2015)

People who are older than the age of 40 years, overweight, have a family history of diabetes, and are physically inactive are at greater risk of developing type 2 diabetes. There is an increased prevalence of diabetes with age. The percentage of people over the age of 65 years (21.8%) who had diagnosed cases of diabetes in 2015 was more than nine times as high as for people aged 18 to 44 years (2.3%). (See Figure 5.6.)

The prevalence of diabetes is higher when undiagnosed diabetes is included. Andy Menke et al. report in "Prevalence of and Trends in Diabetes among Adults in the United States, 1988–2012" (*Journal of the American Medical Association*, vol. 314, no. 10, September 8, 2015) that in a representative sample of U.S. adults, the prevalence of diabetes, diagnosed and undiagnosed, was between 12% and 14% and the prevalence of prediabetes was between 37% and 38%.

Causes of Diabetes

The causes of both type 1 and type 2 diabetes are unknown, but a family history of diabetes increases the risk for both types, which strongly suggests a genetic component in the genesis of the disease. Some scientists believe that a flaw in the body's immune system may be a factor in type 1 diabetes. Other researchers believe that physical inactivity and the resulting poor cardiovascular fitness is a risk factor for developing diabetes.

In type 2 diabetes heredity may be a factor, but because the pancreas continues to produce insulin, the disease is considered to be more of a problem of insulin resistance, in which the body is not using the hormone efficiently. In people who are prone to type 2 diabetes, being overweight can set off the disease because excess fat prevents insulin from working correctly. Maintaining a healthy weight and keeping physically fit can usually prevent type 2 diabetes. To date, type 1 diabetes cannot be prevented.

"Diabesity" and "Double Diabetes"

The recognition of obesity-dependent diabetes prompted scientists and physicians to coin a new term to describe this condition: diabesity. The term was first used during the 1990s and has gained widespread acceptance. Although diabesity is attributed to the same causes as type 2 diabetes (insulin resistance and pancreatic cell dysfunction), researchers are beginning to link the inflammation that is associated with obesity to the development of diabetes and cardiovascular disease.

Another recently recognized and increasingly prevalent problem is posed by patients who are diagnosed with both type 1 and type 2 diabetes simultaneously. Called "double diabetes," it has been diagnosed in both children and adults. It occurs when children with type 1 diabetes who rely on insulin injections to control their diabetes gain weight and develop the insulin resistance that is the hallmark of type 2 diabetes. Among adults who have been diagnosed with type 2 diabetes, those who fail to respond to conventional treatment have been found to also suffer from the type 1, insulin-dependent form of the disease.

In "Double Diabetes: A Mixture of Type 1 and Type 2 Diabetes in Youth" (*Endocrine Involvement in Developmental Syndromes*, vol. 14, 2009), Paolo Pozzilli and Chiara Guglielmi of the University Campus Bio-Medico in Rome, Italy, observe that there was an increase in type 1 diabetes, especially in children younger than five years old, during the previous decade that may be attributed to changes in environmental factors, rather than to genetic factors. They assert that the marked increase in the incidence of type 2 diabetes in children and adolescents is very likely the result of the increase in obesity and sedentary lifestyle that is occurring in developed countries. Pozzilli and Guglielmi opine that the "current classification of diabetes should be revised taking into account this new form of diabetes which [is] called double diabetes or hybrid diabetes."

Deaths Resulting from Diabetes

The risk of death among people with diabetes is about twice that of their age peers without diabetes. In 2013 diabetes was the seventh-leading cause of death in the United States. The NCHS notes in *Health, United States, 2014* that 75,578 people died from it in 2013. (See Table 1.5 in Chapter 1.) In *National Diabetes Statistics Report, 2014*, the National Institute of Diabetes and Digestive and Kidney Diseases asserts that diabetes is likely to be underreported as a cause of death. The institute notes that only about 35% to 40% of the deceased with diabetes had diabetes listed on their death certificate, and just 10% to 15% had it listed as the underlying cause of death.

FOOD ALLERGIES

Food allergies are immune reactions that strike shortly after eating a certain food. Symptoms of food allergies include digestive problems, hives, or trouble breathing. Some people experience severe or life-threatening symptoms including a reaction known as anaphylaxis, in which airways tighten and constrict.

Kristen D. Jackson, LaJeana D. Howie, and Lara J. Akinbami of the NCHS observe in *Trends in Allergic Conditions among Children: United States, 1997–2011* (May 2013, http://www.cdc.gov/nchs/data/databriefs/db121.pdf) that the prevalence of food allergies among children under the age of 18 years increased between 1997 and 2011. Hispanic children had a lower prevalence of food allergy, compared with non-Hispanic white and non-Hispanic African American children.

The reasons for the increasing prevalence of food allergies are as yet unknown. According to M. Cecilia Berin and Hugh A. Sampson, in "Food Allergy: An Enigmatic Epidemic" (*Trends in Immunology*, vol. 34, no. 8, August 2013), food allergies affect between 2% and 10% of the U.S. population and the most common food allergies are to milk, eggs, peanuts, fish, and shellfish. The researchers observe that peanut allergies appear to have tripled between 1997 and 2008 in Australia, the United Kingdom, and the United States. They hypothesize that a variety of factors may explain this rise, such as maternal consumption of certain foods during pregnancy or breast-feeding. Environmental influences may also be contributing to the rise. Potential environmental influences include nutritional factors, such as varying levels of vitamins A and D, which may suppress or promote allergies, and a high-fat diet, which is known to promote allergies. Antibiotic use may also contribute to food allergy by altering the flora that live in the intestines.

The results of a clinical trial to prevent food allergy in a group of high-risk infants were reported by George Du Toit et al. in "Randomized Trial of Peanut Consumption in Infants at Risk for Peanut Allergy" (*New England Journal of Medicine*, vol. 372, no. 9, February 26, 2015). The researchers tested the premise that regular consumption of foods containing peanuts beginning during the first year of life might elicit a protective immune response rather than an allergic reaction. The study followed more than 600 children aged four to 11 months who were considered at high risk for developing peanut allergy because they had severe eczema and/or egg allergy. The researchers then compared the incidence of peanut allergy among the children who ate peanuts with the children who avoided peanuts until age five.

The children exposed to peanuts ate a peanut-containing snack at least three times per week while the other group did not eat any foods containing peanuts. By age five, just 3% of the children who ate the peanut snack developed peanut allergies, compared with 17% in the group who did not consume peanuts. Du Toit et al. conclude, "Our findings showed that early, sustained consumption of peanut products was associated with a substantial and significant decrease in the development of peanut allergy in high-risk infants. Conversely, peanut avoidance was associated with a greater frequency of clinical peanut allergy than was peanut consumption, which raises questions about the usefulness of deliberate avoidance of peanuts as a strategy to prevent allergy."

CHAPTER 6

DEGENERATIVE DISEASES

Degenerative diseases are noninfectious disorders that are characterized by progressive disability. Patients can often live for years with their diseases. Although they may not die from degenerative diseases, patients' symptoms usually grow more disabling, and they often succumb to complications of their disorders.

ARTHRITIS AND OTHER RHEUMATIC DISEASES

The word *arthritis* literally means joint inflammation, and it is applied to more than 100 related diseases that are known as rheumatic diseases. When a joint (the point where two bones meet) becomes inflamed, swelling, redness, pain, and loss of motion occur. In the most serious forms of the disease, the loss of motion can be physically disabling.

Normally, inflammation is part of the body's response to an injury or a disease. It leads to pain, redness, swelling, and warmth in the inflamed body part. Once the injury is healed or the disease is cured, the inflammation stops. In arthritis, however, the inflammation does not subside. Instead, it becomes part of the problem, damaging healthy tissues. This generates more inflammation and more damage, and the painful cycle continues. The damage can change the shape of bones and other tissues of the joints, making movement difficult and painful.

Types of Arthritis

More than 100 types of arthritis have been identified, but four major types affect large numbers of Americans:

- Osteoarthritis—the most common type of arthritis, osteoarthritis generally affects people as they grow older. Sometimes called degenerative arthritis, it causes the breakdown of bones and cartilage (connective tissue that attaches to bones) and usually causes pain and stiffness in the fingers, knees, feet, hips, and back. The Arthritis Foundation notes in "What Is Osteoarthritis?" (2016, http://www.arthritis.org/about-arthritis/types/osteoarthritis/what-is-osteoarthritis.php) that osteoarthritis affects about 27 million Americans.
- Fibromyalgia—fibromyalgia affects the muscles and connective tissues and causes widespread pain, fatigue, sleep problems, and stiffness. Fibromyalgia also causes "tender points" that are more sensitive to pain than other areas of the body. According to the National Fibromyalgia Association, in "Prevalence" (2015, http://www.fmaware.org/about-fibromyalgia/prevalence/), about 10 million Americans, mostly women, have this condition.
- Rheumatoid arthritis—rheumatoid arthritis is caused by a flaw in the body's immune system that results in inflammation and swelling in joint linings, followed by damage to bone and cartilage in the hands, wrists, feet, knees, ankles, shoulders, or elbows. The Arthritis Foundation reports in "What Is Rheumatoid Arthritis?" (2016, http://www.arthritis.org/about-arthritis/types/rheumatoid-arthritis/what-is-rheumatoid-arthritis.php) that 1.5 million Americans, mostly women, have this form of arthritis.
- Gout—gout is an inflammation of a joint that is caused by an accumulation of uric acid (a natural substance) in the joint, usually the big toe, knee, or wrist. The uric acid forms crystals in the affected joint, causing severe pain and swelling. According to the Arthritis Foundation, in "What Is Gout" (2016, http://www.arthritis.org/about-arthritis/types/gout/what-is-gout.php), about 6 million men and 2 million women have had at least one gout attack. A gout attack lasts from days to two weeks.

Lupus

Another less common, but potentially life-threatening, form of rheumatic disease is systemic lupus erythematosus (SLE; also called lupus), an inflammatory autoimmune disease (a disease in which the immune system mistakenly attacks the body's own tissues) that affects skin, joints, blood, and the kidneys. The Centers for Disease Control and Prevention (CDC) reports in "Systemic Lupus Erythematosus" (April 23, 2015, http://www.cdc.gov/arthritis/basics/lupus.htm) that SLE occurs more frequently among females than among males (approximately four to 12 females for every male) and that African Americans are more likely to be affected than whites. U.S. prevalence estimates vary from about 322,000 to more than 1.5 million. Generally diagnosed in women of childbearing age, the symptoms of SLE include:

- Painful or swollen joints, muscle pain, and fatigue
- Fever, weight loss, hair loss, and skin rashes
- Cold, pale, or blue fingers, also known as Raynaud's phenomenon
- Swollen legs or glands
- Nephritis (inflammation of the kidneys)
- Pleuritis (inflammation of the lungs) that may produce chest pain or increase the risk of developing pneumonia
- Myocarditis, endocarditis, or pericarditis (inflammation of the heart muscle, the heart valves, and the membrane around the heart, respectively) and vasculitis (inflammation of blood vessels)

As with other inflammatory and autoimmune disorders, each patient experiences the disease differently. SLE symptoms ranging from mild to severe flare up and subside throughout the course of the illness. Some patients with SLE also experience headaches, vision disturbances, strokes, or behavior changes as a result of the effects of the disease on the central nervous system.

No cure exists for SLE, and treatment aims to relieve symptoms and reduce the potential for organ damage and complications. Most patients are treated with immunosuppressive drugs, such as hydroxychloroquine, and corticosteroids, such as prednisone and dexamethasone. In 2011 the U.S. Food and Drug Administration (FDA) approved a new drug for lupus: belimumab. Patients with SLE are also treated with nonsteroidal anti-inflammatory drugs (NSAIDs) such as ibuprofen, naproxen, and indomethacin along with other drugs to combat pain, swelling, and fever.

Many chronic degenerative diseases, especially autoimmune diseases, are thought to occur when a genetically susceptible individual encounters an environmental trigger. For example, some researchers believe viruses may be the environmental triggers for diseases such as SLE and scleroderma (an illness in which skin and internal organs thicken and harden).

Prevalence of Arthritis

Arthritis is a common problem. In "Arthritis-Related Statistics" (January 25, 2016, http://www.cdc.gov/arthritis/data_statistics/arthritis_related_stats.htm), the CDC's National Center for Chronic Disease Prevention and Health Promotion reports that in 2012 an estimated 52.5 million U.S. adults had been diagnosed with arthritis. By 2030 the total number is expected to increase to nearly 67 million U.S. adults suffering from some form of arthritis. (See Table 6.1.)

The CDC indicates in "About Arthritis Disabilities and Limitations" (January 25, 2016, http://www.cdc.gov/arthritis/data_statistics/disabilities-limitations.htm) that arthritis is the leading cause of disability among Americans. As of 2012, 22.7 million people reported activity limitations because of arthritis. This was nearly 10% of all adults and 43% of the 52.5 million adults with diagnosed arthritis at that time. By 2030 about 25 million adults will likely have arthritis-attributable activity limitations. The CDC notes that in 2013 arthritis-attributable activity limitations affected at least one out of every three arthritis sufferers. (See Figure 6.1.)

In *Arthritis Foundation Scientific Strategy 2015–2020* (February 2015, http://www.arthritis.org/Documents/arthritis-foundation-scientific-strategy.pdf), the Arthritis Foundation indicates that about 34% of people older than age 65 have osteoarthritis. However, although some think of it as only an older person's disease, it can also affect children. The Arthritis Foundation reports that arthritis is one of the most common childhood diseases in the United States. Approximately 294,000 children and teenagers, or one out of 250 youth under the age of 18 years, suffer from arthritis.

Developments in Arthritis Research

According to Anja Schwenzer et al., in "Identification of an Immunodominant Peptide from Citrullinated Tenascin-C as a Major Target for Autoantibodies in Rheumatoid Arthritis" (*Annals of the Rheumatic Diseases*, December 9, 2015), a blood test that recognizes

TABLE 6.1

Projected prevalence of physician-diagnosed arthritis among adults aged 18 and older, selected years 2020–30

	Estimated number of adults with doctor-diagnosed arthritis (in 1,000s)		
Year	Men	Women	Total
2020	23,164	36,244	59,409
2025	24,622	38,587	63,209
2030	26,053	40,915	66,969

SOURCE: Adapted from "Figure 1. Projected Prevalence of Doctor-Diagnosed Arthritis among US Adults Aged 18 Years and Older, 2005–2030," in *NHIS Arthritis Surveillance—National Statistics Text Description*, Centers for Disease Control and Prevention, National Center for Chronic Disease Prevention and Health Promotion, October 20, 2010, http://www.cdc.gov/arthritis/data_statistics/national_nhis_text.htm#1 (accessed December 30, 2015)

FIGURE 6.1

Proportion of adults with arthritis who have arthritis-attributable activity limitations, 2013

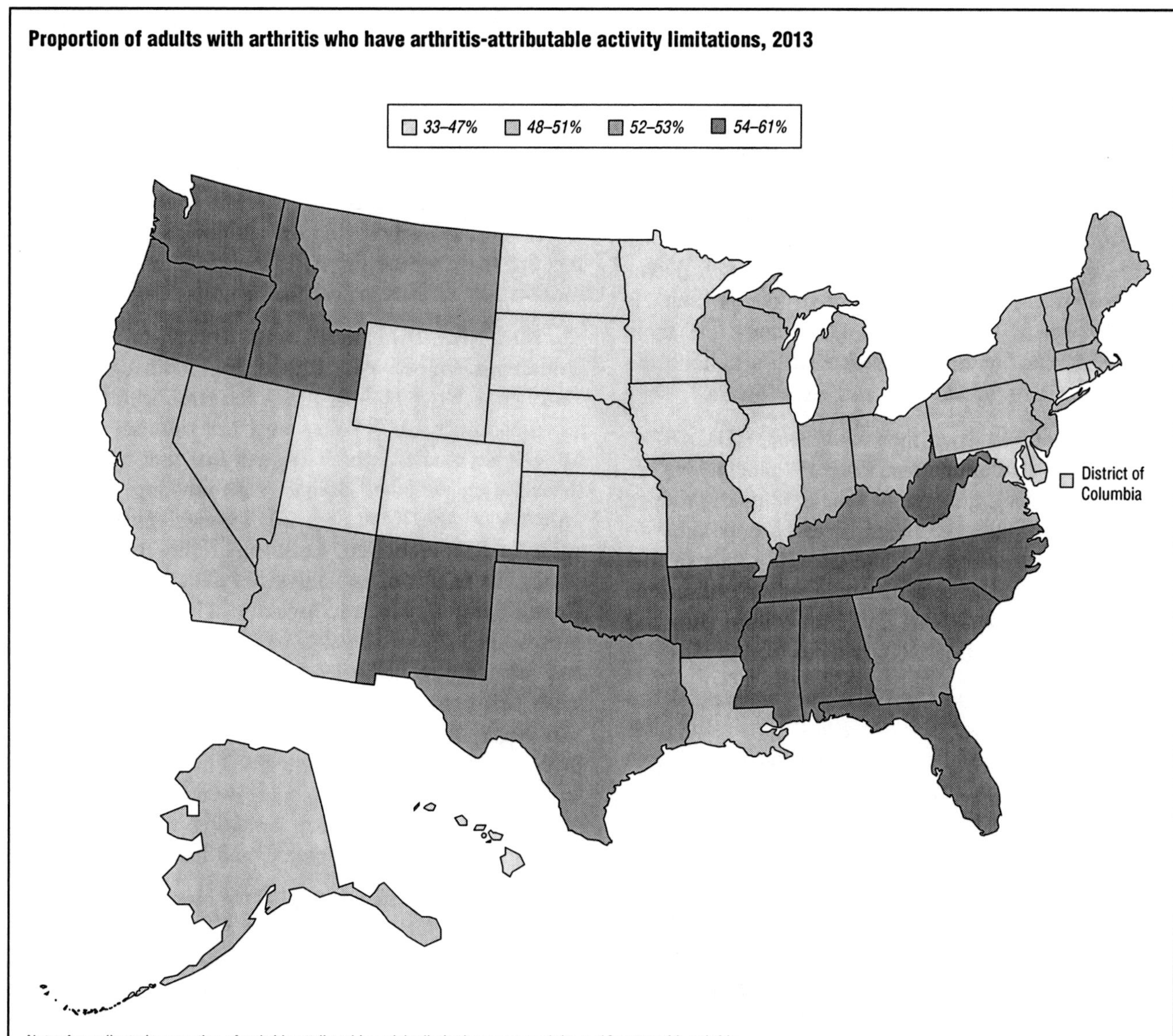

Note: Age-adjusted proportion of arthritis-attributable activity limitation among adults ≥ 18 years with arthritis.

SOURCE: "Arthritis-Attributable Activity Limitations Affect at Least 1 in 3 Adults with Arthritis in Every State," in *Arthritis: Disabilities and Limitations*, Centers for Disease Control and Prevention, National Center for Chronic Disease Prevention and Health Promotion, Division of Population Health, November 2, 2015, http://www.cdc.gov/arthritis/data_statistics/disabilities-limitations.htm (accessed December 29, 2015)

altered proteins that can cause rheumatoid arthritis can be used to predict who will suffer from the disease years before it becomes evident. The researchers find the test is able to detect rheumatoid arthritis up to 16 years before it begins. Because the test detects the disease so early, it can enable early diagnosis and prompt treatment, which result in better clinical outcomes.

As researchers learn more about inflammation and the body's immune system, they come closer to finding new drugs that can relieve the pain of arthritis and block the degenerative process of these diseases. Researchers are investigating ways to improve treatment with the body's own biologic response modifiers (products that modify immune responses). They expect that these substances can be used to control the destructive processes of autoimmune diseases without weakening the whole immune system.

Another study reports a promising new method of drug delivery. In "Neutrophil-Derived Microvesicles Enter Cartilage and Protect the Joint in Inflammatory Arthritis" (*Science Translational Medicine*, vol. 7, no. 315, November 25, 2015), Sarah E. Headland et al. explain that until recently, arthritic cartilage was believed to be impenetrable to therapy. Recent research reveals that microvesicles (tiny fluid-filled structures [0.05 to 1 micrometer in diameter] in white blood cells) are able to penetrate cartilage cells and deliver therapies for arthritis. The researchers posit that in the not-too-distant future, patients suffering from cartilage damage as a result of osteoarthritis or rheumatoid arthritis could be given therapy using their body's own transport system.

Treatment

Medications that are used to help relieve the symptoms of joint pain, stiffness, and swelling include NSAIDs, aspirin, analgesics, and corticosteroids. These drugs may be used in combination. Among recent advances are more effective pain-relief drugs with fewer adverse side effects than those already on the market. This is important because NSAIDs, among the most widely used class of drugs for osteoarthritis, have the potential to irritate the stomach and cause ulcers.

Disease-modifying antirheumatic drugs (DMARDs) help reduce joint inflammation. They are generally effective but take as long as three to four months to produce benefits, so they must be started as early as possible to help prevent joint deformities and disability later in life. Doctors often prescribe an additional medication, such as a corticosteroid or an NSAID, to help control pain and inflammation while a DMARD starts to work.

DMARDs include low doses of methotrexate, leflunomide, penicillamine, sulfasalazine, auranofin (also known as oral gold), gold sodium thiomalate (also known as injectable gold), minocycline, azathioprine, hydroxychloroquine sulfate (and other antimalarials), cyclosporine, and biologic agents. DMARDs are used most often for rheumatoid arthritis, but some DMARDs can also be used for juvenile rheumatoid arthritis, ankylosing spondylitis, psoriatic arthritis, and SLE.

The Arthritis Foundation describes in "Rheumatoid Arthritis Treatment" (2016, http://www.arthritistoday.org/about-arthritis/types-of-arthritis/rheumatoid-arthritis/treatment-plan/medication-overview/ra-medications.php) a subset of DMARDs known as biologic response modifiers (biologics). These genetically engineered drugs block specific steps in the process of inflammation, which in turn slows the progression of joint damage. In 2016 there were a number of biologics approved for the treatment of rheumatoid arthritis. Abatacept blocks the activation of T cells. Adalimumab, infliximab, certolizumab pegol, etanercept, and golimumab block tumor necrosis factor-alpha. Anakinra blocks interleukin-1, rituximab blocks B cells, and tocilizumab blocks interleukin-6.

In 2012 the FDA approved tofacitinib, a drug that inhibits the production of Janus kinase, which is involved in inflammation. Unlike biologics, which must be injected, tofacitinib may be taken orally (by mouth).

Other therapies are also available. For example, patients with moderate to severe rheumatoid arthritis who have not responded well to DMARDs may try Prosorba therapy. This involves drawing blood, separating plasma from red blood cells, and treating plasma through a Prosorba column (a cylinder the size of a soup can that holds a sandlike substance coated with protein A, a molecule that binds antibodies). The treated plasma is then rejoined with red blood cells and returned to the body. Treatments are given in 12 weekly sessions that last about two and a half hours each. The therapy works in much the same way that dialysis does. It cleans and filters the blood, removing the antibodies that are attacking the body's own joints. It may take as long as four months for patients to feel the benefits of the therapy.

DIET AND RHEUMATOID ARTHRITIS. In "Diet May Determine Your Risk for Rheumatoid Arthritis" (ScienceDaily.com, November 8, 2015), the American College of Rheumatology (ACR) discusses the findings from two large-scale studies, which suggest that diet has a role in determining whether people will develop rheumatoid arthritis. At the November 2015 annual meeting of the ACR in San Francisco, California, Bing Lu et al. presented the results of an analysis of data from the Nurses' Health Study II, which followed 93,859 female registered nurses aged 25 to 42 years without rheumatoid arthritis and who completed dietary questionnaires every four years between 1991 and 2011. The researchers identified two major dietary patterns they described as "Western" (a diet high in red meat, processed meat, refined grains, fried food, high-fat dairy, and sweets) and "Prudent" (a largely plant-based diet including fruit, vegetables, legumes, whole grains, poultry, and fish).

During the study period, 347 women developed rheumatoid arthritis. After controlling for other potential risk factors such as body mass index (a measure that incorporates height and weight to categorize adult body weight as underweight, healthy weight, overweight, or obese), smoking, level of physical activity, alcohol consumption, and total caloric intake, the researchers found that women on Prudent diets had less risk of developing rheumatoid arthritis than did those consuming a Western diet.

Another study conducted by the same research team and presented at the ACR meeting considered the same population but looked at how closely study subjects adhered to the 2010 Dietary Guidelines for Americans. The results of this study were consistent with the first one: subjects who closely followed the guidelines were 33% less likely to develop rheumatoid arthritis than those who did not closely adhere to the guidelines.

OSTEOPOROSIS

Osteoporosis is a skeletal disorder that is characterized by compromised bone strength, which predisposes affected individuals to increased risk of fracture. Some bone loss occurs naturally with age, but in "Having a Bone Density Test" (2016, http://nof.org/articles/743) the National Osteoporosis Foundation (NOF) defines osteoporosis as about 25% bone loss compared with a healthy young adult, or, on a bone density test, 2.5 standard deviations below normal.

Nicole C. Wright et al. estimate in "The Recent Prevalence of Osteoporosis and Low Bone Mass in the United States Based on Bone Mineral Density at the Femoral Neck or Lumbar Spine" (*Journal of Bone and Mineral Research*, vol. 29, no, 11, November 2014) that 10.3% of U.S. adults over the age of 50 years, or 10.2 million older adults, had osteoporosis in 2010. An estimated 43.9% (43.4 million older adults) had low bone mass. Taken together, osteoporosis and low bone mass affected an estimated 54 million older adults in 2010. Not surprisingly, the majority of people with osteoporosis were women. Women who have gone through menopause (the natural end of their fertility due to aging, which typically occurs around age 50) are at particularly high risk of osteoporosis because of associated hormonal changes.

Wright et al. find that the prevalence of osteoporosis increases with age and differs by sex, race, and ethnicity. For example, women and non-Hispanic whites had the highest rates of osteoporosis and low bone mass, and non-Hispanic African Americans had the lowest prevalence of osteoporosis and low bone mass. Not unexpectedly, the prevalence of osteoporosis was three times higher in men over the age of 80 years than in men aged 50 to 59 years.

Bone density builds during childhood growth and reaches its peak in early adulthood. From then on, bone loss gradually increases, outpacing the body's natural ability to replace bone. The denser bones are during the growth years, the less likely they will be to develop osteoporosis. A healthy, balanced diet, especially one that contains foods rich in calcium and vitamin D long before the visible symptoms of osteoporosis appear, is vitally important.

The body needs vitamin D to absorb calcium. Vitamin D–rich foods include fortified dairy products, liver, saltwater fish, and egg yolks. Table 6.2 lists some calcium-rich foods. In "Calcium and Vitamin D: Important at Every Age" (May 2015, http://www.niams.nih.gov/Health_Info/Bone/Bone_Health/Nutrition/calcium_vit_d_important.pdf), the National Institutes of Health's Osteoporosis and Related Bone Diseases National Resource Center provides the recommended calcium intake for people of all ages as well as information about the role of diet in preventing osteoporosis.

Screening tests for bone density can identify people who are in need of additional testing. Often performed at health fairs, such tests are also known as peripheral tests and measure bone density in the lower arm, wrist, finger, or heel. Peripheral bone density tests may be performed using:

TABLE 6.2

Selected calcium-rich foods

Food	Calcium (mg)
Fortified oatmeal, 1 packet	350
Sardines, canned in oil, with edible bones, 3 oz.	324
Cheddar cheese, 1 1/2 oz. shredded	306
Milk, nonfat, 1 cup	302
Milkshake, 1 cup	300
Yogurt, plain, low-fat, 1 cup	300
Soybeans, cooked, 1 cup	261
Tofu, firm, with calcium, 1/2 cup	204
Orange juice, fortified with calcium, 6 oz.	200–260 (varies)
Salmon, canned, with edible bones, 3 oz.	181
Pudding, instant (chocolate, banana, etc.) made with 2% milk, 1/2 cup	153
Baked beans, 1 cup	142
Cottage cheese, 1% milk fat, 1 cup	138
Spaghetti, lasagna, 1 cup	125
Frozen yogurt, vanilla, soft-serve, 1/2 cup	103
Ready-to-eat cereal, fortified with calcium, 1 cup	100–1,000 (varies)
Cheese pizza, 1 slice	100
Fortified waffles, 2	100
Turnip greens, boiled, 1/2 cup	99
Broccoli, raw, 1 cup	90
Ice cream, vanilla, 1/2 cup	85
Soy or rice milk, fortified with calcium, 1 cup	80–500 (varies)

SOURCE: "Selected Calcium-Rich Foods," in *Calcium and Vitamin D: Important at Every Age*, The National Institutes of Health, Osteoporosis and Related Bone Diseases, May 2015, http://www.niams.nih.gov/Health_Info/Bone/Bone_Health/Nutrition/ (accessed December 29, 2015)

- Peripheral dual energy x-ray absorptiometry—this is a portable machine that uses very low doses of radiation to measure the density of bones in the arms or legs
- Quantitative ultrasound—this technique assesses mineral bone density without using radiation
- Peripheral quantitative computed tomography—this technique is often used to measure bone density and strength in the wrist

Full-scale bone density testing is generally performed using dual energy x-ray absorptiometry to measure bone density in the hip and spine. The painless test takes less than 15 minutes and uses very little radiation. Bone density testing is generally recommended for women aged 65 years and older, men aged 70 years and older, anyone who breaks a bone after the age of 50 years as well as postmenopausal women under the age of 65 years and men aged 50 to 69 years with risk factors for osteoporosis (e.g., a family history of osteoporosis, people with low bone density known as osteopenia, and so on).

Osteoporosis worsens with age, leaving its sufferers at risk of broken hips or other bones, curvature of the spine, and other disabilities. In severe cases the disease may cause patients to experience spontaneous (without external causes) fractures, generally in the vertebrae of the spine. The stooped posture (kyphosis) and loss of height (greater than 1 to 2 inches [2.5 to 5.1 cm]) experienced by many older adults result from vertebral fractures that are caused by osteoporosis.

The National Institute of Arthritis and Musculoskeletal and Skin Diseases (NIAMS) reports that, like other chronic conditions that disproportionately affect older adults, the prevalence of bone disease and fractures is projected to increase markedly as the population ages. In "Preventing Falls and Related Fractures" (April 2015, http://www.niams.nih.gov/Health_Info/Bone/Osteoporosis/Fracture/prevent_falls.asp), the NIAMS reports that the majority of hip fractures are associated with osteoporosis. Older adults who have a hip fracture are more likely to die in the year following the fracture than their age peers, and among people living independently before a hip fracture, many will remain in long-term care institutions a year after their fractures.

The 1994 discovery of a gene linked to bone density was hailed as the most important finding in osteoporosis research in a decade. Two forms of the gene, B and b, exist. People with two b genes, one from each parent, have the highest bone density and are the least likely to develop osteoporosis, whereas those with one of each, the Bb genotype, have intermediate bone density. People with two B genes have the lowest bone density and the highest risk of osteoporosis. Women with the BB genotype may be four times as likely to experience hip fractures as those with the bb genotype. According to Interleukin Genetics, Inc., in "Bone Health" (2015, http://ilgenetics.com/content/products-services/inherent-health/bone-health/), it offers a Bone Health Genetic Test that detects genetic patterns associated with the development of osteoporosis. The test analyzes gene variations that are associated with an increased risk for spinal fracture and low bone mineral density.

Table 6.3 summarizes the factors that predispose a person to osteoporosis and fractures. Apart from genetics, the risk factors—poor nutrition, lack of physical activity (especially weight-bearing exercise), and choosing to smoke—are all modifiable.

TABLE 6.3

Causes of bone loss and fractures in osteoporosis

Failure to develop a strong skeleton
Genetics—limited growth or abnormal bone composition
Nutrition—calcium, phosphorous and vitamin D deficiency, poor general nutrition
Lifestyle—lack of weight-bearing exercise, smoking
Loss of bone due to excessive breakdown (resorption)
Decreased sex hormone production
Calcium and vitamin D deficiency, increased parathyroid hormone
Excess production of local resorbing factors
Failure to replace lost bone due to impaired formation
Loss of ability to replenish bone cells with age
Decreased production of systemic growth factors
Loss of local growth factors
Increased tendency to fall
Loss of muscle strength
Slow reflexes and poor vision
Drugs that impair balance

SOURCE: "Table 2-2. Causes of Bone Loss and Fractures in Osteoporosis," in *Bone Health and Osteoporosis: A Report of the Surgeon General 2004*, U.S. Department of Health and Human Services, Public Health Service, Office of the Surgeon General, 2004, http://www.ncbi.nlm.nih.gov/books/NBK45513/pdf/TOC.pdf (accessed December 30, 2015)

Treatment of Osteoporosis

One of the goals of osteoporosis treatment is to maintain bone health by preventing bone loss and by building new bone. Another is to minimize the risk and impact of falls because they can cause fractures. Figure 6.2 shows the pyramid for prevention and treatment of osteoporosis. At its base are lifestyle changes. These include good nutrition, with adequate intake of calcium, vitamin D, and other minerals; physical exercise; and preventive measures to reduce the risk of falls (such as wearing rubber-soled shoes for traction and reducing clutter). The second layer of the pyramid involves identifying drugs (e.g., aluminum-coated antacids, some antiseizure medications, and steroids) and diseases (e.g., thyroid disease) that can cause osteoporosis. The peak of the pyramid involves drug therapy for osteoporosis.

There are two primary types of drugs that are used to treat osteoporosis. Antiresorptive agents act to reduce bone loss, and anabolic agents act to build bone. Antiresorptive therapies include use of bisphosphonates, estrogen, selective estrogen receptor modulators, and calcitonin. Antiresorptive therapies reduce bone loss, stabilize the architecture of the bone, and decrease bone turnover. Bisphosphonates (alendronate, risedronate, ibandronate, and zoledronic acid) are FDA approved for the prevention or treatment of osteoporosis as is a synthetic form of parathyroid hormone known as teriparatide that is administered by injection. In 2005 the FDA approved raloxifene, and in 2010 it approved denosumab, another injected agent, for postmenopausal women with osteoporosis who are at high risk for fractures. Denosumab is a monoclonal antibody that binds to a protein involved in the formation, function, and survival of osteoclasts, the cells that are responsible for bone resorption.

At the dawn of the 21st century it was typical for postmenopausal women who had osteoporosis or were at risk for the disease to include hormone replacement therapy (HRT) in their treatment regimen. HRT supplements a woman's natural supply of estrogen and other hormones that typically decrease as a woman ages. It can slow the advance of osteoporosis and help prevent fractures and disability. However, serious side effects of HRT were recognized in 2002, including increased risks of cardiovascular disease and certain types of cancer, so many women discontinued HRT treatment. For some women at heightened risk for osteoporosis who also have fewer risk factors for cardiovascular disease, HRT remains a treatment option.

FIGURE 6.2

The osteoporosis pyramid for prevention and treatment

Pharmacotherapy (antiresorptives and anabolics)

Address secondary factors (drugs and diseases)

Lifestyle changes (nutrition, physical activity, and fall prevention)

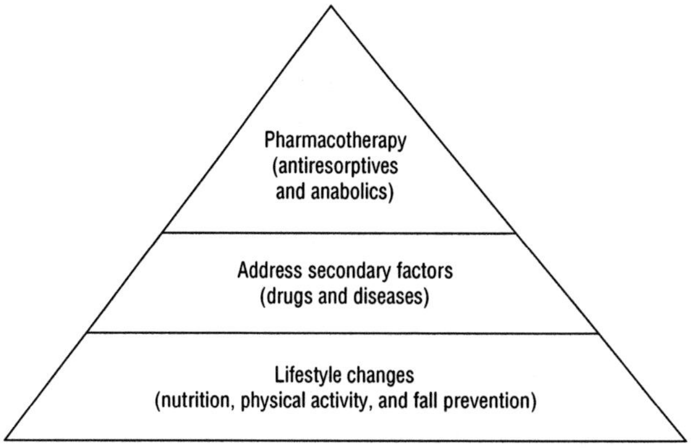

Note: **The base of the pyramid:** The first step in the prevention and treatment of osteoporosis and the prevention of fractures is to build a foundation of nutrition and lifestyle measures that maximize bone health. The diet should not only be adequate in calcium and vitamin D, but should have a healthy balance of other nutrients. A weight-bearing exercise program should be developed. Cigarette smoking and excessive alcohol use must be avoided. In the older individual, at high risk for fractures, the changes in lifestyle would include a plan not only to maximize physical activity, but also to minimize the risk of falls. The use of hip protectors can be considered in some high-risk patients. Diseases that increase the risk of falls by causing visual impairment, postural hypotension (a drop in blood pressure on standing, which leads to dizziness), or poor balance should be treated. Drugs that cause bone loss or increase the risk of falls should be avoided or given at the lowest effective dose.
The second level of the pyramid: The next step is to identify and treat diseases that produce secondary osteoporosis or aggravate primary osteoporosis. These measures are the foundation upon which specific pharmacotherapy is built and should never be forgotten.
The third level of the pyramid: If there is sufficiently high risk of fracture to warrant pharmacotherapy, the patient is usually started on antiresorptives. Anabolic agents are used in individuals in whom antiresorptive therapy is not adequate to prevent bone loss or fractures.

SOURCE: "Figure 9-1. The Osteoporosis Pyramid for Prevention and Treatment, in *Bone Health and Osteoporosis: A Report of the Surgeon General 2004*, U.S. Department of Health and Human Services, Public Health Service, Office of the Surgeon General, 2004, http://www.ncbi.nlm.nih.gov/books/NBK45513/pdf/TOC.pdf (accessed December 30, 2015)

In 2013 the FDA approved conjugated estrogens/bazedoxifene for the treatment of osteoporosis in postmenopausal women (and other conditions). It warned that, as with other medications containing estrogen, it should be used with caution.

EXERCISE AND BONE HEALTH IN CHILDREN AND OLDER ADULTS. In "Effects of Weight-Bearing Activities on Bone Mineral Content and Density in Children and Adolescents: A Meta-analysis" (*Journal of Bone and Mineral Research*, vol. 29, no. 2, February 2014), Michael Behringer et al. review 27 studies on the effects of weight-bearing activities on bone mineral content and density during childhood and adolescence. The researchers find that weight-bearing exercise and high calcium intake are associated with bone mineral accrual and opine that calcium intake and weight-bearing activities should be encouraged to enhance peak bone mass early in life. Improving bone mineral content in youth can help prevent or minimize the effects of osteoporosis in later life.

Evidence that exercise has measurable positive effects on bone structure continues to mount. Karen L. Bolton et al. explain in "Effects of Exercise on Bone Density and Falls Risk Factors in Post-menopausal Women with Osteopenia: A Randomised Controlled Trial" (*Journal of Science and Medicine in Sport*, vol. 15, no. 2, March 2012) that they followed postmenopausal women with osteopenia who were enrolled in an exercise program that met three times per week for 52 weeks. The researchers compared the health-related quality of life and bone mineral density of these women to that of a control group of women who did not exercise. The researchers find that the participants who exercised had small increases in bone mineral density, endurance, and health-related quality of life. In contrast, those who did not exercise experienced a slight loss of bone mineral density.

MULTIPLE SCLEROSIS

Multiple sclerosis (MS) is a chronic, degenerative, and often intermittent disease of the central nervous system. It eventually destroys the myelin protein sheaths that surround and insulate nerve fibers in the brain and spinal cord. Myelin is a fatty substance that aids the flow of electrical impulses from the brain through the spinal cord. These nerve impulses control all conscious and unconscious movements. In MS the myelin sheath disintegrates and is replaced by hard sclerotic plaques (scar tissue) that distort or prevent the flow of electrical impulses along the nerves to various parts of the body.

MS usually appears in young adulthood and is common enough to have earned the title "the great crippler of young adults." Many problems and symptoms are associated with the disease, but the major problem is lost mobility. Symptoms can range from mild problems, such as numbness and muscle weakness, to uncontrollable tremors, slurred speech, loss of bowel and bladder control, memory lapses, and paralysis. Although almost all parts of the nervous system may become involved, the spinal cord is the most vulnerable. Wild mood swings, from euphoria to depression, are another manifestation of the disease. The disease is not fatal in itself, but it weakens its victims and makes them far more susceptible to infection.

The disease is called "multiple" because it usually affects many parts of the nervous system and is often characterized by relapses (exacerbations or flare-ups) followed by periods of partial and sometimes complete recovery. Therefore, it is multiple both in how it affects the body and in how often it strikes.

Prevalence

In "Who Gets MS (Epidemiology)?" (2016, http://www.nationalmssociety.org/What-is-MS/Who-Gets-MS), the

National Multiple Sclerosis Society (NMSS) estimates that MS affects more than 2.3 million people worldwide. The disease is most often diagnosed in patients between the ages of 20 and 50 years old and is more than twice as common in men. Although it occurs in most ethnic groups, it is more common in people of north European ancestry.

A possible clue to the cause of MS is that it is more common in areas farthest from the equator and in cold, damp climates. In Europe it is found most often in the Scandinavian countries, the Baltic region, northern Germany, and Great Britain. It is rare in the Mediterranean countries, China, and Japan. It is also rare among Native Americans and African Americans and practically unheard of in other groups, suggesting that the disease is attributable to a relationship between genetic susceptibility and an as yet unidentified environmental trigger. In the United States most cases are found in the northern areas, and it is more common in Canada than in the southern United States.

Diagnosing MS

MS can be difficult to diagnose and detect because the early symptoms vary considerably from one individual to another, and may disappear entirely for years at a time. Therefore, a diagnosis of MS is generally made only after a thorough history and physical examination and the results of diagnostic tests are evaluated. Among the tests are magnetic resonance imaging (MRI; this provides a detailed view of the brain), spinal tap (to examine spinal fluid for signs of the disease), and evoked potentials (which measure how quickly and accurately a person's nervous system responds to certain stimulation). No single test can detect MS; several must be done and compared.

The neurologic examination for MS focuses on detecting hyperactive (as opposed to normal) reflexes and balance and gait disturbances. An eye examination evaluates damage to the optic nerve. Although some cases of MS are readily diagnosed by physicians based on the history and physical examination, most physicians confirm the diagnosis by using an imaging study to document evidence of plaques in at least two locations of the central nervous system.

Causes of MS

The exact cause of MS is unknown. Many theories about its cause have been proposed—genetics, gender, or exposure to environmental triggers such as viruses, trauma, or heavy metals—but none has been proven. The most widely accepted theory is that damage to myelin results from an abnormal response by the body's immune system. Normally, the immune system defends the body against foreign invaders such as viruses or bacteria. However, in an autoimmune disease the body attacks its own tissue. Some believe that MS is an autoimmune disease in which myelin is attacked.

The NMSS explains in "Who Gets MS (Epidemiology)?" that like other diseases, genetic factors, in a complex interplay with environmental influences such as exposure to viruses, very likely play a significant role in determining who develops MS. This is most clearly demonstrated by the fact that an identical twin of someone with MS has a one in four chance of developing the disease. This is much higher than the prevalence in the general population, indicating that genes do play a role. However, if genes alone caused MS, then the rate would be 100%, so other factors are also important. Other close relatives of people with MS—such as their children and siblings—are also more likely to develop the disease than those without a family history of MS.

Treatment of MS

No known treatment halts the disease process. Once nerve fibers have been destroyed, they cannot recover their function. Current methods of treatment include powerful immunosuppressive drugs that often leave patients vulnerable to secondary infections. In "Medications" (http://www.nationalmssociety.org/Treating-MS/Medications), the NMSS explains that as of 2016 the FDA had approved 13 disease-modifying medications that can reduce disease activity and progression for many people with relapsing forms of MS, including relapsing-remitting MS.

The NMSS recommends that people who are diagnosed with the disease start drug treatment immediately, before symptoms worsen. The society recommends prompt treatment with medication because it appears that patients who receive early treatment will probably have fewer disabling symptoms than those who do not. The drugs used to treat MS act by reducing the inflammation of MS lesions and reducing the accumulation of the lesions. All have demonstrated effectiveness in reducing the number and severity of relapses.

When relapses of the disease occur, which may last from a few days to several months, they are commonly treated with high doses of corticosteroids (to reduce inflammation). Other medications can help manage symptoms such as bladder and bowel problems, emotional changes, pain, tremors, dizziness, fatigue, and itching. Rehabilitation programs help people with MS maintain fitness and pace themselves to conserve their energy during their daily activities. People with MS are advised to build general resistance and avoid fatigue and exposure to extremes in temperature. Physical therapy and psychotherapy are useful in helping patients and their families cope with the limitations that are caused by MS. Other therapy programs provide strategies to maintain independence, to use assistive technologies in the workplace, and to adjust to changes in speech, swallowing, and cognitive abilities.

PROMISING RESEARCH. Danielle E. Harlow, Justin M. Honce, and Augusto A. Miravalle of the University of Colorado explain in "Remyelination Therapy in Multiple Sclerosis" (*Frontiers in Neurology*, vol. 6, no. 257, 2015) that approved treatments for MS act to reduce immune system activity or block entry of immune cells into the central nervous system. These treatments reduce relapse rates and severity of attacks, but do not repair damage to the myelin sheaths surrounding axons (long nerve cell fibers that conduct electrical impulses from cell to cell). Chronic demyelination leads to loss of neurons, which in turn produces the disability associated with MS. The researchers suggest that drugs that exert a positive impact on remyelination and neuroprotection could be used along with drugs that modify immune responses, but note that one of the challenges in the development of remyelination therapies is assessing remyelination in patients. Indirect measures such as an electroencephalogram suggest but do not confirm remyelination, but in the future, analysis biomarkers in serum and cerebrospinal fluid as well as advanced imaging techniques that enable the detection of myelin-specific changes may provide important information about remyelination and repair.

In "Fingolimod Real World Experience: Efficacy and Safety in Clinical Practice" (*Neuroscience Journal*, November 26, 2015), Joaquim Fonseca of the University of Aveiro in Portugal reports the promising results of the use of fingolimod, an MS treatment that has been used in the United States since 2010 and in Europe since 2011. Fonseca reviews nearly 100 studies and concludes that the drug's "real world experience seems to confirm that fingolimod is effective and well tolerated and with a safety profile that is very similar to what was observed on clinical trials."

PARKINSON'S DISEASE

Despite its name, Parkinson's disease (PD) refers not to a particular disease but to a disorder that is marked by a characteristic set of symptoms. According to the Parkinson's Disease Foundation, in "Statistics on Parkinson's" (http://www.pdf.org/en/parkinson_statistics), as many as 1 million people in the United States were affected by PD in 2016 and about 60,000 Americans are diagnosed with it each year. Both men and women can develop PD, with the probability of doing so increasing with advancing age. PD usually strikes people older than age 62, but an estimated 4% of patients are under the age of 50 years.

PD is caused by the progressive deterioration of about half a million brain cells in the portion of the brain that controls certain types of muscle movement. These cells secrete dopamine, a neurotransmitter (chemical messenger). Dopamine's function is to allow nerve impulses to move smoothly from one nerve cell to another. These nerve cells, in turn, transmit messages to the muscles of the body to begin movement. When the normal supply of dopamine is reduced, the messages are not correctly sent, and the symptoms of PD appear.

The four early warning signs of PD are tremors, muscle stiffness, unusual slowness, and a stooped posture. Medications can control initial symptoms, but as time goes on they become less effective. As the disease worsens, patients develop tremors, causing them to fall or jerk uncontrollably. (The jerky body movements that patients with PD experience are known as dyskinesias.) At other times rigidity sets in, rendering patients unable to move. About one-third of patients also develop dementia, an impairment of cognition (thought processes). These and other complications of PD can ultimately lead to death.

Treatment of PD

The management of PD is individualized and includes drug therapy and a program that stresses daily exercise. Medication and therapy may modify the progression of PD. Exercise can often reduce the rigidity of muscles, prevent weakness, and improve the ability to walk.

The main goal of drug treatment is to restore the chemical balance between dopamine and another neurotransmitter, acetylcholine. The standard treatment for most patients is levodopa (L-dopa)—a compound that the body converts into dopamine, replacing the supply missing due to damaged cells and thereby helping alleviate symptoms. However, treatment with L-dopa does not slow the progressive course of the disease or even delay the changes in the brain that PD produces, and it may produce some unpleasant side effects if the body converts it to dopamine before it reaches the brain. Simultaneously administering substances that inhibit this change allows a higher concentration of L-dopa to reach the brain and considerably decreases the side effects.

Along with L-dopa and other drugs called dopamine agonists, which mimic the action of dopamine, four other classes of drugs are used to treat the symptoms of PD: anticholinergics, COMT inhibitors, MAO-B inhibitors, and amantadine. Anticholinergics work to relieve tremor and rigidity. COMT inhibitors act by prolonging the effectiveness of a dose of L-dopa by preventing its breakdown. MAO-B inhibitors slow the breakdown of dopamine in the brain. Amantadine, which was initially developed as an antiviral drug, has demonstrated effectiveness in reducing dyskinesias.

In "Surgical Treatments" (2016, http://www.pdf.org/en/surgical_treatments), the Parkinson's Disease Foundation explains that surgical treatment consisting of deep brain stimulation has been used by an estimated 30,000 people worldwide. It can be an effective treatment option for various symptoms of PD; however, only symptoms that previously improved while a specific patient was on L-dopa have the potential to improve after the surgery.

Genetic Link to PD

Two studies, Suzanne Lesage et al.'s "LRRK2 G2019S as a Cause of Parkinson's Disease in North African Arabs" and Laurie J. Ozelius et al.'s "LRRK2 G2019S as a Cause of Parkinson's Disease in Ashkenazi Jews" (both published in *New England Journal of Medicine*, vol. 354, no. 4, January 26, 2006), describe the discovery of a single genetic mutation on a gene called leucine-rich repeat kinase 2 (LRRK2) that accounts for as many as 30% of all cases of PD in Arabs, North Africans, and Jews. People with the mutation make an abnormal version of a protein called dardarin (a form of the Basque word for "tremor") in which a single amino acid—number 2019—is glycine instead of serine. This finding may help direct the development of a drug that modifies the impact of this mutation to prevent or substantially delay onset of the disease.

Subsequent studies, such as Jeanne C. Latourelle et al.'s "Genomewide Association Study for Onset Age in Parkinson Disease" (*BMC Medical Genetics*, September 22, 2009) and Laura Brighina et al.'s "Analysis of Vesicular Monoamine Transporter 2 Polymorphisms in Parkinson's Disease" (*Neurobiology of Aging*, vol. 34, no. 6, June 2013), find that in addition to the identification of five single genes that are associated with PD, there are multiple genes and gene interactions that increase and reduce susceptibility to PD. The researchers note that the age at which PD begins is also a highly heritable trait. This finding is especially important because by identifying the genes that are related to the age of onset, it may be possible to identify ways to delay the onset of PD symptoms. Effectively postponing disease onset could reduce the prevalence of PD.

Experimental Therapies

GENE THERAPY. In 2011 the first successful rigorous clinical study of gene therapy for PD was completed. The results were published by Peter A. LeWitt et al. in "AAV2-*GAD* Gene Therapy for Advanced Parkinson's Disease: A Double-Blind, Sham-Surgery Controlled, Randomised Trial" (*Lancet Neurology*, vol. 10, no. 4, April 2011). The researchers report that patients who received a gene therapy called NLX-P101 via infusion into a region of the brain that is involved in motor function experienced "a significant reduction in the motor symptoms of Parkinson's, including tremor, rigidity and difficulty initiating movement." Half of the patients receiving gene therapy achieved dramatic symptom improvements, compared with just 14% of untreated patients in the control group. Patients receiving gene therapy had nearly twice the improvement in motor score, 23.1%, compared with a 12.7% improvement in the control group.

As of 2016, the use of gene therapy for PD patients remained highly experimental. In "Gene Therapy for Parkinson's Disease: Still a Hot Topic?" (*Neuropsychopharmacology Reviews*, vol. 40, no. 1, January 2015), Jeffrey H. Kordower of the Rush University Medical Center in Chicago, Illinois, explains that the first gene therapy attempts were aimed at relieving PD symptoms. Since then, disease-modifying gene therapy strategies have focused on the glial cell. Gene delivery of derived neurotrophic factor, a protein that appears to strengthen brain cells and helps prevent the death of sick cells, has been shown to be effective in animal studies, stopping the progression of PD and perhaps even reversing it. Research has not yet replicated these results in humans.

Kordower asserts that gene therapy is still a very promising treatment, but observes that none of the clinical trials to date has shown significant clinical benefit. He also notes that current approaches to gene therapy have only targeted physical, motor symptoms and opines that a different gene therapy approach will be necessary to address the psychiatric symptoms associated with PD.

ELECTRODE IMPLANTS. Another approach is the use of electrical implants, which create deep brain stimulation. Electrodes are surgically implanted in the brain and connected to a battery-operated device, which is also implanted in the body. The device allows patients to "turn off" the tremors that prevent them from performing the activities of daily living such as pouring a glass of milk and feeding themselves. One shortcoming is that the device's batteries must be surgically replaced periodically.

Paul J. Mattis, Chaya B. Gopin, and Kathryn Lombardi Mirra observe in "Neuropsychological Considerations for Parkinson's Disease Patients Being Considered for Surgical Intervention with Deep Brain Stimulation" (*Handbook on the Neuropsychology of Aging and Dementia*, 2013) that deep brain stimulation not only improves motor function in PD but also may help improve cognitive function and mood. In "Effect of Frequency on Subthalamic Nucleus Deep Brain Stimulation in Primary Dystonia" (*Parkinsonism and Related Disorders*, vol. 20, no. 4, April 2014), Jill L. Ostrem et al. indicate that deep brain stimulation for the involuntary muscle contractions that cause slow repetitive movements or abnormal postures characteristic of PD that does not respond to drug or other treatment is now considered a well-established treatment option.

STEM CELL RESEARCH. The excitement and optimism about stem cells centers on the capacity of these cells to renew themselves and develop into specialized cell types. Unlike other cells that have predetermined roles and functions, such as heart or brain cells, stem cells can develop into nearly all the specialized cells of the body—with the potential to replace cells for the nervous system, heart, pancreas, kidneys, skin, bone, or blood.

Research is under way that uses stem cells to treat neurologic disorders by replacing diseased or malfunctioning cells in the brain and spinal cord. The results of this research could have life-changing consequences for people suffering from PD, MS, Alzheimer's disease, and spinal cord injuries. Other research focuses on developing organs and tissues for transplantation, because there is an urgent need for donor organs. Still other researchers are looking at ways to induce stem cells to become insulin-producing cells of the pancreas to treat diabetes.

Hideki Mochizuki, Chi-Jing Choong, and Toru Yasuda explain in "The Promises of Stem Cells: Stem Cell Therapy for Movement Disorders" (*Parkinsonism and Related Disorders*, vol. 20, suppl. 1, January 2014) that pluripotent stem cells offer an opportunity to replace specific types of degenerating neurons. Induced pluripotent stem cell–derived neurons (cells that are artificially derived from adult cells and behave like natural pluripotent stem cells—they are able to differentiate into specialized cell types and self-renew to generate more stem cells) may also be used to translate the genetic basis for an individual's risk of developing PD into clinically meaningful information. Furthermore, stem cell–derived neurons may be a renewable source of replacement cells for damaged neurons in other movement disorders.

ALZHEIMER'S DISEASE

Alzheimer's disease (AD) is a progressive, degenerative disease that affects the brain and results in severely impaired memory, thinking, and behavior. According to the Alzheimer's Association, in *2015 Alzheimer's Disease Facts and Figures* (2015, https://www.alz.org/facts/downloads/facts_figures_2015.pdf), in 2015 it was the sixth-leading cause of death among American adults and the fifth-leading cause of death for those aged 65 years and older. Approximately 5.3 million Americans were afflicted with AD in 2015. The overwhelming majority of AD sufferers (5.1 million) were aged 65 years and older. AD usually begins after age 60, and risk goes up with age. In 2015, 4% of people with AD were under the age of 65 years, 15% were aged 65 to 74 years, 43% were aged 75 to 84 years, and the remaining 38% were aged 85 years and older. About two-thirds of Americans with AD are women. Women have a higher lifetime risk of developing the disease because, on average, they live longer than men.

The German physician Alois Alzheimer (1864–1915) first described the disease in 1907, after he had cared for a patient with an unusual mental illness. Alzheimer observed anatomic changes in his patient's brain and described them as abnormal clumps and tangled bundles of fibers. Nearly a century later these abnormal findings, now described as amyloid plaques and neurofibrillary tangles, along with abnormal clusters of proteins in the brain, are recognized as the characteristic markers of AD.

Suspected Causes

AD is not a normal consequence of healthy aging, and researchers continue to seek its cause. Like most other chronic, progressive diseases, it is believed to be influenced by some combination of genetic and nongenetic factors.

Researchers have identified different patterns of inheritance, ages of onset (when symptoms begin), genes, chromosomes, and proteins that are linked to the development of AD. Mutations in at least four genes, situated on chromosomes 1, 14, 19, and 21, and possibly as many as 14 genes are thought to be involved in the disease.

The first genetic breakthrough—the discovery that a mutation in a single gene could cause this progressive neurological illness—was reported in 1991 by Alison Goate et al. in "Segregation of a Missense Mutation in the Amyloid Precursor Protein Gene with Familial Alzheimer's Disease" (*Nature*, vol. 349, no. 6311, February 21, 1991). The researchers identified the defect in the gene that directs cells to produce a substance called amyloid protein. Goate et al. found that low levels of the brain chemical acetylcholine contribute to the formation of plaques, the hard deposits of amyloid protein that accumulate in the brain tissue of AD patients. In healthy people, these protein fragments are broken down and excreted. Because amyloid protein is found in cells throughout the body, the question is: Why and how does it become a deadly substance in the brain cells of some people and not others?

In 1995 three more genes linked to AD were identified. One gene is linked to a rare, devastating form of early-onset AD, which occurs as early as the third decade of life. When defective, this gene may prevent brain cells from correctly processing a substance called beta amyloid precursor protein. The second gene, which is also involved in the production of beta amyloid, is associated with another early-onset form of AD that strikes people younger than age 65.

The third gene, known as apolipoprotein E (apoE), was initially linked to AD in 1993, but its role in the body was not immediately identified. Researchers have since discovered that the gene regulates lipid metabolism within the organs and helps redistribute cholesterol. In the brain, apoE plays a key role in repairing nerve tissue that has been injured. There are three forms (alleles) of the gene: apoE-2, apoE-3, and apoE-4. Between one-half and one-third of all AD patients have at least one apoE-4 gene, whereas only 15.5% of the general population carries an apoE-4 gene. In 1998 Marion R. Meyer et al. noted in "APOE Genotype Predicts When—Not Whether—One Is Predisposed to Develop Alzheimer Disease" (*Nature Genetics*, vol. 19, no. 4, August 1998) that the apoE-4 gene does not determine whether an individual will develop the disease; instead, it appears to affect when AD will strike—the age when AD symptoms are likely to begin. The National Institute on Aging (February 18, 1998, http://www.nia.nih.gov/newsroom/1998/02/26-national-alzheimers-disease-centers-collaborate-study-utility-genetic-testing) confirmed that although this gene occurs in 40% of people who develop late-onset AD, one-third of people with AD do not have the form of apoE-4 gene that is associated with AD.

Also in 1998 Deborah Blacker et al. found in "Alpha-2 Macroglobulin Is Genetically Associated with Alzheimer Disease" (*Nature Genetics*, vol. 19, no. 4, August 1998) that A2M-2, another gene variant, appears to affect whether a person will develop AD. An estimated one-third of Americans may carry this gene, potentially tripling their risk of developing late-onset AD, compared with their siblings with the normal version of the A2M gene.

Between 2009 and 2016 additional genes that may increase the risk for AD were identified. The identification of new genes that are associated with AD improves understanding of the causes of the disease and informs drug discovery.

In "The Genetics of Alzheimer's Disease" (*Clinical Interventions in Aging*, vol. 9, April 1, 2014), Eva Bagyinszky et al. explain that although AD is the most common form of dementia, distinguishing it from other neurodegenerative diseases is challenging. Therefore, using genetic testing and other diagnostic disease markers may help establish the diagnosis. Identifying the genes involved in the progression of AD is also important because treatment is more likely to be effective during the early stages of AD, before symptoms appear.

Symptoms of AD

AD begins slowly. The symptoms include difficulty with memory and a loss of cognition. The patient with AD may also experience confusion; language problems, such as trouble finding words; impaired judgment; disorientation in place and time; and changes in mood, behavior, and personality. How quickly these changes occur varies from person to person, but eventually the disease leaves its victims unable to care for themselves. In their terminal stages, patients with AD require care 24 hours per day. They no longer recognize family members or themselves, and they need help with daily activities such as eating, dressing, bathing, and using the toilet. Eventually, they may become incontinent, blind, and unable to communicate. Finally, their bodies may "forget" how to breathe or make the heart beat. Many patients die from pneumonia.

Updated Diagnostic Criteria

In 2011 the National Institute on Aging and the Alzheimer's Association proposed new diagnostic criteria for AD. Rather than describing AD as mild/early-stage, moderate/mid-stage, or severe/late-stage, as the existing diagnostic criteria do, the proposed new criteria identify three stages of AD, with the first occurring before symptoms such as memory loss develop and before the ability to perform everyday activities is affected. As described in *2015 Alzheimer's Disease Facts and Figures*, the three stages are:

- Preclinical AD—there are measurable changes in the brain, cerebrospinal fluid, and/or blood of people in this stage, but there are no symptoms such as memory loss. This presymptomatic stage may be as long as 20 years because brain changes are thought to precede the appearance of other symptoms. The new criteria call for additional biomarker research to effectively diagnose this stage of AD.
- MCI due to AD—people with mild cognitive impairment (MCI) have measurable changes in their thinking abilities. These changes are noticeable to affected individuals and those who know them, but affected individuals are still able to perform everyday activities. Research suggests that as many as 20% of people aged 65 years and older have MCI due to AD and nearly half of all people who visit a doctor about MCI symptoms develop dementia in three or four years.
- Dementia due to AD—people in this stage of AD have significant memory, thinking, and behavioral symptoms that prevent them from maintaining a normal life.

Testing for AD

A complete physical, psychiatric, and neurologic evaluation can usually produce a diagnosis of AD that is about 90% accurate. For many years the only sure way to diagnose the disease was to examine brain tissue under a microscope, which was not possible while a potential AD victim was still alive. An autopsy of someone who has died of AD reveals a characteristic pattern that is the hallmark of the disease: tangles of fibers (neurofibrillary tangles) and clusters of degenerated nerve endings (neuritic plaques) in areas of the brain that are crucial for memory and intellect. Also, the cortex of the brain is shrunken.

In 2000 John C. Mazziotta of the University of California, Los Angeles, School of Medicine reported in "Window on the Brain" (*Archives of Neurology*, vol. 57, no. 10) that the use of MRI techniques could measure the volume of brain tissue in areas of the brain that are used for memory, organizational ability, and planning. In addition, the use of these measurements could accurately identify people with AD and predict which people would develop AD. That same year, in "Using Serial Registered Brain Magnetic Resonance Imaging to Measure Disease Progression in Alzheimer Disease: Power Calculations and Estimates of Sample Size to Detect Treatment Effects" (*Archives of Neurology*, vol. 57, no. 3, March 2000), Nick C. Fox et al. reported using MRI to identify parts of the brain that are affected by AD before symptoms appear and to measure brain atrophication to monitor the progression of AD.

In 2005 Dimitra G. Georganopoulou et al. announced in "Nanoparticle-Based Detection in Cerebral Spinal Fluid of a Soluble Pathogenic Biomarker for Alzheimer's Disease" (*Proceedings of the National Academy of Sciences*, vol. 102, no. 7, February 15, 2005) the development of another diagnostic test, one that detects small amounts of protein in spinal fluid. Called a bio-barcode assay, the test is as much as a million times more sensitive than other tests. The test is used to detect a protein in the brain called amyloid-beta-derived diffusible ligand (ADDL). ADDLs are small soluble proteins. To detect them the researchers used nanoscale particles that had antibodies specific to ADDL.

In 2009 a test debuted that accurately detects AD in its earliest stages, before the onset of memory problems and other symptoms of cognitive impairment. Leslie M. Shaw et al. explain in "Cerebrospinal Fluid Biomarker Signature in Alzheimer's Disease Neuroimaging Initiative Subjects" (*Annals of Neurology*, vol. 65, no. 4, April 2009) that the test measures the concentration of specific biomarkers, in this case proteins (tau protein and amyloid beta42 polypeptide) in spinal fluid that can indicate AD. The researchers report that subjects with low concentrations of amyloid beta42 and high levels of tau in their spinal fluid were more likely to develop AD. The test had an 87% accuracy rate when predicting which subjects would be diagnosed with AD.

In 2010 John L. Woodard et al. reported that the combination of a test for the apoE-4 gene and a functional MRI (fMRI shows how areas of the brain are activated during mental processes) effectively predicted near-term cognitive decline. In "Prediction of Cognitive Decline in Healthy Older Adults Using fMRI" (*Journal of Alzheimer's Disease*, vol. 21, no. 3, January 2010), the researchers indicate that in 75% of study subjects the genetic test and fMRI accurately predicted which healthy older adults would experience cognitive decline within 18 months of testing.

Wayne R. Leifert et al. report in "Buccal Cell Cytokeratin 14 Correlates with Multiple Blood Biomarkers of Alzheimer's Disease Risk" (*Journal of Alzheimer's Disease*, vol. 48, no. 2, 2015) that in addition to biomarkers for AD in blood and cerebrospinal fluid, it may be possible to detect AD in peripheral cells. The researchers analyze buccal cells (from the side of the mouth) for cytokeratin 14 (CK14; a biomarker for neurodegenerative disorders) and find that changes in buccal cell CK14 expression may be a biomarker that can help identify people with increased risk of developing MCI and AD.

Researchers continue to look at other biological markers and at neuropsychological tests, which measure memory, orientation, judgment, and problem solving, to see if they can accurately predict whether healthy, unaffected older adults will develop AD or whether those with MCI will go on to develop AD. However, the availability of tests raises ethical and practical questions about patients' desires or needs to know their risk of developing AD. Is it helpful or useful to predict a condition that is not yet considered preventable or curable?

Treatments for AD

As of 2016, there was no cure or method of prevention for AD, and treatment focused on managing symptoms. Medication can reduce some of the symptoms, such as agitation, anxiety, unpredictable behavior, and depression. Physical exercise and good nutrition are important, as is a calm and highly structured environment. The object is to help the patient with AD maintain as much comfort, normalcy, and dignity as possible.

In 2016 there were five FDA-approved prescription drugs for the treatment of AD. The first four drugs to be approved were cholinesterase inhibitors, which are drugs designed to prevent the breakdown of acetylcholine. Cholinesterase inhibitors keep levels of this chemical messenger high, even while the cells that produce acetylcholine continue to become damaged or die. About half of the people who take cholinesterase inhibitors see modest improvement in cognitive symptoms. Until 1997 tacrine was the nation's only AD medication, but it is rarely prescribed today because of associated side effects, including possible liver damage. However, there are three other cholinesterase inhibitors currently used that produce some delay in the deterioration of memory and other cognitive skills: donepezil, approved in 1996; rivastigmine, approved in 2000; and galantamine, approved in 2001.

Memantine was approved by the FDA in 2003 for the treatment of moderate to severe AD. It is classified as an uncompetitive low-to-moderate affinity N-methyl-D-aspartate receptor antagonist, and it is the first Alzheimer drug of this type to be approved in the United States. According to the Alzheimer's Association, memantine acts by regulating the activity of glutamate, one of the brain's specialized messenger chemicals that are involved in information processing, storage, and retrieval.

The National Institutes of Health (http://www.clinicaltrials.gov/ct2/results?term=Alzheimer%27s+disease&;pg=19) notes that in early 2016 there were more than 1,800 clinical trials of new treatments for AD under way. Some research involved the use of drugs and vaccines to block the production of beta amyloid, which is thought to be the source of the problem, or to help rid the body of it quickly. Researchers are also looking at antiamyloid antibodies (proteins made by the immune system that counter the effects of beta amyloid) as a way to halt the progress of the disease early in its course. All the drugs being tested were intended to decrease the frequency or severity of the symptoms of AD and slow its progression, but none was expected to cure AD. Investigational drugs aim to address three aspects of AD: improve cognitive function in people with early AD; slow or postpone the progression of the disease; and control behavioral problems such as wandering, aggression, and agitation of patients with AD.

Sylvie Claeysen, Joël Bockaert, and Patrizia Giannoni of the Institut de Génomique Fonctionnelle in Montpellier, France, posit in "Serotonin: A New Hope in Alzheimer's Disease?" (*ACS Chemical Neuroscience*, vol. 6, no. 7, July 15, 2015) that increasing extracellular serotonin (a naturally occurring neurotransmitter that is partly responsible for mood) may be a promising therapeutic strategy for treatment of AD. The researchers suggest that the use of selective serotonin reuptake inhibitors (prescription drugs that are often used to treat depression) may reduce production of toxic beta amyloid proteins, which is a hallmark of AD.

The Impact of AD on Caregivers' Health and Well-Being

The suffering of a patient with AD is only part of the devastating emotional, physical, and financial trauma of the disease. According to the Alzheimer's Association, in *2015 Alzheimer's Disease Facts and Figures*, more than 15 million Americans served as unpaid caregivers for people with AD in 2012. People who care for loved ones with AD are considered to be the "second patients" of the disease. Caring for someone with AD can be very demanding, and caregivers often neglect their own needs, including their health and social lives, and the needs of other family members. As a result, they may develop more stress-related illnesses and are at a greater risk for depression.

Research demonstrates that caregivers are more likely than their peers who do not provide care for people suffering from AD or other forms of dementia to suffer from health problems as well as mood and sleep disorders such as insomnia, at least in part because they are awakened by their care-recipients at night. In "Caregiver Health: Health of Caregivers of Alzheimer's and Other Dementia Patients" (*Current Psychiatry Reports*, vol. 15, no. 7, July 2013), Todd J. Richardson et al. assert that "caring for a person with AD and other dementias is associated with significant risk to the caregiver's health and well-being. Healthcare providers must recognize that family caregivers often present as secondary patients." Health professionals assert that in view of caregivers' risks of developing health problems, there is an urgent need to exhort family caregivers to engage in activities such as regular exercise and preventive medical care that will benefit their own health, well-being, and longevity.

CHAPTER 7
INFECTIOUS DISEASES

Pursue him to his house, and pluck him thence;

Lest his infection, being of a catching nature,

Spread further.

—William Shakespeare, *Coriolanus* (1607–08)

Infectious (contagious) diseases are caused by microorganisms—viruses, bacteria, parasites, or fungi—that are transmitted from one person to another through casual contact, such as influenza; through bodily fluids, such as the human immunodeficiency virus (HIV; the virus that produces acquired immunodeficiency syndrome [AIDS]); or via contaminated air, food, or water supplies. Infectious diseases may also spread by vectors (small organisms) of disease such as insects or ticks that carry the infectious agent.

According to the World Health Organization (WHO), infectious diseases are a leading cause of death worldwide. Not long ago, the U.S. government and medical experts believed that the widespread use of vaccines, antibiotics, and public health measures had effectively eliminated the public health threat of infectious diseases in the United States. Throughout the world, however, new and rare diseases were emerging, and old diseases were resurfacing. Some of these infections reflected changes that were associated with increasing population, growing poverty, urban migration, drug-resistant microbes, and expanding international travel.

The mistaken belief that infectious diseases were problems of the past prompted the governments of many countries, including the United States, to neglect public health programs that were aimed at preventing and treating infectious disease. By the dawn of the 21st century, however, enough troubling new diseases had arisen and old ones recurred that the United States resurrected and intensified efforts to respond to and contain infections.

The National Notifiable Diseases Surveillance System (NNDSS) is a public health surveillance information system that provides the U.S. Centers for Disease Control and Prevention (CDC) with data to track certain infectious diseases (notifiable diseases). The CDC (July 5, 2013, http://www.cdc.gov/mmwr/preview/mmwrhtml/mm6053a1.htm) defines a notifiable disease as "one for which regular, frequent, timely information on individual cases is considered necessary to prevent and control that disease." As such, it does not include every infectious disease. The list of nationally notifiable diseases is revised periodically. For instance, a disease might be added to the list as a new pathogen (an organism that causes disease) emerges, or a disease might be deleted as its incidence declines. Physicians, clinics, and hospitals must report any occurrences of notifiable diseases to the CDC each week. Table 7.1 shows the nationally notifiable infectious diseases that were tracked in 2016.

MOST FREQUENTLY REPORTED DISEASES

Table 7.2 shows that, of the CDC's notifiable diseases, among the top-10 most frequently reported infectious diseases in the United States in 2013 were four sexually transmitted infections (STIs): chlamydia (1,401,906 cases); gonorrhea (333,004 cases); syphilis, all stages (56,471 cases)—an infection that occurs in three stages; it can also be congenital (an infant can be born with the disease); and HIV diagnoses (34,969 cases). The remaining notifiable infectious diseases in the top 10 were:

- Salmonellosis (50,634 cases)—a food-borne disease that causes fever and intestinal disorders
- Lyme disease (36,307 cases)—a disease that is spread by ticks
- Pertussis (28,639 cases)—a respiratory infection caused by the bacterium *Bordetella pertussis* or *Bordetella parapertussis*, which is more commonly called whooping cough

TABLE 7.1

Nationally notifiable infectious diseases, 2016

Anthrax
Arboviral diseases, neuroinvasive and non-neuroinvasive
  California serogroup virus diseases
  Chikungunya virus disease* (not OMB PRA approved)
  Eastern equine encephalitis virus disease
  Powassan virus disease
  St. Louis encephalitis virus disease
  West Nile virus disease
  Western equine encephalitis virus disease
  Zika virus disease
Babesiosis
Botulism/*c. botulinum*
  Botulism, foodborne
  Botulism, infant
  Botulism, other
  Botulism, wound
Brucellosis
Campylobacteriosis
Cancer
Carbon monoxide poisoning
Chancroid
Chlamydia trachomatis infection
Cholera
Coccidioidomycosis/Valley fever
Congenital syphilis
Cryptosporidiosis
Cyclosporiasis
Dengue virus infections
  Dengue
  Dengue fever (DF)
  Dengue hemorrhagic fever (DHF)
  Dengue shock syndrome (DSS)
  Dengue-like illness* (not OMB PRA approved)
  Severe dengue
Diphtheria
Ehrlichiosis and anaplasmosis
  Anaplasma phagocytophilum infection
  Ehrlichia chaffeensis infection
  Ehrlichia ewingii infection
  Undetermined human ehrlichiosis/anaplasmosis
Foodborne disease outbreak
Giardiasis
Gonorrhea
Haemophilus in fluenzae, invasive disease
Hansen's disease/leprosy
Hantavirus infection, non-Hantavirus pulmonary syndrome* (not OMB PRA approved)
Hantavirus pulmonary syndrome (HPS)
Hemolytic uremic syndrome, post-diarrheal (HUS)
Hepatitis A, acute
Hepatitis B, acute
Hepatitis B, chronic
Hepatitis B, perinatal infection
Hepatitis C, acute
Hepatitis C, chronic
HIV infection (AIDS has been reclassified as HIV Stage III) (AIDS/HIV)
Influenza-associated pediatric mortality
Invasive pneumococcal disease (IPD)/*Streptococcus pneumoniae,* invasive disease
Lead, elevated blood levels
  Lead, elevated blood levels, adult (≥16 years)
  Lead, elevated blood levels, children (<16 years)
Legionellosis/Legionnaire's disease or pontiac fever
Leptospirosis
Listeriosis
Lyme disease
Malaria
Measles/rubeola
Meningococcal disease
Mumps
Novel influenza A virus infections

TABLE 7.1

Nationally notifiable infectious diseases, 2016 [CONTINUED]

Pertussis/whooping cough
Pesticide-related illness and injury, acute
Plague
Poliomyelitis, paralytic
Poliovirus infection, nonparalytic
Psittacosis/ornithosis
Q fever
  Q fever, acute
  Q fever, chronic
Rabies, animal
Rabies, human
Rubella/German measles
Rubella, congenital syndrome (CRS)
Salmonellosis
Severe acute respiratory syndrome-associated coronavirus disease (SARS)
Shiga toxin-producing *Escherichia coli* (STEC)
Shigellosis
Silicosis
Smallpox/variola
Spotted fever rickettsiosis
Streptococcal toxic shock syndrome (STSS)
Syphilis
  Syphilis, early latent
  Syphilis, late latent
  Syphilis, late with clinical manifestations (including late benign syphilis and cardiovascular syphilis)
  Syphilis, primary
  Syphilis, secondary
  Syphilitic stillbirth
Tetanus/*c. tetani*
Toxic shock syndrome (other than streptococcal) (TSS)
Trichinellosis/trichinosis
Tuberculosis (TB)
Tularemia
Typhoid fever
Vancomycin-intermediate *Staphylococcus aureus* and vancomycin-resistant *Staphylococcus aureus* (VISA/VRSA)
Varicella/chickenpox
Varicella deaths
Vibriosis
Viral hemorrhagic fever (VHF)
  Crimean-Congo hemorrhagic fever virus
  Ebola virus
  Lassa virus
  Lujo virus
  Marburg virus
  New World arenavirus—Guanarito virus
  New World arenavirus—Junin virus
  New World arenavirus—Machupo virus
  New World arenavirus—Sabia virus
Waterborne disease outbreak
Yellow fever

SOURCE: "2016 National Notifiable Conditions," in *National Notifiable Diseases Surveillance System (NNDSS)*, U.S. Department of Health and Human Services, Centers for Disease Control and Prevention, January 2016, http://wwwn.cdc.gov/nndss/conditions/notifiable/2016/ (accessed March 23, 2016)

- Giardiasis (15,106 cases)—a common protozoal infection of the small intestine that is spread via contaminated food and water and direct person-to-person contact
- Shigellosis (12,729 cases)—caused by a group of bacteria called *Shigella* that cause fever and intestinal disorders
- Varicella (11,359 cases)—commonly known as chicken pox, it is caused by varicella zoster virus, a member of the herpesvirus group

INFECTIOUS DISEASE OUTBREAKS

The CDC investigates infectious disease outbreaks and in 2015 reported more than 10 multistate food-borne outbreak investigations. One of the most notable was an

TABLE 7.2

Reported cases of notifiable diseases, by month, 2013

Disease	Jan.	Feb.	Mar.	Apr.	May	June	July	Aug.	Sept.	Oct.	Nov.	Dec.	Month not stated	Total
Arboviral diseases[a]														
California serogroup viruses														
Neuroinvasive	—	—	—	—	1	10	14	37	26	6	1	—	—	95
Nonneuroinvasive	1	—	—	—	—	4	4	5	3	—	—	—	—	17
Eastern equine encephalitis virus														
Neuroinvasive	2	—	1	—	—	1	—	2	—	2	—	—	—	8
Powassan virus														
Neuroinvasive	—	—	—	—	3	1	2	2	1	2	1	—	—	12
Nonneuroinvasive	—	—	—	—	—	1	—	1	—	—	1	—	—	3
St. Louis encephalitis virus														
Neuroinvasive	—	—	—	—	—	—	—	—	—	1	—	—	—	1
West Nile virus														
Neuroinvasive	1	—	2	1	2	16	131	440	523	139	11	1	—	1,267
Nonneuroinvasive	1	—	1	2	3	22	150	496	448	71	6	2	—	1,202
Babesiosis, total	7	6	14	7	22	222	513	481	176	143	81	124	—	1,796
Confirmed	3	4	2	3	11	185	463	420	136	110	59	86	—	1,482
Probable	4	2	12	4	11	37	50	61	40	33	22	38	—	314
Botulism, total	12	10	21	11	11	12	10	11	10	12	13	19	—	152
Foodborne	—	—	—	—	—	2	—	—	—	—	1	1	—	4
Infant	11	8	20	10	10	9	9	11	10	12	10	16	—	136
Other, (wound and unspecified)	1	2	1	1	1	1	1	—	—	—	2	2	—	12
Brucellosis	8	3	7	6	7	13	8	10	8	11	8	10	—	99
Chancroid[b]	—	—	—	1	3	—	1	2	1	—	1	1	—	10
Chlamydia trachomatis infection[b]	101,875	110,849	138,658	109,846	109,008	130,607	102,560	141,065	108,877	111,788	131,504	105,269	—	1,401,906
Cholera	3	1	—	1	—	—	—	4	1	1	—	3	—	14
Coccidioidomycosis	814	794	572	597	697	889	669	889	645	688	1,202	982	—	9,438
Cryptosporidiosis, total	373	378	465	442	354	533	1,134	2,111	1,288	858	653	467	—	9,056
Confirmed	242	240	291	275	232	364	703	1,239	807	598	421	286	—	5,698
Probable	131	138	174	167	122	169	431	872	481	260	232	181	—	3,358
Cyclosporiasis	2	4	1	4	4	156	253	276	29	19	5	31	—	784
Dengue virus infection[a]														
Dengue fever	68	29	48	38	27	51	95	198	67	79	101	36	—	837
Dengue hemorrhagic fever	—	1	—	—	—	2	—	3	—	—	—	—	—	6
Ehrlichiosis/anaplasmosis														
Anaplasma phagocytophilum	11	16	23	44	160	675	661	458	218	213	190	113	—	2,782
Ehrlichia chaffeensis	7	3	6	13	82	292	381	309	147	85	64	129	—	1,518
Ehrlichia ewingii	—	—	—	—	1	5	7	15	2	1	—	—	—	31
Undetermined	1	3	1	2	11	34	56	48	24	22	11	7	—	220
Giardiasis	853	958	1,151	957	961	1,238	1,333	1,992	1,682	1,448	1,377	1,156	—	15,106
Gonorrhea[b]	24,460	25,220	30,938	24,944	24,554	30,910	25,478	34,360	26,818	27,119	31,448	26,755	—	333,004
Haemophilus influenzae, invasive disease														
All ages, all serotypes	370	349	352	332	314	409	258	289	213	273	276	357	—	3,792
Age <5 years														
Serotype[b]	1	5	3	3	2	1	1	2	3	3	3	4	—	31
Nonserotype[b]	16	24	19	22	24	22	9	12	15	19	18	22	—	222
Unknown serotype	14	25	20	12	19	18	15	8	14	9	14	17	—	185
Hansen disease (leprosy)	4	5	3	4	15	5	6	9	3	9	5	13	—	81
Hantavirus pulmonary syndrome	—	—	1	2	5	3	1	—	4	2	1	2	—	21
Hemolytic uremic syndrome postdiarrheal	15	7	16	13	21	37	51	52	33	38	27	19	—	329

TABLE 7.2

Reported cases of notifiable diseases, by month, 2013 [CONTINUED]

Disease	Jan.	Feb.	Mar.	Apr.	May	June	July	Aug.	Sept.	Oct.	Nov.	Dec.	Month not stated	Total
Hepatitis virus, acute														
A	86	119	127	104	188	227	152	185	191	146	141	115	—	1,781
B	194	238	240	226	234	295	249	280	224	264	330	276	—	3,050
C	115	146	199	169	167	209	140	225	195	141	217	215	—	2,138
Hepatitis B perinatal infection	2	3	6	6	4	7	4	6	3	2	3	2	—	48
Human immunodeficiency virus (HIV) diagnoses[c]	3,658	3,350	3,441	3,566	3,350	3,272	3,331	3,352	2,952	2,756	1,568	373	—	34,969
Influenza-associated pediatric mortality[d]	27	36	30	27	12	5	4	3	3	3	5	5	—	160
Invasive pneumococcal disease														
All ages	2,237	1,842	2,277	1,717	1,458	1,260	606	690	685	955	1,511	1,955	—	17,193
Age <5 years	94	103	160	115	122	80	53	50	69	79	120	126	—	1,171
Legionellosis	175	203	194	142	212	892	816	787	481	402	324	326	—	4,954
Listeriosis	30	25	42	37	41	71	93	124	87	68	63	54	—	735
Lyme disease, total	784	746	849	898	1,454	6,082	8,985	7,087	3,292	2,559	2,093	1,478	—	36,307
Confirmed	496	457	550	552	988	4,918	7,221	5,504	2,350	1,774	1,447	946	—	27,203
Probable	288	289	299	346	466	1,164	1,764	1,583	942	785	646	532	—	9,104
Malaria	88	80	82	99	117	203	181	222	173	96	126	127	—	1,594
Measles, total	7	6	13	23	33	36	15	28	6	—	16	4	—	187
Indigenous	4	3	8	20	29	30	2	22	4	—	13	—	—	135
Imported	3	3	5	3	4	6	13	6	2	—	3	4	—	52
Meningococcal disease														
All serogroups	60	69	63	59	45	30	36	38	29	32	51	44	—	556
Serogroup ACWY	11	14	14	16	17	7	13	13	5	9	11	12	—	142
Serogroup B	10	17	11	14	14	4	4	4	3	3	5	10	—	99
Serogroup other	1	3	3	2	—	—	1	1	—	—	3	3	—	17
Serogroup unknown	38	35	35	27	14	19	18	20	21	20	32	19	—	298
Mumps	19	22	61	106	137	38	20	49	61	38	22	11	—	584
Novel influenza A virus infection	—	—	—	—	—	5	9	4	2	1	—	—	—	21
Pertussis	1,650	1,697	2,047	1,771	2,053	2,706	2,591	3,237	2,309	2,225	3,217	3,136	—	28,639
Plague	—	—	—	—	—	—	—	2	1	1	—	—	—	4
Poliomyelitis, paralytic	—	—	—	—	—	—	1	—	—	—	—	—	—	1
Psittacosis	—	—	—	1	1	—	—	1	2	—	—	1	—	6
Q fever, total	5	7	11	7	10	22	20	25	22	7	8	26	—	170
Acute	4	6	7	6	7	18	14	21	18	6	6	24	—	137
Chronic	1	1	4	1	3	4	6	4	4	1	2	2	—	33
Rabies														
Animal	156	281	320	365	403	411	351	610	466	322	291	272	—	4,248
Human	—	—	1	—	1	—	—	—	—	—	—	—	—	2
Rubella	1	—	1	1	—	—	3	—	—	—	1	2	—	9
Rubella, congential syndrome	—	—	—	—	—	—	—	—	—	—	—	1	—	1
Salmonellosis	1,807	1,802	2,881	2,855	3,554	5,440	5,728	7,292	5,562	5,297	4,697	3,719	—	50,634
Shiga toxin-producing *Escherichia coli* (STEC)	244	213	361	353	568	800	820	1,140	720	552	492	400	—	6,663
Shigellosis	511	622	706	620	673	994	1,008	1,520	1,210	1,329	1,747	1,789	—	12,729
Spotted fever rickettsiosis, total	30	47	50	69	219	573	569	739	419	295	159	190	—	3,359
Confirmed	2	3	5	8	17	31	31	34	18	17	3	5	—	174
Probable	28	44	44	60	202	542	538	704	401	277	156	185	—	3,181
Streptococcal toxic-shock syndrome	26	21	24	26	22	17	11	12	19	7	18	21	—	224
Syphilis, total all stages[b, e]	3,729	4,188	5,423	4,427	4,381	5,168	4,133	5,504	4,689	4,607	5,297	4,925	—	56,471
Congenital[b]	25	20	31	27	33	32	31	36	22	26	31	34	—	348
Primary and secondary[b]	1,072	1,261	1,652	1,318	1,322	1,593	1,279	1,744	1,548	1,378	1,656	1,552	—	17,375

TABLE 7.2

Reported cases of notifiable diseases, by month, 2013 [CONTINUED]

Disease	Jan.	Feb.	Mar.	Apr.	May	June	July	Aug.	Sept.	Oct.	Nov.	Dec.	Month not stated	Total
Tetanus	4	2	—	2	1	1		2	5	2	4	3	—	26
Toxic-shock syndrome (other than streptococcal)	6	8	3	8	9	4	7	11	8	1	4	2	—	71
Trichinellosis	—	4	5	2	—	1	—	—	2	1	5	2	—	22
Tuberculosis[f]	493	611	668	795	789	892	882	783	768	895	769	1,237	—	9,582
Tularemia	2	2	3	5	16	63	33	38	14	14	7	6	—	203
Typhoid fever	24	17	30	30	24	39	39	28	28	21	32	26	—	338
Vancomycin-intermediate *Staphylococcus aureus* (VISA)	9	14	17	36	21	25	18	15	27	29	15	22	—	248
Varicella (Chickenpox)														
Morbidity	710	941	1,206	1,038	1,127	1,018	496	752	1,027	1,015	1,139	890	—	11,359
Mortality[g]	—	—	—	—	2	1	—	—	—	—	—	—	—	3
Vibriosis	15	31	24	33	55	116	271	361	170	119	61	43	—	1,299

[a]Totals reported to the Division of Vector-Borne Diseases, National Center for Emerging and Zoonotic Infectious Diseases (ArboNET Surveillance), as of June 1, 2014.
[b]Totals reported to the Division of STD Prevention, National Center for HIV/AIDS, Viral Hepatitis, STD, and TB Prevention (NCHHSTP), as of June 4, 2014.
[c]Total number of HIV diagnoses reported to the Division of HIV/AIDS Prevention, NCHHSTP through December 28, 2013.
[d]Totals reported to the Influenza Division, National Center for Immunization and Respiratory Diseases (NCIRD), as of December 28, 2013.
[e]Includes the following categories: primary, secondary, latent (including early latent, late latent, and latent syphilis of unknown duration), neurosyphilis, late (including late syphilis with clinical manifestations other than neurosyphilis), and congenital syphilis. Totals reported to the Division of STD Prevention, NCHHSTP, as of June 4, 2014.
[f]Totals reported to the Division of Tuberculosis Elimination, NCHHSTP, as of July 1, 2014.
[g]Totals reported to the Division of Viral Diseases, NCIRD, as of May 30, 2014.
Notes: No cases of anthrax; diphtheria; eastern equine encephalitis, nonneuroinvasive disease; poliovirus infection, nonparalytic; severe acute respiratory syndrome-associated coronavirus disease (SARS-CoV); smallpox; St. Louis encephalitis, nonneuroinvasive disease; western equine encephalitis, neuroinvasive and nonneuroinvasive disease; vancomycin-resistant staphylococcus aureus (VRSA); viral hemorrhagic fevers and Yellow fever were reported in the United States during 2013. Data on chronic hepatitis B and hepatitis C virus infection (past or present) are not included because they are undergoing data quality review.

SOURCE: Deborah A. Adams et al., "Table 1. Reported Cases of Notifiable Diseases, by Month—United States, 2013," in "Summary of Notifiable Diseases and Conditions—United States, 2013," *Morbidity and Mortality Weekly Report*, vol. 62, no. 53, October 23, 2015, http://www.cdc.gov/mmwr/pdf/wk/mm6253.pdf (accessed January 2, 2016)

outbreak of infection with Shiga toxin-producing *Escherichia coli* O26 (STEC O26) linked to Chipotle Mexican Grill restaurants that began in October 2015. Illnesses associated with the case were characterized by gastrointestinal symptoms (diarrhea and abdominal cramps) that began two to six days after ingesting the organism. In its final update on the outbreak (February 1, 2016, http://www.cdc.gov/ecoli/2015/o26-11-15/index.html), the CDC reports that, in all, 55 people in 11 states became ill, resulting in 21 hospitalizations but no deaths.

In "Signs and Symptoms" (December 21, 2015, http://www.cdc.gov/ecoli/2015/o26-11-15/signs-symptoms.html), the CDC states that although most people recover from the STEC 026 infection within a week, some people, especially children under the age of five years, older adults, and people with compromised immune systems, risk developing a type of kidney failure called hemolytic uremic syndrome. Symptoms may include fever, abdominal pain, pale skin tone, fatigue and irritability, small, unexplained bruises or bleeding from the nose and mouth, and decreased urination and require immediate medical attention.

RESISTANT STRAINS OF BACTERIA

Antibiotics have generally been considered "miracle drugs" that control or cure many bacterial infectious diseases. However, since 2000 nearly all the major bacterial infections in the world have become increasingly resistant to the most commonly prescribed antibiotic treatments, primarily because of repeated and improper uses of antibiotics. Decreasing inappropriate antibiotic use is the best way to control this resistance.

Such bacteria as pneumococcus, which can cause common diseases such as pneumonia and children's ear infections that have long been considered treatable, are evolving into strains that are proving to be untreatable with commonly used antibiotics. Pneumococcal bacteria cause many hundreds of thousands of cases of pneumonia and bacterial meningitis (inflammation of the tissue covering the brain and spinal cord). They also cause otitis media (middle-ear infection), which, according to Allan S. Lieberthal in "The Diagnosis and Management of Acute Otitis Media" (*Pediatrics*, vol. 131, no. 3, March 1, 2013), remains the most common indication for antibiotic prescribing in young children despite the fact that it is usually a mild condition that resolves spontaneously without any treatment.

Joseph P. Lynch and George G. Zhanel indicate in "Streptococcus Pneumoniae: Does Antimicrobial Resistance Matter?" (*Seminars in Respiratory and Critical Care Medicine*, vol. 30, no. 2, April 2009) that during the previous three decades antimicrobial resistance among *Streptococcus pneumoniae*, the most common cause of community-acquired pneumonia, escalated significantly, with 15% to 30% of infections being multidrug-resistant (MDR), meaning they were resistant to three or more classes of antibiotics. Lynch and Zhanel explain that previous antibiotic use is the most common risk factor that is associated with antibiotic drug resistance.

To treat patients with penicillin-resistant pneumococcus infections, physicians use a combination of other antibiotics, such as vancomycin, imipenem, and rifampin for resistant pneumonia and clindamycin or cefuroxime for ear infections. Another strategy to combat the illness is the pneumococcal vaccine. One of the reasons that public health professionals advocate widespread use of the pneumococcal vaccine is the hope that it will produce "herd immunity"—when a large proportion of the population is immune, the likelihood of person-to-person spread is so small that the disease does not proliferate and even nonimmune individuals are protected from disease. Nevertheless, Lynch and Zhanel observe that some of the reduction in the occurrence of illness anticipated from the introduction of the pneumococcal vaccine has been offset by the increased prevalence of resistant infections that are not prevented by the current vaccine.

Methicillin-Resistant *Staphylococcus Aureus*

Methicillin-resistant *Staphylococcus aureus* (MRSA) are infections of staph bacteria that resist treatment with customary antibiotics. According to the CDC, they are most common in hospitalized patients with weakened immune systems as well as in nursing home residents. Nevertheless, they can also appear in people living in the community at large. In "General Information about MRSA in the Community" (2015, http://www.cdc.gov/mrsa/community/index.html), the CDC explains that most MRSA infections that happen among the general population are skin infections, but that when MRSA infects someone in a medical facility it may well take the form of a serious bloodstream, pneumonia, or surgical-site infection.

The CDC reports that MRSA is usually spread via direct, physical contact with an infected wound or with something (such as a doctor's hands) that has touched such a wound, but infections can be prevented by following infection control guidelines. In the United States all MRSA infections were in decline as of 2015. In *The State of the World's Antibiotics 2015* (2015, https://cddep.org/sites/default/files/swa_2015_final.pdf), the Center for Disease Dynamics, Economics and Policy (CDDEP) states that there was a 44% decline in such infections in health care settings between 2007 and 2015.

Educating Physicians and the Public about the Appropriate Use of Antibiotics

According to the CDDEP, in *The State of the World's Antibiotics 2015*, antibiotic resistance is a global problem and one of the most urgent public health concerns. In the

United States it is responsible for more than 2 million infections and 23,000 deaths each year. In 1995 the CDC Division of Foodborne Bacterial and Mycotic Diseases began a national campaign to reduce antimicrobial resistance by encouraging the appropriate use of antibiotics.

In *The State of the World's Antibiotics 2015*, the CDDEP presents the following six strategies to reduce antibiotic use to lower the rates of drug-resistant bacteria:

1. Reduce the need for antibiotics through improved water, sanitation, and immunization
2. Improve hospital infection control and antibiotic stewardship—increase hand washing with soap or using alcohol disinfectant between patients
3. Eliminate economic incentives that encourage antibiotic overuse and misuse in hospitals, communities and in agriculture to incentives that encourage antibiotic stewardship
4. Reduce and eventually phase out antibiotic use in agriculture for growth promotion or disease prevention
5. Educate health professionals, policy makers, and the public on sustainable antibiotic use
6. Ensure political commitment to meet the threat of antibiotic resistance

In the United States, by changing and managing how physicians choose and administer antimicrobial drugs, hospitals have been able to prevent or slow the emergence of antimicrobial resistance; optimize the selection, dosing, and duration of antimicrobial therapy; reduce the incidence of drug-related adverse events; and lower rates of morbidity and mortality.

The consequences of the failure of antibiotics to treat formerly treatable illnesses could be dire: longer-lasting illnesses, more physician office visits or longer hospital stays, the need for more expensive and toxic medications, and even death.

More public education about appropriate antibiotic use is needed. In "Prevalence of Parental Misconceptions about Antibiotic Use" (*Pediatrics*, vol. 136, no. 2, August 2015), Louise Elaine Vaz et al. report the results of their research about parents' attitudes and knowledge about childhood illnesses and the need for antibiotics. Vaz et al. surveyed 1,500 parents of young children from diverse socio-demographic backgrounds to determine if specific characteristics predicted particular misconceptions, and compared current knowledge and attitudes with the results of a similar survey conducted in 2000. The researchers find that antibiotic use and misconceptions about antibiotic use were more prevalent among socioeconomically disadvantaged parents than among parents who were not socioeconomically disadvantaged. Younger parents, minority race or ethnicity, and having less than a college degree also were important predictors of less knowledge about antibiotic use in common childhood illnesses. Vaz et al. conclude, "Despite large-scale educational campaigns to decrease antibiotic misuse, deficits in parental knowledge persist. New strategies to change expectations about antibiotic use must be a continued focus of public health initiatives. These initiatives will be more effective if they address local knowledge and attitudes and tailor interventions to combat specific misconceptions."

PREVENTION THROUGH IMMUNIZATION

When someone is affected by an infectious disease, his or her immune system responds by creating antibodies to destroy it. The first time someone is exposed to a particular disease this process can take some time, and an infected individual may have a noticeable illness. However, having been infected with a particular disease once, the immune system in effect learns to recognize and fight that disease very quickly and effectively in the future. This means that once someone has been infected with a disease, that person will likely be immune to it (unaffected by it) if it is encountered again in the future.

Vaccines are medications that contain a version of a disease, such as an influenza virus or tuberculosis bacteria, that has been rendered harmless but that a person's immune system will still recognize as a threat and attack. By exposing someone to a vaccine, he or she can be immunized against an infectious disease(s) without actually becoming ill. In some cases this immunization will last a lifetime, but for other diseases it may be necessary to receive boosters (additional doses of vaccine) from time to time.

According to the CDC's National Immunization Program, in "List of Vaccine-Preventable Diseases" (September 3, 2015, http://www.cdc.gov/vaccines/vpd-vac/vpd-list.htm), there are 25 diseases that can be prevented by vaccination in the United States. However, immunization against only a portion of these diseases is recommended for the general public. See Figure 2.1, Figure 2.2, and Figure 2.3 in Chapter 2 for the CDC's 2015 recommendations on which vaccines should be administered, and on what schedule, for children, adolescents, and adults, respectively.

The following list describes the diseases that the CDC recommends people be immunized against:

- Diphtheria—This bacterial disease causes potentially fatal respiratory infections.
- Haemophilus influenza type b (Hib)—This bacterial infection can cause a variety of serious respiratory infections and other diseases, such as meningitis.

- Hepatitis A—This virus causes acute liver disease.
- Hepatitis B—This virus infects the liver, in some cases becoming a chronic condition causing long-term health problems or death.
- Human papillomavirus (HPV)—These viruses can cause cervical cancer and genital warts.
- Influenza (flu)—This viral infection produces sudden fever, muscle aches, and respiratory infection symptoms.
- Measles—This highly contagious viral disease is characterized by fever, a cough, and red circular spots on the skin. Complications from measles can lead to death.
- Meningococcal diseases—The meningococcal conjugate vaccine protects against a variety of diseases caused by *Neisseria meningitides*. Among the most worrisome is meningitis, inflammation of the meninges (the covering of the brain and the spinal cord) that it is characterized by fever, vomiting, intense headache, and stiff neck.
- Mumps—This highly contagious viral disease produces swelling of the parotid glands (salivary glands that occur below and in front of the ear).
- Pertussis (whooping cough)—This bacterial infection causes illness that is marked by powerful spasms of coughing.
- Pneumococcal—This bacteria causes pneumonia, an inflammation of the lungs.
- Poliomyelitis (polio)—This viral disease causes fever, atrophy (wasting) of skeletal muscles, and paralysis.
- Rotavirus—This virus inflames the stomach and intestines, causing potentially severe diarrhea, vomiting, and abdominal pain.
- Rubella (German measles)—This viral infection is usually mild in children but can seriously harm an unborn child when contracted by a woman early during her pregnancy.
- Tetanus (lockjaw)—The bacteria from this disease produce a toxin that causes victims to have painful muscle spasms. It kills approximately 10% of everyone infected.
- Varicella (chicken pox)—This is a highly contagious viral disease that is marked by skin eruptions of fluid-filled lesions that itch.
- Zoster (chicken pox)—A single dose of zoster vaccine is recommended for adults aged 60 years and older to prevent shingles, a painful rash caused by the chicken pox virus, herpes zoster.

Widespread administration of the other available vaccines is not recommended because the risk of contracting these diseases—such as anthrax and smallpox—is very low.

OUTBREAKS OCCUR LARGELY AMONG THE UNVACCINATED

High rates of vaccination afford communities high population immunity. For example, in 2000 the United States declared measles eliminated (defined as interruption of year-round transmission); however, vulnerable populations such as people who cannot be vaccinated because of underlying medical conditions or infants too young to be vaccinated may still be infected.

In "Measles—United States, January 4 to April 2, 2015" (*Morbidity and Mortality Weekly Report*, vol. 64, no. 14, April 17, 2015), Nakia S. Clemmons et al. report that in early 2015, 70% of reported measles cases were associated with an outbreak that originated in late December 2014 in Disney theme parks in Orange County, California, that was traced to foreign visitors. Clemmons et al. observe that since worldwide about 20 million measles cases occur annually, "importations to the U.S. will continue to place unvaccinated populations at risk for measles."

INFLUENZA

Influenza (the flu) is a contagious respiratory disease that is caused by a virus. When a person infected with the flu sneezes or coughs, the virus is expelled into the air via droplets and may be inhaled by anyone nearby. It can also be transmitted by direct hand contact. The flu primarily affects the lungs, but the whole body experiences symptoms. The infected person usually becomes acutely ill, with fever, chills, weakness, loss of appetite, and aching muscles in the head, back, arms, and legs. Someone with an influenza infection may also have a sore throat, a dry cough, nausea, and burning eyes. The accompanying fever increases quickly—sometimes reaching 104 degrees Fahrenheit (40 degrees C)—but usually subsides after two or three days. Influenza leaves the patient exhausted.

For healthy individuals, the flu is typically a moderately severe illness, with most adults and children back to work or school within a week. However, for the very young, the very old, and people who are not in good general health, the flu can be extremely severe and even fatal. Complications such as secondary bacterial infections may develop, taking advantage of the body's weakened condition and lowered resistance. The most common bacterial complication is pneumonia, but sinuses, bronchi, or inner ears can also become secondarily infected with bacteria. Less common but very serious complications include viral pneumonia, encephalitis (inflammation of the brain), acute renal (kidney) failure, and nervous system disorders. These complications can be fatal.

Who Gets the Flu?

Anyone can get the flu, especially if there is an epidemic in the community. (An epidemic is a period when the number of cases of a disease exceeds the number that is expected based on past experience.) During an epidemic year, 20% to 30% of the population may contract influenza. Not surprisingly, people who are not healthy are considered to be at high risk for most strains of influenza and their complications. The high-risk population includes people with chronic lung conditions, such as asthma, emphysema, chronic bronchitis, tuberculosis, or cystic fibrosis (an inherited disease that is characterized by chronic respiratory and digestive problems); people with heart disease, chronic kidney disease, diabetes, or severe anemia; people residing in nursing homes; people over the age of 65 years; and some health care workers.

Vaccines

Influenza can be prevented by inoculation with a current influenza vaccine. Influenza vaccine must be formulated annually so that it contains the strains of influenza virus that are expected to cause the most cases of flu during the upcoming year. The viruses are killed or inactivated to prevent those who are vaccinated from getting influenza from the vaccine. After being immunized, the person develops antibodies to the influenza viruses. The antibodies are most effective after one or two months. High-risk people should be vaccinated early during the fall because peak flu activity usually occurs around the beginning of the new calendar year. The flu season usually runs from October to May and peaks in December and January.

Each year's flu vaccine protects against only the viruses that were included in its formulation. If another strain of flu appears, people can still catch the new strain even though they were vaccinated for the primary expected strains.

Most people have little or no noticeable reaction to the vaccine; about a quarter may have a swollen, red, tender area where the vaccination was injected. Children may suffer a slight fever for 24 hours or have chills or a headache. Those who already suffer from a respiratory disease may experience worsened symptoms. Usually, these reactions are temporary. Because the virus used in influenza vaccines is grown in eggs, people with egg protein allergies should consult their physician before receiving the vaccine and, if vaccinated, should be closely observed for any indications of an allergic reaction.

OLDER ADULTS BENEFIT FROM FLU VACCINATIONS. Influenza is a major cause of illness and death among people aged 65 years and older. According to Walter E. P. Beyer et al., in "Cochrane Re-arranged: Support for Policies to Vaccinate Elderly People against Influenza" (*Vaccine*, vol. 31, no. 50, December 2013), older adults are at much greater risk than younger adults of developing complications of influenza. Because recent research questioned whether adults aged 65 years and older who obtain influenza vaccinations significantly reduce their risk of contracting influenza, the researchers reviewed the data from a large number of studies. Beyer et al. conclude "that vaccination of the elderly is efficacious in reducing infection, disease, and death, caused by influenza virus infection; is worthwhile as a public health intervention; and that there is a sound scientific basis for the recommendations made by the World Health Organization, and multiple international and national bodies."

Antiviral Drugs

According to the U.S. Food and Drug Administration (FDA), in "Influenza (Flu) Antiviral Drugs and Related Information" (December 16, 2015, http://www.fda.gov/drugs/drugsafety/informationbydrugclass/ucm100228.htm), antiviral drugs can be used to shorten the duration of a flu infection. In some cases they can also be used to reduce the chance that someone who was exposed to influenza virus will become ill. However, they cannot cure the flu, nor are they as effective as a vaccine at preventing it. They are recommended primarily for people who are at risk of complications from the flu.

As of March 2016 three influenza antiviral medications—Rapivab (peramivir), Relenza (zanamivir), and Tamiflu (oseltamivir phosphate)—had been approved by the FDA for the treatment and/or prevention of influenza and were recommended by the CDC. Flumadine (rimantadine) and Symmetrel (amantadine) also are FDA-approved for the treatment of influenza, but in 2016 the CDC advised against their use because recent influenza strains, including the 2009 H1N1 strain (commonly known as "swine flu"), have proved resistant to them. However, even approved drugs are not always effective because influenza virus strains can become resistant to one or more of these medications.

Pandemic Influenza

In "CDC Resources for Pandemic Flu" (October 20, 2015, http://www.cdc.gov/flu/pandemic-resources/), the CDC describes pandemic flu as occurring "when a nonhuman (novel) influenza virus gains the ability for efficient and sustained human-to-human transmission and then spreads globally." Pandemics are different from seasonal outbreaks or even epidemics of influenza. Seasonal outbreaks are caused by influenza viruses that already move from person to person, whereas pandemics are caused by new viruses, subtypes of viruses that have never passed between people, or subtypes that have not circulated among people for a very long time.

In the past, influenza pandemics produced high levels of illness, death, social disruption, and economic loss. The 20th century saw three pandemics. The CDC reports that the 1918–19 "Spanish flu" claimed a half-million lives in the United States and as many as 50 million people throughout the world. Nearly half of the deaths were young, healthy adults. In 1957–58 the "Asian flu" was responsible for 70,000 deaths in the United States. The 1968–69 "Hong Kong flu" proved fatal for 34,000 people in the United States. All three pandemics involved avian influenza, or bird flu. The 1957–58 and 1968–69 pandemics were caused by viruses that contained a combination of genes from a human influenza virus and an avian influenza virus; the 1918–19 pandemic virus also appears to have been an avian flu. The 2009 H1N1 "swine flu" pandemic of 2009–10 is estimated to have killed between 150,000 and 575,000 people worldwide.

AVIAN INFLUENZA. Avian influenza is an infectious disease of birds that is caused by type A strains of the influenza virus. The disease, which was first identified in Italy more than 100 years ago, occurs worldwide. Because these viruses usually do not infect humans, there is little or no immune protection against them. If an avian influenza virus infects people and gains the ability to spread easily from person to person, an influenza pandemic can begin, as those that occurred in 1918, 1957, and 1968.

More commonly, an individual who was in contact with infected birds or surfaces that were contaminated with excretions from infected birds will contract a version of avian flu that cannot easily be transmitted from one human to another. The CDC indicates in "Highly Pathogenic Asian Avian Influenza A (H5N1) in People" (June 11, 2015, http://www.cdc.gov/flu/avianflu/h5n1-people.htm) that between November 2003 and June 2015 more than 700 human cases of H5N1 strain avian influenza virus were reported. They primarily occurred in 15 countries in Asia, Africa, the Pacific, Europe, and the Near East. The first report of a human infection and death in North America was in Canada in January 2014 and was diagnosed in a traveler returning from China.

The CDC indicates that human infection with H5N1 is rare, but about 60% of infected individuals have died. In an effort to prepare for a possible avian flu pandemic, in 2007 the FDA approved the first human H5N1 vaccine, which could help protect people at the highest risk of exposure during the early critical months of a pandemic. In November 2013 the FDA approved another vaccine for the prevention of H5N1 influenza, which also could be used to prevent a pandemic should H5N1 virus develop the capacity to spread efficiently from human to human. According to the FDA news release "FDA Approves First Adjuvanted Vaccine for Prevention of H5N1 Avian Influenza" (November 22, 2013, http://www.fda.gov/NewsEvents/Newsroom/PressAnnouncements/ucm376444.htm), it is intended to "supplement the national stockpile" to have on hand should a pandemic arise and is not commercially available.

The U.S. Department of Health and Human Services (HHS) supports pandemic influenza activities in the areas of surveillance, vaccine development and production, strategic stockpiling of antiviral medications, research, and risk communications. The HHS aims to have sufficient antiviral courses of drug treatment on hand in anticipation of a possible pandemic. There are also plans in place for pandemic preparedness for health care facilities, schools, local governments, businesses, and law enforcement agencies. Individuals and families can prepare for a pandemic flu by stockpiling nonperishable food and regular prescription medication.

SWINE FLU. In April 2009, H1N1, sometimes called "swine flu" because it has two genes from flu viruses that normally circulate in pigs (as well as avian and human flu genes), was detected in people in the United States. On June 11, 2009, the WHO declared that the 2009 H1N1 influenza was a pandemic. The pandemic lasted into 2010 and is estimated to have killed as many as 575,000 people worldwide.

After the 2009 H1N1 pandemic ran its course, this variant of influenza (and its descendants) became part of the group of influenza viruses that commonly circulate in humans. It is no longer of particular concern compared with other flu viruses, and current flu vaccines provide protection against it. As with avian flu, however, there are occasional cases of other forms of swine flu being transmitted from animals to humans. In "Key Facts about Human Infections with Variant Viruses (Swine Origin Influenza Viruses in Humans)" (August 19, 2014, http://www.cdc.gov/flu/swineflu/keyfacts-variant.htm), the CDC describes the illness caused by such cases of swine flu as ranging from mild to severe, with symptoms that include "fever, lethargy, lack of appetite and coughing. Some people also have reported runny nose, sore throat, eye irritation, nausea, vomiting, and diarrhea."

Preventing Flu

Along with annual influenza vaccinations, the CDC encourages several general preventive measures, including:

- Covering the nose and mouth with a tissue when coughing or sneezing and throwing the tissue in the trash after using it
- Washing hands often with soap and water and, when soap and water are unavailable, using an alcohol-based hand sanitizer
- Avoiding touching the eyes, nose, and mouth to prevent the spread of virus
- Staying home from work or school when sick to limit contact with others and keep from infecting them

TUBERCULOSIS

Tuberculosis (TB), a communicable disease that is caused by the bacterium *Mycobacterium tuberculosis*, is spread from person to person through the inhalation of airborne particles containing *M. tuberculosis*. The particles, called droplet nuclei, are produced when a person with infectious TB of the lungs or larynx forcefully exhales, such as when coughing, sneezing, speaking, or singing. These infectious particles can remain suspended in the air and may be inhaled by someone sharing the same air.

The CDC notes in the fact sheet "Questions and Answers about TB" (December 18, 2014, http://www.cdc.gov/tb/publications/faqs/qa_introduction.htm) that most TB occurs in the lungs (pulmonary TB). The risk of transmission is increased where ventilation is poor and when susceptible people share air for prolonged periods with a person who has untreated pulmonary TB. However, the disease may occur at any site of the body, such as the larynx, the lymph nodes, the brain, the kidneys, or the bones. This type of TB infection, which occurs outside the lungs, is referred to as extrapulmonary. Except for laryngeal TB, people with extrapulmonary TB are usually not considered infectious to others.

In the fact sheet "The Difference between Latent TB Infection and TB Disease" (November 21, 2014, http://www.cdc.gov/tb/publications/factsheets/general/LTBIandActiveTB.htm), the CDC explains that TB does not develop in everyone who is infected with the bacteria. In the United States about 90% of infected people never show symptoms of TB, but they are considered to have latent TB infections. The only indication of a latent TB infection is a positive reaction to the tuberculin skin test or special TB blood test. Between 5% and 10% of those infected develop active disease later in life, and about half of those who develop active TB do so within the first two years of infection. Table 7.3 shows the differences between latent TB infection and TB disease. People with compromised immune systems are at greater risk of developing TB than those with healthy immune systems. For example, the WHO notes in the fact sheet "Tuberculosis" (March 2016, http://www.who.int/mediacentre/factsheets/fs104/en/) that an individual who is HIV-positive and infected with TB bacilli is 20 to 30 times more likely to become sick with TB than someone infected with TB who is HIV-negative.

Continuing Threat

The CDC reports in the fact sheet "Data and Statistics" (September 24, 2015, http://www.cdc.gov/tb/statistics/default.htm) that TB is among the world's deadliest diseases. Overall, one-third of the world's population is infected with the TB bacillus, many of them latent carriers. In 2014 about 9.6 million people worldwide became sick with TB, and approximately 1.5 million people died from it. The numbers of people who become infected with and die from TB have increased dramatically since the HIV/AIDS epidemic swept through many countries. TB is a leading cause of death among people who are infected with HIV.

After several decades of decline, TB made a comeback in the United States during the early 1990s. (See Figure 7.1.) In 1992 the CDC reported 26,673 cases of TB, up from 22,201 in 1985. Subsequently, the number of infections decreased 5% to 7% each year. From 2002 to 2003, TB cases decreased just 1.4%, but from 2008 to 2009, the total number of TB cases decreased more than 10%. In 2014 a total of 9,421 cases were reported, which represents a decline of 1.5% from 2013 and 64.7% from the 1992 peak.

In *Tuberculosis in the United States: National Tuberculosis Surveillance System Highlights from 2014* (September 15, 2015, http://www.cdc.gov/tb/statistics/surv/surv2014/default.htm), the CDC reports that the proportion of TB cases in foreign-born people has increased steadily since 1993 and that in 2014 it accounted for 66% of all TB cases in the United States. (See Figure 7.2.) People born outside the United States have accounted for

TABLE 7.3

Distinguishing latent TB infection from TB disease

A person with latent TB infection	A person with TB disease
• Does not feel sick	• Usually feels sick
• Has no symptoms	• Has symptoms that may include:—a bad cough that lasts 3 weeks or longer—pain in the chest—coughing up blood or sputum—weakness or fatigue—weight loss—no appetite—chills—fever—sweating at night
• Cannot spread TB bacteria to others	• May spread TB bacteria to others
• Usually has a positive TB skin test or positive TB blood test	• Usually has a positive TB skin test or positive TB blood test
• Has a normal chest x-ray and a negative sputum smear	• May have an abnormal chest x-ray, or positive sputumsmear or culture
• Should consider treatment for latent TB infection to prevent TB disease	• Needs treatment for TB disease

TB = Tuberculosis.

SOURCE: "The Difference between Latent TB Infection and TB Disease," in *Questions and Answers about TB*, Centers for Disease Control and Prevention, Division of Tuberculosis Elimination, December 18, 2014, http://www.cdc.gov/tb/publications/faqs/qa_introduction.htm (accessed January 2, 2016)

FIGURE 7.1

Reported TB cases, 1982–2014

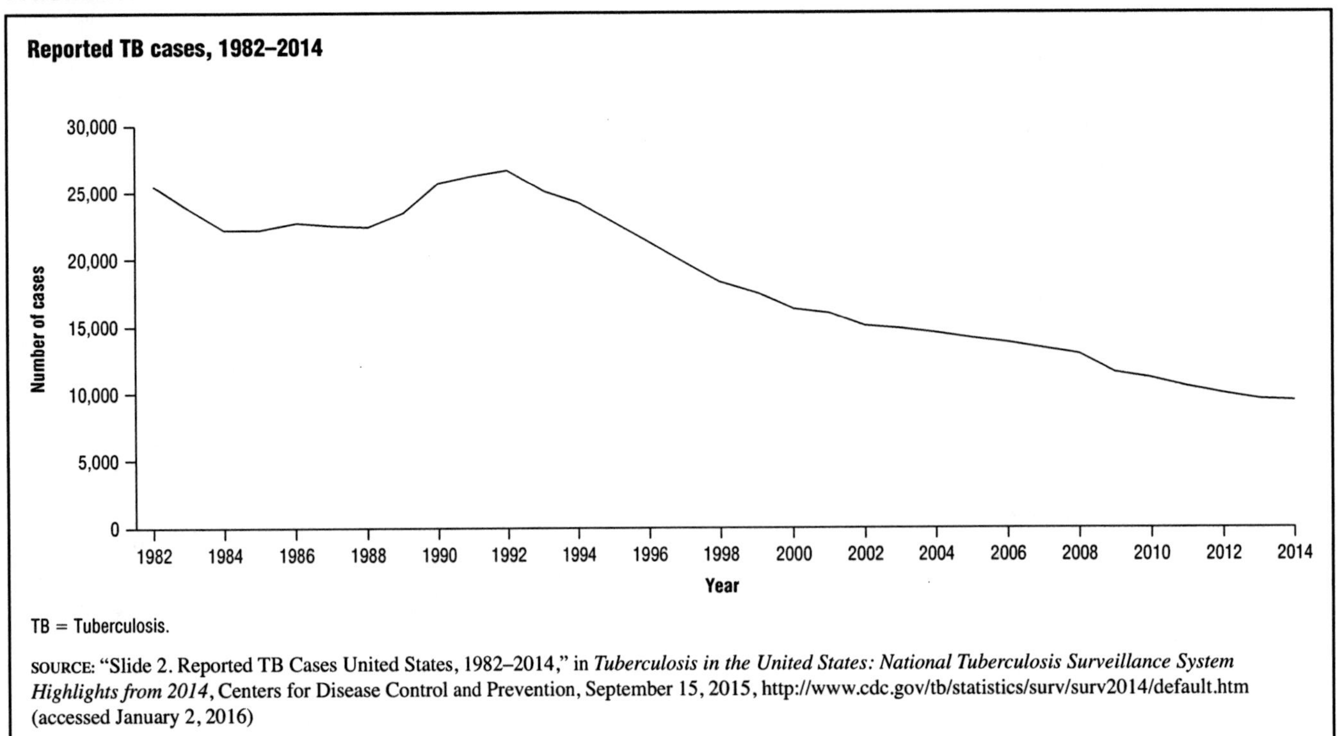

30,000
25,000
20,000
15,000
10,000
5,000
0
Number of cases
1982 1984 1986 1988 1990 1992 1994 1996 1998 2000 2002 2004 2006 2008 2010 2012 2014
Year

TB = Tuberculosis.

SOURCE: "Slide 2. Reported TB Cases United States, 1982–2014," in *Tuberculosis in the United States: National Tuberculosis Surveillance System Highlights from 2014*, Centers for Disease Control and Prevention, September 15, 2015, http://www.cdc.gov/tb/statistics/surv/surv2014/default.htm (accessed January 2, 2016)

FIGURE 7.2

Number of TB cases in U.S.-born versus foreign-born people, 1993–2014

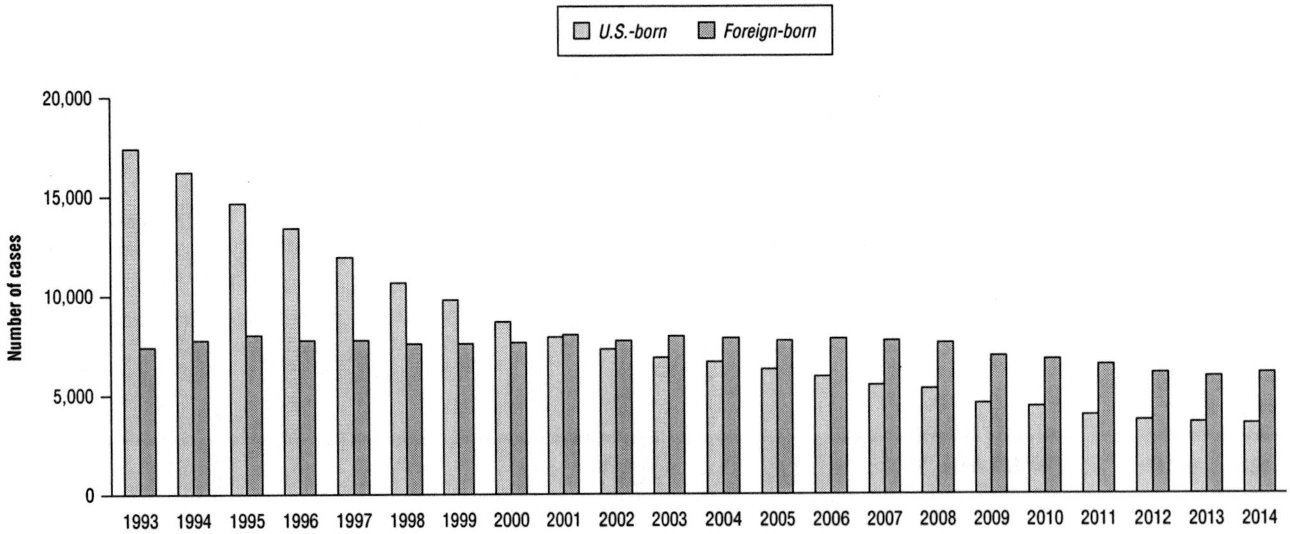

U.S.-born
Foreign-born
20,000
15,000
10,000
5,000
0
Number of cases
1993 1994 1995 1996 1997 1998 1999 2000 2001 2002 2003 2004 2005 2006 2007 2008 2009 2010 2011 2012 2013 2014

TB = Tuberculosis.

SOURCE: "Slide 13. Number of TB Cases in U.S.-Born vs. Foreign-Born Persons, United States, 1993–2014," in *Tuberculosis in the United States: National Tuberculosis Surveillance System Highlights from 2014*, Centers for Disease Control and Prevention, September 15, 2015, http://www.cdc.gov/tb/statistics/surv/surv2014/default.htm (accessed January 2, 2016)

the majority of TB cases in the United States every year since 2001. Given that people can have latent TB infections for many years and that TB is more common outside the United States, it seems likely that many foreign-born individuals who developed active TB disease in the United States contracted TB before they arrived.

Treatment has become increasingly difficult because new strains of MDR TB have developed. If the disease is not properly treated or if treatment is not completed, some TB can become resistant to drugs, making it much harder to cure. According to the CDC, in *Tuberculosis in the United States*, in 1994 roughly 2% of all TB cases in the United States were MDR. This percentage declined to roughly 1% by 2003 but increased slightly beginning in 2009 and was 1.3% in 2014. The percentage of foreign-born TB patients with MDR TB was higher than among the native-born population in 2014.

March 24 of each year has been designated World TB Day by the CDC to recognize and increase awareness of the global threat to health posed by the disease. This annual event, first sponsored by the WHO, honors the date in 1882 when Robert Koch (1843–1910) announced his discovery of *M. tuberculosis*.

HIV/AIDS

AIDS is the late stage of an infection caused by HIV, a retrovirus that attacks and destroys certain white blood cells, which weakens the body's immune system and makes it susceptible to infections and diseases that ordinarily would not be life threatening. AIDS is considered to be a blood-borne STI because HIV is spread through contact with blood, semen, or vaginal fluids from an infected person.

Around the World

AIDS and HIV were virtually unknown before 1981, when testing and reporting of the disease became mandatory, but awareness grew as the annual number of diagnosed cases and deaths steadily increased. In *Fact Sheet 2015* (2015, http://www.unaids.org/en/resources/campaigns/HowAIDSchangedeverything/factsheet), the Joint United Nations Programme on HIV/AIDS notes that there were about 2 million new HIV infections in 2014, down from 3.1 million in 2000. Another 36.9 million people worldwide were estimated to be living with HIV/AIDS. About 1.2 million deaths were attributable to AIDS-related causes in 2014.

In the United States

The CDC reports in *HIV Surveillance Report: Diagnoses of HIV Infection and AIDS in the United States and Dependent Areas, 2013* (February 2015, http://www.cdc.gov/hiv/pdf/library/reports/surveillance/cdc-hiv-surveillance-report-vol-25.pdf) that at the end of 2012 there were an estimated 508,845 people living with AIDS in the United States. In 2013 an estimated 47,352 diagnoses of HIV infection were made. Of these cases, 187 were among children aged 12 years and younger, 9,278 were among adult or adolescent females, and 37,887 were among adult or adolescent males. (See Table 7.4.)

The CDC indicates that the rate of HIV diagnoses in the United States was 15 per 100,000 population in 2013. (See Table 7.4.) Between 2009 and 2013 the rate of HIV diagnoses among people aged 20 to 29 and 60 to 64 years increased, while the rates of those aged 15 to 19 and 30 to 59 years decreased, and the rates among children and adults over the age of 65 years were essentially unchanged.

In 2013, 80% of HIV diagnoses (an estimated 37,887 of 47, 352) were made among adult and adolescent males. (See Table 7.4.) Between 2009 and 2013 the annual number of HIV infections attributed to male-to-male sexual contact increased. In contrast, infections attributed to injection drug use, infections attributed to heterosexual contact, and infections attributed to male-to-male sexual contact and injection drug use decreased during the same period.

The CDC's analysis of the groups most affected by HIV/AIDS confirms that the majority of infections are diagnosed in men who have sex with men. The analysis also identifies the racial and ethnic distribution of new HIV infections. For example, African Americans are the most affected by HIV/AIDS. (See Table 7.4.) In 2013 African Americans accounted for an estimated 46% of all diagnoses of HIV infection. The rates per 100,000 population were 55.9 in the African American population, 18.7 in the Hispanic population, 12.7 in the Native Hawaiian or Pacific Islander population, 16.8 in people reporting multiple races, 9.4 in the Native American or Alaskan Native population, 6.6 in the white population, and 6 in the Asian American population.

The CDC reports that in 2013 the overall rate of AIDS diagnoses was 8.4 per 100,000 population. (See Table 7.5.) Between 2009 and 2013 AIDS diagnoses among people aged 20 to 24 years and aged 60 to 64 years and older increased somewhat, whereas the rates for people aged 35 to 59 years decreased and the rates remained stable for children aged 12 years and younger and teens aged 13 to 19.

In *HIV Surveillance Report*, the CDC indicates that from the beginning of the AIDS epidemic through 2013, an estimated 1,194,039 people in the United States and dependent areas had been reported as having AIDS, and 658,992 people had died from the disease by the end of 2012.

How Is AIDS Spread?

HIV/AIDS is not transmitted through casual contact with an infected person. More than 30 years of research and observation have definitively concluded that the HIV infection can be transmitted by only the following methods:

- By oral, anal, or vaginal sex with an infected person; worldwide, heterosexual sex is the most common mode of transmission

TABLE 7.4

HIV infections, by selected characteristics, 2009–13

	2009			2010			2011			2012			2013		
		Estimated[a]			Estimated[a]			Estimated[a]			Estimated[a]			Estimated[a]	
	No.	No.	Rate	No.	No.	Rate	No.	No.	Rate	No.	No.	Rate	No.	No.	Rate
Age at diagnosis (yr)															
<13	218	223	0.4	225	232	0.4	187	196	0.4	232	250	0.5	164	187	0.4
13–14	30	31	0.4	40	41	0.5	44	47	0.6	49	53	0.6	39	45	0.5
15–19	2,187	2,228	10.3	2,069	2,123	9.7	1,988	2,074	9.6	1,846	1,989	9.3	1,652	1,863	8.8
20–24	6,741	6,875	31.9	7,064	7,265	33.5	7,066	7,386	33.3	7,196	7,752	34.3	7,059	8,053	35.3
25–29	6,510	6,641	30.6	6,342	6,533	30.9	6,366	6,658	31.3	6,556	7,083	33.1	6,844	7,825	36.3
30–34	5,714	5,835	29.3	5,481	5,652	28.2	5,262	5,508	26.9	5,589	6,037	28.9	5,404	6,165	29.0
35–39	5,659	5,779	28.1	5,028	5,184	25.8	4,456	4,673	23.8	4,264	4,611	23.7	4,246	4,858	24.8
40–44	5,991	6,120	29.2	5,233	5,402	25.8	4,800	5,032	23.9	4,554	4,923	23.4	4,217	4,820	23.1
45–49	5,297	5,413	23.7	4,860	5,014	22.1	4,628	4,859	21.9	4,449	4,822	22.2	4,311	4,961	23.4
50–54	3,659	3,742	17.2	3,512	3,629	16.2	3,364	3,532	15.6	3,274	3,554	15.7	3,254	3,747	16.6
55–59	2,163	2,212	11.7	2,065	2,137	10.8	1,992	2,095	10.3	1,975	2,146	10.3	2,151	2,467	11.6
60–64	1,007	1,031	6.5	1,073	1,109	6.5	1,069	1,123	6.3	1,066	1,164	6.5	1,150	1,316	7.3
≥65	823	842	2.1	789	815	2.0	812	858	2.1	825	901	2.1	896	1,045	2.3
Race/ethnicity															
American Indian/Alaska Native	167	169	7.2	180	183	8.1	172	177	7.8	194	202	8.8	197	218	9.4
Asian	718	734	5.4	717	742	5.0	787	827	5.4	833	901	5.8	862	973	6.0
Black/African American	21,661	22,136	58.7	20,510	21,148	55.6	19,453	20,436	53.3	19,079	20,803	53.7	18,803	21,836	55.9
Hispanic/Latino[b]	9,411	9,620	19.9	9,009	9,317	18.4	8,852	9,299	17.9	8,980	9,710	18.3	8,878	10,117	18.7
Native Hawaiian/other Pacific Islander	64	65	14.5	59	61	12.1	56	59	11.5	71	75	14.4	61	67	12.7
White	12,518	12,750	6.4	11,957	12,290	6.2	11,465	11,923	6.0	11,593	12,372	6.3	11,672	13,101	6.6
Multiple races	1,460	1,497	32.8	1,349	1,395	24.7	1,249	1,318	22.6	1,125	1,223	20.4	914	1,039	16.8
Transmission category															
Male adult or adolescent															
Male-to-male sexual contact	21,811	27,394	—	21,712	27,106	—	21,791	27,357	—	21,962	28,967	—	21,498	30,689	—
Injection drug use	1,507	2,501	—	1,306	2,205	—	1,076	1,879	—	922	1,799	—	887	1,942	—
Male-to-male sexual contact and injection drug use	1,251	1,611	—	1,177	1,507	—	1,024	1,346	—	978	1,316	—	851	1,270	—
Heterosexual contact[c]	3,120	4,501	—	2,871	4,176	—	2,725	3,959	—	2,452	3,776	—	2,199	3,887	—
Other[d]	7,625	56	—	6,935	55	—	6,415	53	—	6,953	79	—	7,745	99	—
Subtotal	**35,314**	**36,062**	**29.1**	**34,001**	**35,049**	**28.0**	**33,031**	**34,595**	**27.4**	**33,267**	**35,937**	**28.2**	**33,180**	**37,887**	**29.4**
Female adult or adolescent															
Injection drug use	931	1,687	—	777	1,426	—	661	1,288	—	599	1,227	—	510	1,154	—
Heterosexual contact[c]	5,014	8,943	—	4,669	8,382	—	4,200	7,905	—	3,800	7,811	—	3,446	8,031	—
Other[d]	4,522	56	—	4,109	46	—	3,955	57	—	3,977	61	—	4,087	93	—
Subtotal	**10,467**	**10,686**	**8.3**	**9,555**	**9,855**	**7.5**	**8,816**	**9,250**	**7.0**	**8,376**	**9,099**	**6.8**	**8,043**	**9,278**	**6.9**
Child (<13 yrs at diagnosis)															
Perinatal	175	179	—	175	180	—	135	142	—	154	165	—	93	107	—
Other[e]	43	44	—	50	52	—	52	54	—	78	85	—	71	80	—
Subtotal	**218**	**223**	**0.4**	**225**	**232**	**0.4**	**187**	**196**	**0.4**	**232**	**250**	**0.5**	**164**	**187**	**0.4**
Region of residence															
Northeast	9,006	9,209	16.7	8,421	8,711	15.7	7,865	8,307	14.9	7,829	8,629	15.5	7,499	8,908	15.9
Midwest	5,812	5,917	8.9	5,559	5,698	8.5	5,444	5,634	8.4	5,608	5,906	8.8	5,600	6,109	9.0
South	23,032	23,513	20.7	21,895	22,564	19.6	21,244	22,285	19.2	20,804	22,629	19.3	21,066	24,323	20.5
West	8,149	8,332	11.6	7,906	8,163	11.3	7,481	7,814	10.7	7,634	8,122	11.0	7,222	8,013	10.8
Total[f]	**45,999**	**46,971**	**15.3**	**43,781**	**45,136**	**14.6**	**42,034**	**44,040**	**14.1**	**41,875**	**45,287**	**14.4**	**41,387**	**47,352**	**15.0**

TABLE 7.4

HIV infections, by selected characteristics, 2009–13 [CONTINUED]

[a]Estimated numbers resulted from statistical adjustment that accounted for reporting delays and missing transmission category, but not for incomplete reporting. Rates are per 100,000 population. Rates are not calculated by transmission category because of the lack of denominator data.
[b]Hispanics/Latinos can be of any race.
[c]Heterosexual contact with a person known to have, or to be at high risk for, HIV infection.
[d]Includes hemophilia, blood transfusion, perinatal exposure, and risk factor not reported or not identified.
[e]Includes hemophilia, blood transfusion, and risk factor not reported or not identified.
[f]Because column totals for estimated numbers were calculated independently of the values for the subpopulations, the values in each column may not sum to the column total.
Note: Data include persons with a diagnosis of HIV infection regardless of stage of disease at diagnosis.

SOURCE: "Table 1a. Diagnoses of HIV infection, by Year of Diagnosis and Selected Characteristics, 2009–2013—United States," in "Diagnoses of HIV Infection in the United States and Dependent Areas, 2013," *HIV/AIDS Surveillance Report*, vol. 25, Centers for Disease Control and Prevention, February 2015, http://www.cdc.gov/hiv/pdf/library/reports/surveillance/cdc-hiv-surveillance-report-vol-25.pdf (accessed January 2, 2016)

TABLE 7.5

AIDS diagnoses, by selected characteristics, 2009–13 and cumulative

	2009			2010			2011			2012			2013			Cumulative[b]	
		Estimated[a]			Estimated[a]			Estimated[a]			Estimated[a]			Estimated[a]			
	No.	No.	Rate	No.	No.	Rate	No.	No.	Rate	No.	No.	Rate	No.	No.	Rate	No.	Est. No.[a]
Age at diagnosis (yr)																	
<13	14	14	0.0	23	24	0.0	15	16	0.0	10	10	0.0	7	8	0.0	9,399	9,421
13–14	45	46	0.6	47	49	0.6	37	39	0.5	28	29	0.4	25	30	0.4	1,442	1,461
15–19	439	450	2.1	454	470	2.1	428	447	2.1	340	361	1.7	381	435	2.1	8,636	8,793
20–24	1,947	1,996	9.3	1,987	2,062	9.5	1,971	2,064	9.3	1,863	1,982	8.8	1,996	2,239	9.8	50,040	50,787
25–29	3,140	3,220	14.9	2,884	2,993	14.2	2,763	2,896	13.6	2,701	2,877	13.4	2,787	3,123	14.5	138,724	139,957
30–34	3,651	3,743	18.8	3,302	3,423	17.1	3,129	3,276	16.0	3,218	3,424	16.4	2,927	3,268	15.4	222,750	224,308
35–39	4,335	4,442	21.6	3,708	3,844	19.1	3,179	3,329	17.0	2,891	3,074	15.8	2,869	3,200	16.3	241,443	243,169
40–44	4,989	5,116	24.4	4,304	4,463	21.3	3,753	3,930	18.7	3,424	3,640	17.3	3,121	3,496	16.8	202,176	204,006
45–49	4,813	4,935	21.6	4,273	4,431	19.6	3,953	4,138	18.7	3,614	3,843	17.7	3,386	3,781	17.8	137,405	139,062
50–54	3,492	3,578	16.4	3,180	3,298	14.8	2,900	3,043	13.5	2,863	3,045	13.5	2,803	3,135	13.9	81,518	82,718
55–59	1,939	1,987	10.5	1,759	1,826	9.2	1,793	1,874	9.2	1,756	1,872	9.0	1,789	1,998	9.4	44,927	45,628
60–64	917	939	5.9	933	967	5.7	910	950	5.3	984	1,049	5.9	1,019	1,144	6.3	23,899	24,274
≥65	777	796	2.0	741	767	1.9	724	754	1.8	721	766	1.8	740	831	1.9	20,169	20,455
Race/ethnicity																	
American Indian/Alaska Native	104	106	4.5	119	122	5.4	114	117	5.1	101	105	4.5	96	104	4.5	3,486	3,514
Asian[c]	374	384	2.8	365	380	2.6	367	384	2.5	358	382	2.4	374	415	2.6	9,560	9,712
Black/African American	14,326	14,687	39.0	13,440	13,951	36.7	12,353	12,946	33.7	11,949	12,735	32.9	11,678	13,172	33.7	491,715	497,267
Hispanic/Latino[d]	6,454	6,629	13.7	5,599	5,817	11.5	5,215	5,469	10.5	4,981	5,307	10.0	4,814	5,336	9.9	213,246	215,685
Native Hawaiian/other Pacific Islander	37	38	8.4	39	40	8.1	32	33	6.5	30	32	6.1	34	37	6.9	845	855
White	7,917	8,097	4.1	6,979	7,208	3.7	6,505	6,786	3.4	6,079	6,429	3.3	6,090	6,759	3.4	433,681	436,557
Multiple races	1,286	1,322	29.0	1,054	1,097	19.4	969	1,020	17.5	915	984	16.4	764	867	14.0	29,995	30,448
Transmission category																	
Male adult or adolescent																	
Male-to-male sexual contact	12,574	15,530	—	11,635	14,575	—	11,157	13,958	—	10,700	13,821	—	10,542	14,611	—	520,784	577,403
Injection drug use	1,741	2,432	—	1,482	2,152	—	1,242	1,825	—	1,105	1,705	—	932	1,610	—	164,750	187,218
Male-to-male sexual contact and injection drug use	1,322	1,595	—	1,130	1,389	—	977	1,232	—	860	1,115	—	716	1,026	—	77,304	83,828
Heterosexual contact[e]	2,626	3,549	—	2,239	3,155	—	2,093	2,918	—	1,891	2,790	—	1,774	2,865	—	64,842	82,447
Other[f]	4,398	125	—	4,138	116	—	3,696	122	—	3,821	115	—	4,164	144	—	106,136	11,545
Subtotal	**22,661**	**23,232**	**18.7**	**20,624**	**21,387**	**17.1**	**19,165**	**20,055**	**15.9**	**18,377**	**19,546**	**15.3**	**18,128**	**20,256**	**15.7**	**933,816**	**942,440**
Female adult or adolescent																	
Injection drug use	1,160	1,734	—	959	1,472	—	839	1,313	—	755	1,225	—	645	1,143	—	74,970	89,790
Heterosexual contact[e]	4,108	6,156	—	3,584	5,599	—	3,265	5,240	—	3,003	5,077	—	2,696	5,109	—	111,561	146,521
Other[f]	2,555	125	—	2,405	136	—	2,271	132	—	2,268	114	—	2,374	172	—	52,782	5,868
Subtotal	**7,823**	**8,016**	**6.2**	**6,948**	**7,206**	**5.5**	**6,375**	**6,684**	**5.0**	**6,026**	**6,417**	**4.8**	**5,715**	**6,424**	**4.8**	**239,313**	**242,178**
Child (<13 yrs at diagnosis)																	
Perinatal	13	13	—	17	18	—	12	13	—	9	9	—	6	7	—	8,532	8,553
Other[g]	1	1	—	6	6	—	3	3	—	1	1	—	1	1	—	867	869
Subtotal	**14**	**14**	**0.0**	**23**	**24**	**0.0**	**15**	**16**	**0.0**	**10**	**10**	**0.0**	**7**	**8**	**0.0**	**9,399**	**9,421**

TABLE 7.5

AIDS diagnoses, by selected characteristics, 2009–13 and cumulative [CONTINUED]

	2009			2010			2011			2012			2013			Cumulative[b]	
		Estimated[a]			Estimated[a]			Estimated[a]			Estimated[a]			Estimated[a]			
	No.	No.	Rate	No.	No.	Rate	No.	No.	Rate	No.	No.	Rate	No.	No.	Rate	No.	Est. No.[a]
Region of residence																	
Northeast	6,516	6,750	12.2	5,639	5,923	10.7	5,119	5,449	9.8	4,771	5,173	9.3	4,301	4,872	8.7	348,674	352,167
Midwest	3,652	3,714	5.6	3,369	3,456	5.2	3,249	3,356	5.0	3,130	3,283	4.9	2,944	3,221	4.8	125,360	126,372
South	14,718	15,036	13.3	13,715	14,183	12.3	12,908	13,466	11.6	12,382	13,109	11.2	12,769	14,345	12.1	473,007	477,964
West	5,612	5,761	8.0	4,872	5,054	7.0	4,279	4,484	6.2	4,130	4,408	6.0	3,836	4,251	5.7	235,487	237,536
Total[h]	**30,498**	**31,262**	**10.2**	**27,595**	**28,616**	**9.3**	**25,555**	**26,755**	**8.6**	**24,413**	**25,973**	**8.3**	**23,850**	**26,688**	**8.4**	**1,182,528**	**1,194,039**

[a]Estimated numbers resulted from statistical adjustment that accounted for reporting delays and missing transmission category, but not for incomplete reporting. Rates are per 100,000 population. Rates are not calculated by transmission category because of the lack of denominator data.
[b]From the beginning of the epidemic through 2013.
[c]Includes Asian/Pacific Islander legacy cases.
[d]Hispanics/Latinos can be of any race.
[e]Heterosexual contact with a person known to have, or to be at high risk for, HIV infection.
[f]Includes hemophilia, blood transfusion, perinatal exposure, and risk factor not reported or not identified.
[g]Includes hemophilia, blood transfusion, and risk factor not reported or not identified.
[h]Because column totals for estimated numbers were calculated independently of the values for the subpopulations, the values in each column may not sum to the column total.
Note: Reported numbers less than 12, as well as estimated numbers (and accompanying rates and trends) based on these numbers, should be interpreted with caution.

SOURCE: "Table 2a. Stage 3 (AIDS), by Year of Diagnosis and Selected Characteristics, 2009–2013 and Cumulative—United States," in "Diagnoses of HIV Infection in the United States and Dependent Areas, 2013," *HIV/AIDS Surveillance Report*, vol. 25, Centers for Disease Control and Prevention, February 2015, http://www.cdc.gov/hiv/pdf/library/reports/surveillance/cdc-hiv-surveillance-report-vol-25.pdf (accessed January 2, 2016)

- By sharing drug needles or syringes with an infected person
- From an infected mother to her baby at the time of birth and possibly through breast milk
- By receiving a transplanted organ or bodily fluids, such as blood transfusions or blood products, from an infected person

Because avoiding these methods of transmission virtually eliminates the possibility of becoming infected with HIV, unlike some other infectious diseases, AIDS is considered to be almost entirely preventable.

High concentrations of HIV have been found in blood, semen, and cerebrospinal fluid. Concentrations 1,000 times less have been found in saliva, tears, vaginal secretions, breast milk, and feces. There have been no published reports, however, of HIV transmission from saliva, tears, or human bites.

Table 7.6 shows the estimated number of people diagnosed with AIDS in the United States in 2013, as well as throughout the course of the HIV/AIDS epidemic to that date, and how they contracted HIV. In 2013 male-to-male sexual contact was the most common transmission category in the United States, followed by heterosexual contact, injection drug use alone, and injection drug use and male-to-male sexual contact (i.e., people who engaged in both behaviors and who might have been exposed to HIV through either or both of them).

Opportunistic Infections

Once HIV has destroyed the immune system, the body can no longer protect itself against bacterial, fungal, parasitic, or viral agents that take advantage of the compromised condition, causing opportunistic infections (OIs). OIs are illnesses caused by organisms that would not normally harm a healthy person. Because the patient is considered to have AIDS if at least one OI appears, OIs are considered to be AIDS-defining events. OIs are not the only AIDS-defining events; the diagnosis of malignancies such as Kaposi's sarcoma (a rare skin carcinoma that is capable of spreading to internal organs), Burkitt's lymphoma, invasive cervical cancer, and primary brain lymphoma are also considered to be AIDS-defining events.

One of the most common OIs is *Pneumocystis carinii* pneumonia, a lung infection that is caused by a fungus. Other infections that AIDS patients are susceptible to are toxoplasmosis (a contagious disease that is caused by a one-cell parasite), oral candidiasis (thrush), esophageal candidiasis (an infection of the esophagus), extrapulmonary cryptococcosis (a systemic fungus that enters the body through the lungs and may invade any organ of the body), pulmonary TB, extrapulmonary TB, *Mycobacterium avium* complex (a serious bacterial infection that can occur in one part of the body, such as the liver, bone marrow, and spleen, or can spread throughout the body), and cytomegalovirus disease (a member of the herpesvirus group).

Treatment of HIV/AIDS

The U.S. National Institute of Allergy and Infectious Diseases (NIAID) explains in "HIV/AIDS" (November 14, 2012, http://www.niaid.nih.gov/topics/HIVAIDS/Understanding/Treatment/Pages/default.aspx) that there is no cure for HIV or AIDS. When the epidemic began in the early 1980s, most people who contracted the disease died within a few years. Over time, antiretroviral drugs were developed that can suppress HIV in a person's body, sometimes to such low levels that it is no longer detectable. This slows or stops progression of the disease but does not eliminate viral reservoirs, so HIV remains present. It can still be transmitted to others, and if someone stops taking their medications, virus levels will rise once again.

According to the FDA, in "Antiretroviral Drugs Used in the Treatment of HIV Infection" (October 8, 2015, http://www.fda.gov/ForPatients/Illness/HIVAIDS/Treatment/ucm118915.htm), as of March 2016, 37 medications were approved to target HIV, and researchers were pursuing novel strategies for prevention and vaccine development. The NIAID notes that these drugs fall into six classes. It recommends that at least two classes of drugs be used in combination to treat an HIV infection, an approach called highly active antiretroviral therapy (HAART). The purpose of HAART is to prevent HIV infections from developing resistance to antiretroviral drugs.

COMPLICATIONS AND SIDE EFFECTS OF TREATMENT. HIV drug regimens are complicated, and many produce severe side effects in a substantial number of patients. The difficulty of dealing with a complicated regimen of daily medication and maintaining the personal resolve to continue the regimen are ongoing issues for many HIV/AIDS patients. When effective AIDS drugs were first introduced, patients sometimes had to wake up in the middle of the night to take pills, and some treatment regimens consisted of as many as 50 or 60 pills administered several times a day. Even with intense pressure to simplify treatment regimens, pharmaceutical companies remained skeptical about an effective once-a-day pill despite the consensus opinion that it would help more people start and stick with treatment. Once-a-day regimens became available in 2006.

The Promise of Prevention and Cure

Despite setbacks and several failed attempts, efforts continue to formulate an effective HIV vaccine to prevent infection. In "HIV/AIDS Clinical Trials" (July 13, 2015, http://aidsinfo.nih.gov/clinical-trials), AIDSinfo, a service of the HHS, notes that 75 clinical trials of HIV vaccines were planned or under way in early 2016.

TABLE 7.6

AIDS diagnoses, by year of diagnosis and selected characteristics, 2009–13 and cumulative

	2009			2010			2011			2012			2013			Cumulative[b]	
		Estimated[a]			Estimated[a]			Estimated[a]			Estimated[a]			Estimated[a]			
	No.	No.	Rate	No.	No.	Rate	No.	No.	Rate	No.	No.	Rate	No.	No.	Rate	No.	Est. No.[a]
Age at diagnosis (yr)																	
<13	14	14	0.0	23	24	0.0	16	17	0.0	10	10	0.0	7	8	0.0	9,820	9,843
13–14	45	46	0.6	47	49	0.6	38	40	0.5	29	31	0.4	26	31	0.4	1,500	1,520
15–19	444	455	2.1	458	474	2.1	436	456	2.1	341	362	1.7	384	439	2.0	8,868	9,027
20–24	1,964	2,013	9.2	2,005	2,080	9.5	1,986	2,080	9.3	1,882	2,003	8.8	2,016	2,266	9.8	51,441	52,204
25–29	3,196	3,277	14.9	2,916	3,026	14.1	2,797	2,932	13.6	2,733	2,912	13.5	2,810	3,152	14.4	142,921	144,180
30–34	3,720	3,813	18.9	3,350	3,473	17.1	3,174	3,324	16.0	3,257	3,467	16.4	2,960	3,311	15.4	229,616	231,215
35–39	4,416	4,525	21.7	3,782	3,921	19.3	3,250	3,404	17.1	2,943	3,132	15.9	2,903	3,244	16.3	248,612	250,387
40–44	5,103	5,232	24.6	4,393	4,555	21.5	3,824	4,005	18.8	3,488	3,710	17.4	3,164	3,551	16.8	207,924	209,804
45–49	4,924	5,048	21.8	4,379	4,540	19.8	4,047	4,238	18.9	3,696	3,934	17.9	3,440	3,853	17.9	141,291	143,001
50–54	3,577	3,665	16.6	3,252	3,373	14.9	2,980	3,128	13.7	2,920	3,107	13.6	2,862	3,213	14.1	83,820	85,064
55–59	1,987	2,036	10.6	1,800	1,868	9.3	1,825	1,908	9.3	1,791	1,910	9.1	1,824	2,045	9.5	46,287	47,014
60–64	943	966	6.0	963	998	5.8	926	967	5.4	1,003	1,070	5.9	1,036	1,167	6.4	24,665	25,054
≥65	804	823	2.1	761	788	1.9	755	787	1.9	748	796	1.8	759	854	1.9	21,098	21,398
Race/ethnicity																	
American Indian/Alaska Native	104	106	—	119	122	—	114	117	—	101	105	—	96	104	—	3,487	3,515
Asian[c]	374	384	—	365	380	—	368	385	—	358	382	—	374	415	—	9,617	9,770
Black/African American	14,341	14,702	—	13,449	13,961	—	12,360	12,953	—	11,960	12,747	—	11,683	13,179	—	492,184	497,742
Hispanic/Latino[d]	7,073	7,262	—	6,120	6,355	—	5,703	5,986	—	5,395	5,763	—	5,148	5,773	—	247,904	250,671
Native Hawaiian/other Pacific Islander	38	39	—	41	42	—	34	35	—	31	33	—	34	37	—	861	872
White	7,921	8,101	—	6,981	7,210	—	6,505	6,786	—	6,081	6,431	—	6,092	6,762	—	433,803	436,681
Multiple races	1,286	1,322	—	1,054	1,097	—	970	1,021	—	915	984	—	764	867	—	30,007	30,460
Transmission category																	
Male adult or adolescent																	
Male-to-male sexual contact	12,708	15,670	—	11,748	14,694	—	11,274	14,084	—	10,817	13,953	—	10,636	14,739	—	526,753	583,510
Injection drug use	1,900	2,599	—	1,610	2,287	—	1,340	1,934	—	1,185	1,796	—	992	1,694	—	178,022	200,761
Male-to-male sexual contact and injection drug use	1,350	1,624	—	1,157	1,417	—	996	1,253	—	877	1,133	—	725	1,036	—	79,800	86,354
Heterosexual contact[e]	2,730	3,662	—	2,335	3,258	—	2,196	3,030	—	1,964	2,874	—	1,853	2,974	—	68,789	86,531
Other[f]	4,415	128	—	4,150	120	—	3,709	125	—	3,832	117	—	4,177	146	—	106,670	11,745
Subtotal	**23,103**	**23,684**	**18.8**	**21,000**	**21,775**	**17.2**	**19,515**	**20,426**	**16.0**	**18,675**	**19,873**	**15.4**	**18,383**	**20,590**	**15.8**	**960,034**	**968,901**
Female adult or adolescent																	
Injection drug use	1,204	1,780	—	989	1,503	—	866	1,342	—	777	1,250	—	661	1,165	—	77,959	92,845
Heterosexual contact[e]	4,255	6,310	—	3,706	5,729	—	3,378	5,362	—	3,100	5,193	—	2,758	5,198	—	116,964	152,110
Other[f]	2,561	127	—	2,411	137	—	2,279	136	—	2,279	117	—	2,382	174	—	53,086	6,011
Subtotal	**8,020**	**8,217**	**6.3**	**7,106**	**7,369**	**5.5**	**6,523**	**6,841**	**5.1**	**6,156**	**6,560**	**4.8**	**5,801**	**6,537**	**4.8**	**248,009**	**250,967**
Child (<13 yrs at diagnosis)																	
Perinatal	13	13	—	17	18	—	13	14	—	9	9	—	6	7	—	8,927	8,948
Other[g]	1	1	—	6	6	—	3	3	—	1	1	—	1	1	—	893	895
Subtotal	**14**	**14**	**0.0**	**23**	**24**	**0.0**	**16**	**17**	**0.0**	**10**	**10**	**0.0**	**7**	**8**	**0.0**	**9,820**	**9,843**

TABLE 7.6

AIDS diagnoses, by year of diagnosis and selected characteristics, 2009–13 and cumulative [CONTINUED]

	2009			2010			2011			2012			2013			Cumulative[b]	
		Estimated[a]			Estimated[a]			Estimated[a]			Estimated[a]			Estimated[a]			
	No.	No.	Rate	No.	No.	Rate	No.	No.	Rate	No.	No.	Rate	No.	No.	Rate	No.	Est. No.[a]
Region of residence																	
Northeast	6,516	6,750	12.2	5,639	5,923	10.7	5,119	5,449	9.8	4,771	5,173	9.3	4,301	4,872	8.7	348,674	352,167
Midwest	3,652	3,714	5.6	3,369	3,456	5.2	3,249	3,356	5.0	3,130	3,283	4.9	2,944	3,221	4.8	125,360	126,372
South	14,718	15,036	13.3	13,715	14,183	12.3	12,908	13,466	11.6	12,382	13,109	11.2	12,769	14,345	12.1	473,007	477,964
West	5,612	5,761	8.0	4,872	5,054	7.0	4,279	4,484	6.2	4,130	4,408	6.0	3,836	4,251	5.7	235,487	237,536
U.S. dependent areas	639	653	14.9	534	552	13.4	499	529	13.0	428	471	11.6	341	447	11.2	35,335	35,672
Total[h]	**31,137**	**31,915**	**10.2**	**28,129**	**29,168**	**9.3**	**26,054**	**27,283**	**8.6**	**24,841**	**26,444**	**8.3**	**24,191**	**27,135**	**8.5**	**1,217,863**	**1,229,711**

[a]Estimated numbers resulted from statistical adjustment that accounted for reporting delays and missing transmission category, but not for incomplete reporting. Rates are per 100,000 population. Rates by race/ethnicity are not provided because U.S. census information for U.S. dependent areas is limited. Rates are not calculated by transmission category because of the lack of denominator data.

[b]From the beginning of the epidemic through 2013.

[c]Includes Asian/Pacific Islander legacy cases (see Technical Notes).

[d]Hispanics/Latinos can be of any race.

[e]Heterosexual contact with a person known to have, or to be at high risk for, HIV infection.

[f]Includes hemophilia, blood transfusion, perinatal exposure, and risk factor not reported or not identified.

[g]Includes hemophilia, blood transfusion, and risk factor not reported or not identified.

[h]Because column totals for estimated numbers were calculated independently of the values for the subpopulations, the values in each column may not sum to the column total.

Note: Reported numbers less than 12, as well as estimated numbers (and accompanying rates and trends) based on these numbers, should be interpreted with caution because the numbers have underlying relative standard errors greater than 30% and are considered unreliable.

SOURCE: "Table 2b. Stage 3 (AIDS), by Year of Diagnosis and Selected Characteristics, 2009–2013 and Cumulative—United States and 6 Dependent Areas," in "Diagnoses of HIV Infection in the United States and Dependent Areas, 2013," *HIV/AIDS Surveillance Report*, vol. 25, Centers for Disease Control and Prevention, February 2015, http://www.cdc.gov/hiv/pdf/library/reports/surveillance/cdc-hiv-surveillance-report-vol-25.pdf (accessed January 2, 2016)

For example, in "Affinity Maturation of a Potent Family of HIV Antibodies Is Primarily Focused on Accommodating or Avoiding Glycans" (*Immunity*, vol. 43, no. 6, December 15, 2015), Fernando Garces et al. report the results of their research about how HIV-fighting antibodies, which can bind to and neutralize many strains of HIV, develop over time. By tracking the evolution of the antibodies, the researchers may be able to prompt a fast antibody response, which could then be generated by a vaccine.

In "Ending the HIV-AIDS Pandemic—Follow the Science" (*New England Journal of Medicine*, December 3, 2015), Anthony S. Fauci and Hilary D. Marston explain that the timing of starting antiretroviral therapy (ART) has been controversial. Until recently, initiating treatment later in the course of HIV infection, when the CD4+ T-cell count fell below a certain critical level, seemed much wiser than early treatment, especially in view of the toxic side effects associated with the first approved antiretroviral drugs. Today, not only is early treatment advised, but ART also is being used to prevent HIV in HIV-negative people. This preventive treatment is termed preexposure prophylaxis (PrEP), and research reveals that people who took PrEP were 86% less likely to acquire HIV than those who took a placebo.

Another promising finding is the cure of Timothy Ray Brown (1966–). In "I Am the Berlin Patient: A Personal Reflection," an article in *AIDS Research and Human Retroviruses* (vol. 31, no. 1, January 2015), Brown describes how a regimen of ART and two stem-cell transplants to treat leukemia (also called bone marrow transplants, these procedures infuse healthy stem cells into the body to replace diseased bone marrow) resulted in his cure. Nicknamed "the Berlin patient" because he was diagnosed with HIV infection in Berlin, Germany, in 1995, Brown was able to discontinue ART, and his HIV has not returned. In 2012 he started the Timothy Ray Brown Foundation to help work on a cure for HIV.

LYME DISEASE

Spread by the bites of infected deer ticks, Lyme disease is the most commonly reported vector-borne disease in the United States. A vector-borne disease is one in which a disease-causing agent is transmitted from one carrier to another by a third organism. In this case, if a deer tick bites a deer, mouse, or human infected with Lyme disease, and then subsequently feeds on another human, it may transmit the disease. Lyme disease is caused by the *Borrelia burgdorferi* organism and produces early symptoms such as skin rashes, headache, fever, and general illness. Untreated, the disease can progress to tertiary, or chronic, Lyme disease—a persistent inflammatory condition characterized by skin changes, neurological and musculoskeletal symptoms, as well as arthritis and heart damage.

Furthermore, in "Post-treatment Lyme Disease Syndrome Symptomatology and the Impact on Life Functioning: Is There Something Here?" (*Quality of Life Research*, vol. 22, no. 1, February 2013), John N. Aucott et al. report that some patients treated for Lyme disease report persistent or recurring symptoms that have been termed "post-treatment Lyme disease syndrome." The researchers followed 63 patients diagnosed with Lyme disease over a period of six months. The patients underwent physical examinations as well as assessments of their daily life functioning and depression. Aucott et al. found that after treatment, signs of Lyme disease disappeared but new patient-reported symptoms increased or plateaued over time. At six months, 36% of patients reported new-onset fatigue, 20% widespread pain, and 45% problems thinking, concentrating, or reasoning. The researchers considered the possibility that these new symptoms were actually caused by depression. However, because less than 10% of the patients reported more than minimal depression during the study period the researchers reasoned that depression was not the likely cause of the new-onset symptoms.

The CDC began tracking Lyme disease in 1982, and the disease was added to the list of nationally notifiable diseases in 1990. In 2014 the CDC received reports of 25,359 confirmed cases of Lyme disease and 8,102 probable cases, with most cases occurring in northeastern and north-central states. (See Figure 7.3 and Table 7.7.)

The FDA and the CDC warn that people should take precautions against ticks. Wearing long-sleeved shirts and long pants, tucking pant legs into socks, and spraying the skin and/or clothing with tick repellent can keep ticks away from the skin. If a tick is found on the body, it should be removed promptly, and the affected individual should be alert for early symptoms of the disease. Immediate medical care, which consists of antibiotic treatment, is imperative to prevent long-term health damage from Lyme disease.

WEST NILE VIRUS

The West Nile virus (WNV) is common in Africa, West Asia, and the Middle East, and it can infect birds, mosquitoes, horses, humans, and other mammals. It is spread by bites from infected mosquitoes, and although most people who become infected have few or no symptoms, some develop serious and even fatal illnesses. The virus was first reported in the United States in 1999, and the CDC has tracked its westward spread across the United States. The CDC reports that in 2015, WNV caused 1,996 cases of human illness and 111 deaths in the United States. (See Table 7.8.)

FIGURE 7.3

Reported cases of Lyme disease, 1995–2014

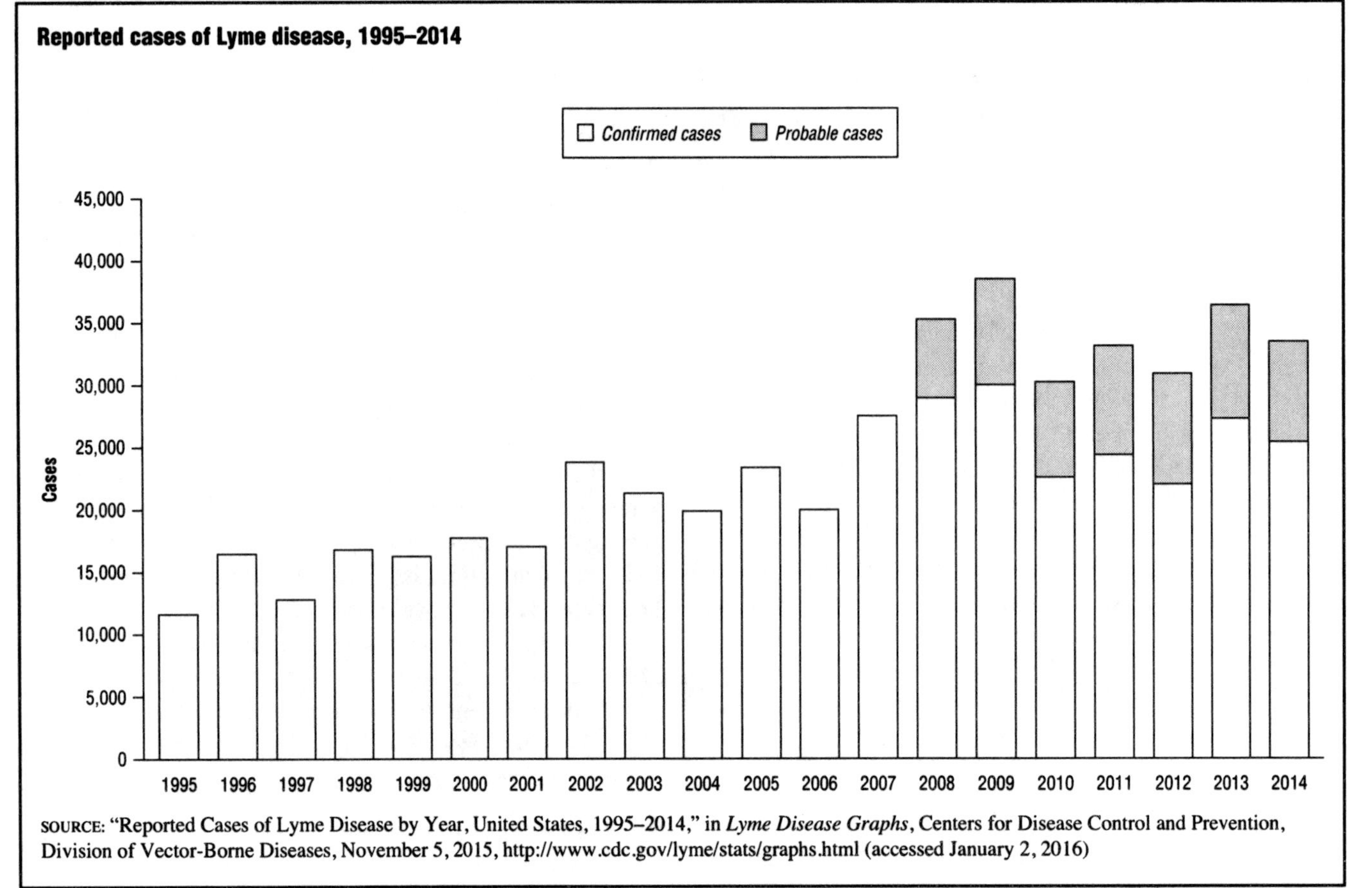

SOURCE: "Reported Cases of Lyme Disease by Year, United States, 1995–2014," in *Lyme Disease Graphs*, Centers for Disease Control and Prevention, Division of Vector-Borne Diseases, November 5, 2015, http://www.cdc.gov/lyme/stats/graphs.html (accessed January 2, 2016)

According to the CDC, the presence of WNV in either humans or infected mosquitoes is permanently established in the United States. Human illness from the virus is relatively rare. The disease is more likely to be fatal in older adults and young children. To avoid contracting West Nile virus, the CDC advises taking precautions against mosquito bites. These include: using insect repellent; wearing long pants and long-sleeved shirts that are treated with insect repellent; remaining indoors during dawn, dusk, and early evening, the hours when mosquitoes are the most likely to bite; and removing standing water to prevent mosquitoes from laying eggs and breeding near homes and other populated areas.

SEVERE ACUTE RESPIRATORY SYNDROME

In "Frequently Asked Questions about SARS" (July 2, 2012, http://www.cdc.gov/sars/about/faq.html), the CDC explains that severe acute respiratory syndrome (SARS) is a viral respiratory illness caused by a coronavirus that was first reported in southern China in November 2002. The illness spread to more than 24 countries in North America, South America, Europe, and Asia before the global outbreak was contained in July 2003. SARS seems to be transmitted primarily by person-to-person contact through respiratory droplets, which travel via coughs or sneezes to the mucous membranes of other people or to surfaces that others touch. Symptoms of the disease may include high fever, body aches, malaise (overall discomfort), diarrhea, and mild respiratory symptoms. After two to seven days the infected person may develop a dry cough and/or difficulty breathing. As many as 20% of infected individuals require mechanical ventilation, and some die.

The CDC reports in "SARS News and Alerts Archive" (December 15, 2011, http://www.cdc.gov/sars/media/index.html) that there has been no known SARS transmission anywhere in the world since April 2004; as of March 2016, this situation remained unchanged. The WHO notes in "Cumulative Number of Reported Probable Cases of Severe Acute Respiratory Syndrome" (2012, http://www.who.int/csr/sars/country/en/index.html) that by the time SARS had run its course a total of 8,096 people were known to have been infected, of whom 774 died. Just 27 cases were reported in the United States, and there were no U.S. SARS-related deaths.

ZIKA VIRUS OUTBREAK

Like West Nile virus, the Zika virus is spread via mosquito bites, and its symptoms include fever, rash, joint pain, and conjunctivitis (red eyes). It was first identified in Uganda in the late 1940s and has occurred in human outbreaks since the 1950s in tropical areas such as Africa,

TABLE 7.7

Reported cases of Lyme disease by state, 2005–14

[Confirmed cases presented for all years except most recent]

										2014		
State	**2005**	**2006**	**2007**	**2008**	**2009**	**2010**	**2011**	**2012**	**2013**	**Confirmed**	**Probable**	**Incidence***
Alabama	3	11	13	6	3	1	9	13	11	28	36	0.6
Alaska	4	3	10	6	7	7	9	4	14	5	3	0.7
Arizona	10	10	2	2	3	2	8	7	22	14	7	0.2
Arkansas	0	0	1	0	0	0	0	0	0	0	0	0.0
California	95	85	75	74	117	126	79	61	90	54	19	0.1
Colorado	0	0	0	2	0	1	0	0	0	0	0	0.0
Connecticut	1,810	1,788	3,058	2,738	2,751	1,964	2,004	1,653	2,111	1,719	641	47.8
Delaware	646	482	715	772	984	656	767	507	400	341	76	36.4
DC	10	62	116	71	53	34	N	N	33	35	5	5.3
Florida	47	34	30	72	77	56	78	67	87	85	70	0.4
Georgia	6	8	11	35	40	10	32	31	8	4	0	0.0
Hawaii	0	0	0	0	0	0	0	0	0	0	0	0.0
Idaho	2	7	9	5	4	6	3	0	14	8	1	0.5
Illinois	127	110	149	108	136	135	194	204	337	233	0	1.8
Indiana	33	26	55	42	61	62	81	64	101	100	10	1.5
Iowa	89	97	123	85	77	68	72	92	153	110	84	3.5
Kansas	3	4	8	16	18	7	11	9	18	12	8	0.4
Kentucky	5	7	6	5	1	5	3	8	17	11	33	0.2
Louisiana	3	1	2	3	0	2	1	3	0	0	2	0.0
Maine	247	338	529	780	791	559	801	885	1,127	1,169	232	87.9
Maryland	1,235	1,248	2,576	1,746	1,466	1,163	938	1,113	801	957	416	16.0
Massachusetts	2,336	1,432	2,988	3,960	4,019	2,380	1,801	3,396	3,816	3,646	1,658	54.1
Michigan	62	55	51	76	81	76	89	80	114	93	34	0.9
Minnesota	917	914	1,238	1,046	1,063	1,293	1,185	911	1,431	896	520	16.4
Mississippi	0	3	1	1	0	0	3	1	0	2	0	0.1
Missouri	15	5	10	6	3	4	5	1	1	7	3	0.1
Montana	0	1	4	6	3	3	9	6	16	5	2	0.5
Nebraska	2	11	7	8	4	7	7	5	7	6	1	0.3
Nevada	3	4	15	9	10	2	3	10	11	4	2	0.1
New Hampshire	265	617	896	1,211	996	830	887	1,002	1,324	622	102	46.9
New Jersey	3,363	2,432	3,134	3,214	4,598	3,320	3,398	2,732	2,785	2,589	697	29.0
New Mexico	3	3	5	4	1	3	2	1	0	0	0	0.0
New York	5,565	4,460	4,165	5,741	4,134	2,385	3,118	2,044	3,512	2,853	883	14.4
North Carolina	49	31	53	16	21	21	18	27	39	27	143	0.3
North Dakota	3	7	12	8	10	21	22	10	12	2	12	0.3
Ohio	58	43	33	40	51	21	36	49	74	94	25	0.8
Oklahoma	0	0	1	1	2	0	2	1	1	0	0	0.0
Oregon	3	7	6	18	12	7	9	5	12	3	42	0.1
Pennsylvania	4,287	3,242	3,994	3,818	4,950	3,298	4,739	4,146	4,981	6,470	1,017	50.6
Rhode Island	39	308	177	186	150	115	111	133	444	570	334	54.0
South Carolina	15	20	31	14	25	19	24	35	33	20	17	0.4
South Dakota	2	1	0	3	1	1	2	4	3	2	0	0.2
Tennessee	8	15	31	7	10	6	5	2	11	7	10	0.1
Texas	69	29	87	105	88	55	28	33	48	20	20	0.1
Utah	2	5	7	3	6	3	6	2	10	5	8	0.2
Vermont	54	105	138	330	323	271	476	386	674	442	157	70.5
Virginia	274	357	959	886	698	911	756	805	925	976	370	11.7
Washington	13	8	12	22	15	12	17	13	11	8	7	0.1
West Virginia	61	28	84	120	143	128	107	82	116	112	24	6.1
Wisconsin	1,459	1,466	1,814	1,493	1,952	2,505	2,408	1,368	1,447	991	370	17.2
Wyoming	3	1	3	1	1	0	1	3	1	2	1	0.3
U.S. total	**23,305**	**19,931**	**27,444**	**28,921**	**29,959**	**22,561**	**24,364**	**22,014**	**27,203**	**25,359**	**8,102**	**7.9**

*Confirmed cases per 100,000 population.
N = not notifiable.

SOURCE: "Reported Cases of Lyme Disease by State or Locality, 2005–2014," in *Lyme Disease Data Tables*, Centers for Disease Control and Prevention, Division of Vector-Borne Diseases, November 9, 2015, http://www.cdc.gov/lyme/stats/tables.html (accessed January 2, 2016)

Southeast Asia, and the Pacific Islands. The Zika virus can spread from a pregnant woman to her fetus and has been linked with serious birth defects affecting vision, hearing, and the development of the brain structures. Of particular concern is a link between maternal Zika virus disease and microcephaly, a birth defect in which an infant's head is much smaller than expected, and thus the growth and development of the brain are also negatively affected.

The CDC notes in "Symptoms, Diagnosis, & Treatment" (March 11, 2016, http://www.cdc.gov/zika/symptoms/index.html) that the illness caused by the Zika virus is generally mild, lasting up to one week and rarely requires hospitalization. However, there is no treatment for Zika virus infections, nor is there a vaccine to prevent them. The CDC reports in "Zika Virus Disease in the United States, 2015–2016" (March 16,

TABLE 7.8

West Nile virus cases, by state, 2015

[Confirmed and probable cases]

State	Neuroinvasive disease cases[a]	Non-neuroinvasive disease cases	Total cases	Deaths
Alabama	5	5	10	0
Arizona	57	35	92	6
Arkansas	16	2	18	1
California	505	176	681	42
Colorado	57	44	101	2
Connecticut	8	2	10	0
Delaware	0	2	2	0
District of Columbia	2	2	4	0
Florida	10	0	10	1
Georgia	13	2	15	0
Idaho	5	8	13	0
Illinois	42	28	70	7
Indiana	16	5	21	3
Iowa	4	10	14	0
Kansas	12	21	33	2
Kentucky	0	0	0	0
Louisiana	36	7	43	4
Maine	1	0	1	0
Maryland	31	15	46	5
Massachusetts	6	3	9	2
Michigan	16	2	18	2
Minnesota	2	4	6	0
Mississippi	26	13	39	1
Missouri	18	10	28	3
Montana	2	1	3	0
Nebraska	17	51	68	2
Nevada	4	3	7	0
New Jersey	22	3	25	2
New Mexico	12	2	14	1
New York	37	15	52	1
North Carolina	4	0	4	1
North Dakota	10	13	23	1
Ohio	23	12	35	2
Oklahoma	47	40	87	7
Oregon	1	0	1	0
Pennsylvania	17	13	30	1
South Carolina	0	0	0	0
South Dakota	11	29	40	0
Tennessee	5	1	6	0
Texas	178	70	248	9
Utah	5	3	8	0
Virginia	14	7	21	1
Washington	8	16	24	1
Wisconsin	4	4	8	1
Wyoming	3	5	8	0
Total	**1,312**	**684**	**1,996**	**111**

[a]Includes cases reported as meningitis, encephalitis, or acute flaccid paralysis.

SOURCE: Adapted from "West Nile Virus Disease Cases and Presumptive Viremic Blood Donors by State—United States, 2015 (as of December 16, 2015)," in "West Nile Virus," Centers for Disease Control and Prevention, Division of Vector-Borne Diseases, December 17, 2015, http://www.cdc.gov/westnile/statsMaps/preliminaryMapsData/histatedate.html (accessed January 4, 2016)

2016, http://www.cdc.gov/zika/geo/united-states.html) that as of March 2016 all 258 cases in the United States had been traced to travelers returning from countries with evidence of past or current virus transmission. These include countries in Central and South America, Africa, Southeast Asia, and the Pacific Islands. As of March 2016 the U.S. territories of American Samoa, Puerto Rico, and U.S. Virgin Islands had confirmed a total of 286 cases, of which three were associated with travel, and 283 had been locally acquired. The disease was added to the list of nationally notifiable diseases in January 2016.

RESPONDING TO BIOLOGIC TERRORISM: INTENTIONAL EPIDEMICS

In September and October 2001, in an unprecedented event, 22 letters containing *Bacillus anthracis* spores that were sent through the U.S. Postal Service caused anthrax outbreaks in seven states. Five of the letters resulted in fatal cases of anthrax.

Anthony S. Fauci (1940–), the director of the NIAID, states in "The Power of Biomedical Research" (WashingtonTimes.com, July 8, 2003) that these anthrax attacks "starkly exposed the vulnerability of the United States—and, indeed, the rest of the world—to bioterrorism." Accordingly, the NIAID devotes considerable attention to accelerated programs to prevent, diagnose, and treat possible bioterrorist attacks. The NIAID explains in "NIAID Emerging Infectious Diseases/Pathogens" (January 25, 2016, http://www.niaid.nih.gov/topics/BiodefenseRelated/Biodefense/Pages/CatA.aspx) that its biodefense research program prioritizes pathogens. Priority A pathogens pose the greatest threat to national security and public health because they "can be easily disseminated or transmitted from person to person; result in high mortality rates and have the potential for major public health impact; might cause public panic and social disruption; and require special action for public health preparedness." Priority A pathogens include anthrax, botulism, plague and smallpox.

The NIAID asserts in "Biodefense and Emerging Infectious Diseases Questions and Answers" October 28, 2011, https://www.niaid.nih.gov/topics/biodefenserelated/biodefense/Pages/qanda.aspx) that "overall, the United States is much better prepared to respond to an infectious disease threat today than it was [in 2001] in part because of the strong investment in basic and applied research, product development, and technology development for biodefense and emerging infectious diseases." For example, in "NIAID Accomplishments in Biodefense and Emerging Infectious Diseases Research," (March 17, 2014, http://www.niaid.nih.gov/topics/BiodefenseRelated/Biodefense/Pages/accomplishments.aspx), the NIAID reports that for anthrax, in addition to supporting vaccine trials in conjunction with HHS Biomedical Advanced Research and Development Authority, it is supporting development of antibody-based therapeutics as anthrax antitoxins to treat patients with anthrax disease.

Collaboration between public health and law enforcement also strengthens bioterrorism investigations and preparation for a biological threat. In the *Joint Criminal and Epidemiological Investigations Handbook* (2015, https://www.fbi.gov/about-us/investigate/terrorism/wmd/criminal-and-epidemiological-investigation-handbook),

TABLE 7.9

Actions and events that may trigger joint public health and law enforcement investigations

- Any specimens (clinical) or samples (environmental) submitted to public health for analysis that test positive for a potential biological threat-related agent
- Large numbers of patients with similar symptoms or disease
- Large numbers of unexplained symptoms, diseases, or deaths
- Disease with an unusual geographic or seasonal distribution (e.g., plague in a non-endemic area)
- Unusual disease presentation (e.g., inhalational vs. cutaneous anthrax)
- Endemic disease with unexplained increase in incidence (e.g., tularemia, plague)
- Higher than expected morbidity and mortality associated with a common disease and/or failure of patients to respond to traditional therapy
- Unusual "typical patient" distribution (i.e., several adults with an unexplained rash)
- Death or illness in humans preceded or accompanied by death or illness in animals that is unexplained or attributed to a zoonotic biological agent
- Any intelligence or indication that any individual or group is unlawfully in possession of any biological agent
- Seizure of bio-processing equipment from any individual, group, or organization
- Seizure of potential dissemination devices from any individual, group, or organization
- Identification or seizure of literature pertaining to the development or dissemination of biological agents
- Any assessments that indicate a credible biological threat exists in an area
- A HAZMAT response that involves the presence of biological agents

SOURCE: Adapted from "Table 2. Public Health Triggers," and "Table 3. Law Enforcement Triggers," in *Joint Criminal and Epidemiological Investigations Handbook: 2015 Domestic Edition*, Centers for Disease Control and Prevention and FBI, WMD Directorate, Biological Countermeasures Unit, 2015, https://www.fbi.gov/about-us/investigate/terrorism/wmd/criminal-and-epidemiological-investigation-handbook (accessed January 4, 2016)

the CDC and Federal Bureau of Investigation explain that they share common goals and, by working together on joint investigations, they can more efficiently respond to a threat, outbreak, or attack. Table 7.9 lists examples of activities and events that may trigger public health and law enforcement agencies to join forces to investigate or counter an emerging threat to public health and safety.

CHAPTER 8
MENTAL HEALTH AND ILLNESS

Mental health can be measured in terms of an individual's ability to think and communicate clearly, to learn and grow emotionally, to deal productively and realistically with change and stress, and to form and maintain fulfilling relationships with others. Mental health is a principal component of wellness. Self-esteem, resilience, and the ability to cope with adversity influence how people feel about themselves and whether they choose lifestyles and behaviors that promote or jeopardize their health.

Mental illness refers to all identifiable mental health disorders and mental health problems. In the landmark study *Mental Health: A Report of the Surgeon General* (1999, http://profiles.nlm.nih.gov/ps/access/NNBBHS.pdf), the Office of the Surgeon General defines mental disorders as "health conditions that are characterized by alterations in thinking, mood, or behavior (or some combination thereof) associated with distress and/or impaired functioning." The surgeon general distinguishes mental disorders from mental problems, describing the signs and symptoms of mental health problems as less intense and of shorter duration than those of mental health disorders. The report, however, acknowledges that both mental health disorders and problems may be distressing and disabling.

The symptoms of mental disorders differentiate one type of problem from another; however, the symptoms of mental illness vary far more widely in both type and intensity than do the symptoms of most physical illnesses. In general, people are usually considered mentally healthy if they are able to maintain their mental and emotional balance in times of crisis and stress and to cope effectively with the problems of daily life. When their coping ability is lost, then there is some degree of mental dysfunction. The goals of diagnosis and treatment of mental disorders are to recognize and understand the conditions, to reduce their underlying causes, and to work toward regaining mental and emotional equilibrium.

HOW MANY PEOPLE ARE MENTALLY ILL?

It is complicated to determine how many people suffer from mental illness due to changing definitions of mental illness and the difficulties in classifying, diagnosing, and reporting mental disorders. Various agencies and organizations attempt to assess the prevalence of mental illness using a variety of survey instruments and methodologies. Table 8.1 shows the surveys and surveillance systems used by the Centers for Disease Control and Prevention (CDC) to collect data about mental illness among adults.

Other factors hinder data collection. There are social stigmas attached to mental illness, such as being labeled "crazy," being treated as a danger to others, or being denied a job, that keep some sufferers from seeking help, and many of those in treatment do not reveal it on surveys. Some people do not realize that their symptoms are caused by mental disorders. Because knowledge about the way the brain works is relatively narrow, mental health professionals must continually reassess how mental illnesses are defined and diagnosed. In addition, what might be considered, for example, delusional thinking in one culture may well be completely acceptable in another. The symptoms of mental illness are notoriously fluid, and diagnosis may be skewed by cultural differences or other biases on the part of both patient and practitioner.

In Healthy People 2020 (March 17, 2016, https://www.healthypeople.gov/2020/leading-health-indicators/2020-lhi-topics/Mental-Health/determinants), a set of 10-year national objectives for improving the health of Americans, the Office of Disease Prevention and Health Promotion estimates that 26% of Americans aged 18 years and older are living with a mental health disorder in any given year, and nearly half (46%) will have a mental health disorder at some point during their lifetime.

TABLE 8.1

Centers for Disease Control and Prevention surveys and surveillance systems that collect data on mental illness among adults

Name, website, and CDC sponsor	Description	Method of data collection	Survey topics	Mental health topics and questions	Population
Behavioral Risk Factor Surveillance System (BRFSS) http://www.cdc.gov/brfss Public Health Surveillance Program Office	BRFSS is a state-based system of health surveys that collects information on health-risk behaviors, preventive health practices, and health-care access primarily related to chronic disease and injury. For many states, BRFSS is the only available source of timely, accurate data on health-related behaviors.	Telephone interviews	Heath-risk behaviors Preventive health practices Health-care access Health-related quality of life Mental illness screening Disability Violence	Anxiety and depression module (PHQ-8, lifetime diagnosis of anxiety and depression) Mental illness and stigma module (K-6, stigma, mental health treatment, and mental illness-related disability) Health-related quality of life (number of days in past 30 days respondent felt that mental health was not good, felt depressed, felt anxious, felt not getting enough sleep, and felt full of energy) Life satisfaction Social support Smoking, alcohol use, physical activity, and body mass index Health-care use and access Sexual and intimate partner violence	National sample of one person (aged ≥18 years) from each household Approximately 450,000 completed interviews, as of 2010
National Health Interview Survey (NHIS) http://www.cdc.gov/nchs/nhis.htm National Center for Health Statistics	NHIS is a national survey on the health of the civilian noninstitutionalized U.S. population. The main objective of NHIS is to monitor the health of the U.S. population through the collection and analysis of data on a broad range of health topics.	In-person household interviews	Health status and limitations Health-care use Family resources Health insurance Health-care access Vaccination Injury Health behaviors Functioning Disability	Activity limitations from physical, mental, or emotional problems External causes and circumstances of injury Mental health-care use Mental health conditions and symptoms (in 2007 survey), including ADHD; schizophrenia; bipolar disorder; depression, anxiety, and emotional problems; dementia and senility; mental retardation; learning disabilities; and general distress symptoms Health-risk behaviors (including tobacco use and alcohol use) K-6 measure of serious psychological distress	Approximately 40,000 households per year, as of 2010 Oversample of blacks, Hispanics, Asians, and adults aged ≥65 years
National Health and Nutrition Examination Survey (NHANES) http://www.cdc.gov/nchs/nhanes.htm National Center for Health Statistics	NHANES is designed to assess the health and nutritional status of adults and children in the United States. The survey combines interviews and physical examinations.	In-person household interviews Physical examinations Laboratory tests Nutritional assessments DNA repository	Numerous diseases, medical conditions, and health indicators Nutrition and nutritional disorders Environmental risk factors Health-care use Mental, behavioral, and emotional problems of children Weight and physical fitness Risk factors	Sleep disorders Alcohol and drug use Social and emotional support Use of mental health-care professionals Activity limitations from poor physical or mental health PHQ-9 depression screening	Approximately 5,000 persons per year, as of 2008 Oversample of blacks, Mexican-Americans, adolescents, and adults aged ≥60 years

TABLE 8.1

Centers for Disease Control and Prevention surveys and surveillance systems that collect data on mental illness among adults [CONTINUED]

Name, website, and CDC sponsor	Description	Method of data collection	Survey topics	Mental health topics and questions	Population
Pregnancy Risk Assessment Monitoring System (PRAMS) http://www.cdc.gov/prams National Center for Chronic Disease Prevention and Health Promotion, Division of Reproductive Health	PRAMS is a surveillance project of CDC and state health departments. PRAMS collects state-specific, population-based data on maternal attitudes and experiences before, during, and shortly after pregnancy.	Mailed surveys with follow-up telephone interviews for nonresponders	Postpartum depressive symptoms Attitudes and feelings about most recent pregnancy Prenatal care Maternal alcohol and tobacco use HIV testing Health insurance coverage Physical abuse before and during pregnancy Pregnancy-related morbidity Infant health care Contraceptive use Breastfeeding practices Health-care provider advice	Whether health-care provider discussed with respondent healthy and risky pregnancy behaviors (including drinking alcohol and smoking during pregnancy) Maternal tobacco and alcohol use before, during, and after pregnancy Difficult or traumatic events before or during pregnancy Pregnancy intention, both of mother and of partner Whether respondent needed and received counseling for substance use or personal problems during or after pregnancy Interpersonal violence before and during pregnancy Injury control and prevention Social support and stress Infant sleeping behaviors Infant and maternal exposure to smoke Feelings, diagnosis, and treatment of postpartum depression, hopelessness, and anxiety	Approximately 50,000 women with live-born infants per year, as of 2008
National Ambulatory Medical Care Survey (NAMCS) http://www.cdc.gov/nchs/ahcd.htm National Center for Health Statistics	NAMCS is a national survey that collects data on the provision and use of ambulatory medical care services in the United States. Findings are based on a sample of visits to nonfederal, employed, office-based physicians who are primarily engaged in direct patient care.	Patient record forms completed by physicians and staff members or survey field representatives	Demographic characteristics of patients Expected payment sources Patients' principal complaints, symptoms, or other reasons for visit Physician diagnoses, diagnostic and screening services Medications Types of health-care providers seen during visit Disposition Causes of injury (if applicable)	Current diagnosed mental health conditions Current depression Cause of injury (including intentional) Health education services ordered or provided at visit (including injury prevention, stress management, and tobacco use and exposure) Nonmedication treatment provided at visit (including psychotherapy and mental health counseling) Type of health-care providers patient visited or was referred to during visit (including providers of mental health services) Medications	Office-based physicians and then visits within the practices. In 2007, data were provided on 32,778 visits.

TABLE 8.1

Centers for Disease Control and Prevention surveys and surveillance systems that collect data on mental illness among adults [CONTINUED]

Name, website, and CDC sponsor	Description	Method of data collection	Survey topics	Mental health topics and questions	Population
National Hospital Ambulatory Medical Care Survey (NHAMCS) http://www.cdc.gov/nchs/ahcd.htm National Center for Health Statistics	NHAMCS is designed to collect data on the use and provision of ambulatory care services in hospital emergency and outpatient departments. Findings are based on a national sample of visits to the emergency departments and outpatient departments of noninstitutional general and short-stay hospitals.	Patient record forms completed by hospital physicians and staff members	Demographic characteristics of patients Expected payment sources Patients' principal complaints, symptoms, or other reasons for visit Physician diagnoses, diagnostic and screening services Procedures (emergency department only) Medications Disposition Types of health-care providers seen during visit Causes of injury (if applicable)	**Emergency department:** Patients' principal complaints, symptoms, or other reasons for visit Causes of injury (including intentional) Health-care provider diagnoses Medications Mental health providers seen during visit Transfer to psychiatric hospital Admission to mental health or detoxification unit **Outpatient department:** Current diagnosed mental health conditions Current depression Cause of injury (including intentional) Health education services ordered or provided at visit (including injury prevention, stress management, and tobacco use and exposure) Nonmedication treatment provided at visit (including psychotherapy and mental health counseling) Type of health-care providers patient visited or was referred to during visit (including providers of mental health services) Medications	Nationally representative sample of 500 nonfederal short-stay (<30 days) hospitals
National Hospital Discharge Survey (NHDS) http://www.cdc.gov/nchs/nhds.htm National Center for Health Statistics	NHDS is a national probability survey of characteristics of inpatients discharged from nonfederal short-stay hospitals in the United States.	Medical record abstraction	Demographic characteristics of patients Expected sources of payment Type and source of admission Disposition Discharge diagnoses (up to seven) Surgical and diagnostic procedures (up to four)	Discharge diagnoses (up to seven) Surgical and diagnostic procedures (up to four)	Nationally representative sample of nonfederal short-stay hospitals and systematic samples of discharges within hospitals

TABLE 8.1

Centers for Disease Control and Prevention surveys and surveillance systems that collect data on mental illness among adults [CONTINUED]

Name, website, and CDC sponsor	Description	Method of data collection	Survey topics	Mental health topics and questions	Population
National Nursing Home Survey (NNHS) http://www.cdc.gov/nchs/nnhs.htm National Center for Health Statistics	NNHS is a continuing series of national sample surveys of nursing homes and their residents and staff members.	Interviews with staff member best acquainted with resident medical records	Demographic characteristics of patients Admitting diagnosis Current diagnoses (up to 16) Health status Activities of daily living Vision and hearing Continence Pain assessment Behavior Mood Medications Falls Services received Sources of payment	Behavioral problems Depressed mood Medications Admitting diagnosis Current diagnoses (up to 16) Current assignment to specialty unit (i.e., dementia or behavioral health) Decision-making ability	Sample of nursing homes (that had at least three beds and were either certified by Medicare or Medicaid or had a state license to operate as a nursing home) and then sample of residents within nursing homes

Notes: ADHD = Attention Deficit Hyperactivity Disorder; HIV = Human Immunodeficiency Virus; K-6 = Kessler-6; PHQ-8 = Patient Health Questionnaire-8; PHQ-9 = Patient Health Questionnaire-9. CDC = Centers for Disease Control and Prevention.

SOURCE: William C. Reeves et al., "CDC Surveys and Surveillance Systems That Collect Data on Mental Illness among Adults," in "Mental Illness Surveillance among Adults in the United States," *Morbidity and Mortality Weekly Report*, suppl. vol. 60, September 2, 2011, http://www.cdc.gov/mmwr/pdf/other/su6003.pdf (accessed January 4, 2016)

How Many Children Suffer from Mental Illness?

Data describing the prevalence of mental disorders in children vary. Ruth Perou et al. estimate in "Mental Health Surveillance among Children—United States, 2005–2011" (*Morbidity and Mortality Weekly Report*, vol. 62, no. 1, May 17, 2013) that between 13% and 20% of children experience a mental disorder, described as "serious deviations from expected cognitive, social, and emotional development," each year and the prevalence of mental disorders in children appears to be increasing.

Attention-deficit/hyperactivity disorder (ADHD) involves problems concentrating, focusing, and paying attention, coupled with excessive restlessness and movement; it was the most frequently reported disorder (6.8%) among children aged three to 17 years. ADHD was followed by behavioral or conduct problems (3.5%), anxiety (3%), depression (2.1%), autism spectrum disorders (developmental disabilities that can cause significant social, communication, and behavioral challenges, 1.1%), and Tourette syndrome (a neurological disorder characterized by repetitive, stereotyped, involuntary movements and vocalizations called tics, 0.2% among children and teens aged six to 17 years).

Nearly 5% of adolescents aged 12 to 17 years reported a drug use disorder, and 4.2% had an alcohol abuse disorder in the past year; 2.8% had cigarette dependence in the past month. About 8% of adolescents aged 12 to 17 years reported 14 or more mentally unhealthy days in the past month. In 2010 the suicide rate for youth aged 10 to 19 years was 4.5 suicides per 100,000 young people.

The Federal Interagency Forum on Child and Family Statistics, a continuing, national survey that is conducted by a consortium of 22 federal government agencies, publishes the annual report *America's Children: Key National Indicators of Well-Being, 2015*. The report notes that in 2013 roughly 5% of children aged four to 17 years reportedly had "serious difficulties with emotions, concentration, behavior, or being able to get along with other people."

Many mental disorders that begin during childhood and adolescence recur or continue into adulthood. Children and teens with mood and anxiety disorders suffer from unfounded fears, prolonged sadness or tearfulness, withdrawal, low self-esteem, and feelings of worthlessness and hopelessness. These children and adolescents often suffer from more than one mental health problem (e.g., symptoms of depression and anxiety together). In 2013 the percentage of adolescents aged 12 to 17 years that had a major depressive episode (defined as a period of at least two weeks of depressed mood or loss of interest or pleasure in daily activities plus at least four additional symptoms of depression such as problems with sleeping, eating, energy, concentration, and feelings of self-worth) was 11%. (See Figure 8.1.) The prevalence of major depressive

FIGURE 8.1

Percentage of youth aged 12–17 who experienced a major depressive episode in the past year, by age and sex, 2004–13

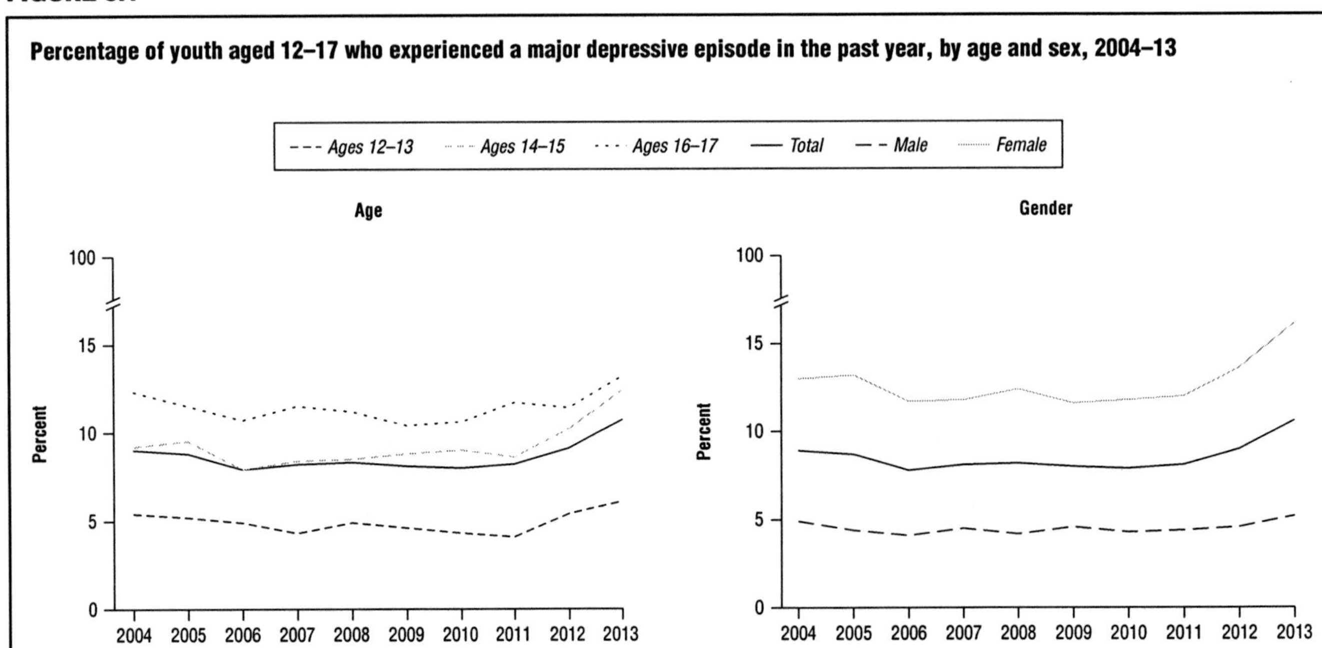

Note: A major depressive episode is defined as a period of at least 2 weeks when a person experienced a depressed mood or loss of interest or pleasure in daily activities plus at least four additional symptoms of depression (such as problems with sleep, eating, energy, concentration, and feelings of self-worth) as described in the fourth edition of the Diagnostic and Statistical Manual of Mental Disorders (DSM-IV).

SOURCE: "Indicator HEALTH4. Percentage of Youth Ages 12–17 Who Experienced a Major Depressive Episode (MDE) in the Past Year by Age and Gender, 2004–2013," in *America's Children: Key National Indicators of Well-Being, 2015*, Federal Interagency Forum on Child and Family Statistics, July 2015, (accessed January 4, 2016)

episode was more than twice as high among girls and higher in older teens than in younger ones.

Some Americans Experience Serious Mental Distress

The National Health Interview Survey (NHIS) poses questions about psychological distress. These questions ask how often a respondent experienced certain symptoms of psychological distress during the 30 days preceding the survey. In the first half of 2015 about 3.4% of adults aged 18 years and older said they had experienced serious psychological distress during the past 30 days. Figure 8.2 shows that the percentage of adults reporting serious psychological distress during the past 30 days was lowest in 1999 (2.4%), rose to 3.4% in 2011 and remained above 3% in 2015.

In surveys conducted between January and June 2015, people aged 45 to 64 years (3.9%) were more likely than people aged 18 to 44 years (3.4%) or 65 years and older (2.5%) to report having experienced serious psychological distress during the 30 days preceding the survey. (See Figure 8.3.) Among people in all age groups, women were more likely than men to report serious psychological distress during the 30 days preceding the survey.

The percentage of adults in the first half of 2015 that experienced serious psychological distress during the 30 days preceding the survey varied by ethnicity. Hispanics were more likely than non-Hispanic whites or non-Hispanic African Americans to report such distress. The age-sex-adjusted prevalence of serious psychological distress was 4.5% for Hispanics, and 3.3% each for non-Hispanic whites and non-Hispanic African Americans. (See Figure 8.4.)

Not All People Need or Seek Treatment

The National Institute of Mental Health (NIMH) observes that not all mental disorders require treatment because many people with mental disorders have relatively brief, self-limiting illnesses that are not disabling enough to warrant treatment. However, in "Service Utilization for Lifetime Mental Disorders in U.S. Adolescents: Results of the National Comorbidity Survey-Adolescent Supplement" (*Journal of the American Academy of Child and Adolescent Psychiatry*, vol. 50, no. 1, January 2011), Kathleen Ries Merikangas et al. report that between 2002 and 2004 just over one-third (36.2%) of adolescents with mental disorders received treatment. Although the likelihood of receiving treatment rose with increasing severity of the disorder, 50% of adolescents with "severely impairing mental disorders had never received mental health treatment for their symptoms." Adolescents with ADHD (59.8%) and behavior disorders (45.4%; inappropriate behaviors that sharply deviate from accepted norms) were the most likely to receive treatment. African American and Hispanic youth were

FIGURE 8.2

Percentage of adults aged 18 and older who experienced serious psychological distress during the previous 30 days, 1997–2015

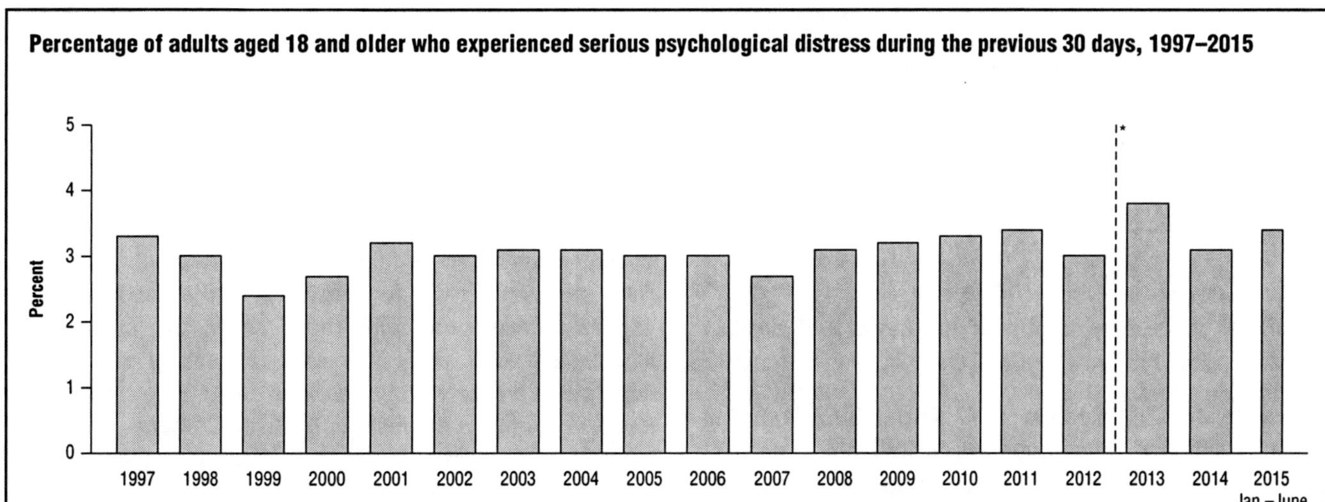

*In 2013, the six psychological distress questions were moved to the Adult Selected Items section of the Sample Adult questionnaire. This change is indicated by a dashed line in the figure. Differences observed in estimates based on the 2012 and earlier National Health Interview Survey (NHIS) and the 2013 and later NHIS may be partially or fully attributable to this change in placement of the six psychological distress questions on the NHIS questionnaire. Due to the higher than usual amount of missing data in the Adult Selected Items section, adults with missing data for any of the six psychological distress questions are excluded from the calculation of the serious psychological distress indicator for 2013 and later.

Notes: Data are based on household interviews of a sample of the civilian noninstitutionalized population. Six psychological distress questions are included in the Sample Adult Core component of the NHIS. These questions ask how often a respondent experienced certain symptoms of psychological distress during the past 30 days. The response codes (0–4) of the six items for each person are summed to yield a scale with a 0–24 range. A value of 13 or more for this scale is used here to define serious psychological distress (9). The analyses excluded those with unknown serious psychological distress status (about 3% of respondents in 2013 and later).

SOURCE: "Figure 13.1. Percentage of Adults Aged 18 Years and over Who Experienced Serious Psychological Distress during the Past 30 Days: United States, 1997–June 2015," in *Early Release of Selected Estimates Based on Data from the January–June 2015 National Health Interview Survey*, Centers for Disease Control and Prevention, National Center for Health Statistics, November 2015, http://www.cdc.gov/nchs/data/nhis/earlyrelease/earlyrelease201511_13.pdf (accessed January 4, 2016)

FIGURE 8.3

Percentage of adults aged 18 and older who experienced serious psychological distress during the previous 30 days, by age group and sex, January–June 2015

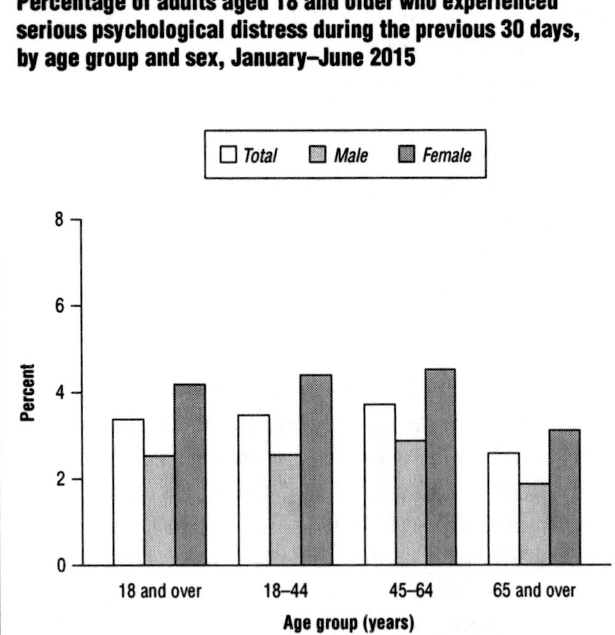

Notes: Data are based on household interviews of a sample of the civilian noninstitutionalized population. Six psychological distress questions are included in the Sample Adult Core component of the National Health Interview Survey (NHIS). These questions ask how often a respondent experienced certain symptoms of psychological distress during the past 30 days. The response codes (0–4) of the six items for each person are summed to yield a scale with a 0–24 range. A value of 13 or more for this scale is used here to define serious psychological distress (9). In 2013, the six psychological distress questions were moved to the Adult Selected Items section of the Sample Adult questionnaire. Differences observed in estimates based on the 2012 and earlier NHIS and the 2013 and later NHIS may be partially or fully attributable to this change in placement of the six psychological distress questions on the NHIS questionnaire. The analyses excluded the 4.0% of persons with unknown serious psychological distress status.

SOURCE: "Figure 13.2. Percentage of Adults Aged 18 Years and over Who Experienced Serious Psychological Distress during the Past 30 Days, by Age Group and Sex: United States, January–June 2015," in *Early Release of Selected Estimates Based on Data from the January–June 2015 National Health Interview Survey*, Centers for Disease Control and Prevention, National Center for Health Statistics, November 2015, http://www.cdc.gov/nchs/data/nhis/earlyrelease/earlyrelease201511_13.pdf (accessed January 4, 2016)

FIGURE 8.4

Age-sex-adjusted percentage of adults aged 18 and older who experienced serious psychological distress during the previous 30 days, by race/ethnicity, January–June 2015

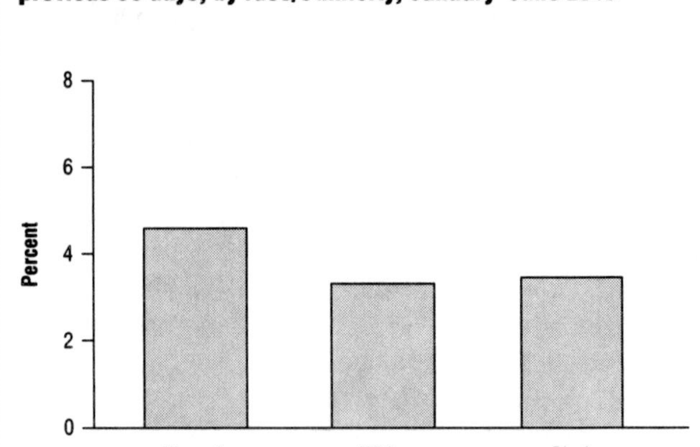

Notes: Data are based on household interviews of a sample of the civilian noninstitutionalized population. Six psychological distress questions are included in the Sample Adult Core component of the National Health Interview Survey (NHIS). These questions ask how often a respondent experienced certain symptoms of psychological distress during the past 30 days. The response codes (0–4) of the six items for each person are summed to yield a scale with a 0–24 range. A value of 13 or more for this scale is used here to define serious psychological distress (9). In 2013 the six psychological distress questions were moved to the Adult Selected Items section of the Sample Adult questionnaire. Differences observed in estimates based on the 2012 and earlier NHIS and the 2013 and later NHIS may be partially or fully attributable to this change in placement of the six psychological distress questions on the NHIS questionnaire. Estimates are age-sex adjusted using the projected 2000 U.S. population as the standard population and using three age groups: 18–44, 45–64, and 65 and over. The analyses excluded the 4.0% of persons with unknown serious psychological distress status.

SOURCE: "Figure 13.3. Age-Sex-Adjusted Percentage of Adults Aged 18 Years and over Who Experienced Serious Psychological Distress during the Past 30 Days, by Race/Ethnicity: United States, January–June 2015," in *Early Release of Selected Estimates Based on Data from the January–June 2015 National Health Interview Survey*, Centers for Disease Control and Prevention, National Center for Health Statistics, November 2015, http://www.cdc.gov/nchs/data/nhis/earlyrelease/earlyrelease201511_13.pdf (accessed January 4, 2016)

less likely to receive treatment for mood and anxiety disorders than were white youth.

The Patient Protection and Affordable Care Act (more commonly known as the Affordable Care Act [ACA] or Obamacare) required insurers to extend dependent coverage eligibility until age 26 in September 2010. In "Effect of the Affordable Care Act's Young Adult Insurance Expansions on Hospital-Based Mental Health Care" (*American Journal of Psychiatry*, vol. 172, no. 2, February 1, 2015), Ezra Golberstein et al. compared inpatient hospitalizations and emergency department visits for psychiatric diagnoses for young adults newly covered by the ACA dependent coverage provision (aged 19 to 25 years) and those who were not (aged 26 to 29) to assess changes in utilization before and after implementation of the dependent coverage provision. The researchers find that after ACA expansion of dependent coverage until age 26, use of inpatient psychiatric care rose modestly faster for young adults targeted by the expansion compared with those above the age cutoff. There also were small increases in rates of emergency department visits with psychiatric diagnoses among 19- to 25-year-olds compared with 26- to 29-year-olds. Golberstein et al. opine, "Increased insurance could lead to more clinically appropriate hospitalizations if necessary services become more affordable because of expanded insurance, or if greater access to outpatient services identifies the need for hospitalization."

Types of Treatment and Treatment Sites Vary over Time

Until the early 20th century, many people with mental illness were cared for by their families, in almshouses supported by local governments or in state hospitals. Over time, the states assumed increasing responsibility for people with mental illness and relocated them to state mental hospitals.

By the 1940s public sentiment began to shift and state mental hospitals were criticized as overcrowded, uncaring, and largely ineffective facilities that served as little more than "warehouses" for the mentally ill. At the same time, psychiatry began to emphasize treatment that considered life experiences and social problems as potential causes of mental illness, and psychiatrists began to assume therapeutic, as opposed to purely custodial, relationships with their patients. Together, changing public opinion, new philosophies about treatment, optimism about the potential for people with mental disorders to function in the community, and financially depleted state governments promoted the shift from inpatient residential treatment to community-based programs.

Community-based treatment received a resounding vote of confidence with passage of the Community Mental Health Centers Act of 1963, which elevated the status of outpatient clinics and community treatment. During this same period, mental hospital population counts began a slow decline. The decline was in part a response to growing enthusiasm for outpatient treatment, but it also arose in response to condemnation of mental hospitals which were assailed as "snake pits"—repressive and dehumanizing institutions that systematically denied the civil rights of patients. Enactment of public entitlement programs (i.e., Medicare and Medicaid) and third-party payers' preference for outpatient treatment also encouraged the exodus from inpatient facilities.

Legislation passed during the 1970s expanded community mental health center funding and services but disagreement about the delivery of mental health treatment persisted. The deinstitutionalization from public mental hospitals that began during the 1960s accelerated during the 1970s as states began to make use of federal funds such as Medicare, Medicaid, and Social Security Disability Insurance that enabled them to support people with serious mental illness in the community. Older adults were among the first to be relocated from mental hospitals to nursing homes, many of which were unprepared to treat mental illnesses. Others were young adults who had grown up in mental institutions and with few coping skills were unable to manage in the community. These young adults often suffered from substance abuse and mental illness; some were homeless or became fixtures in hospital emergency departments, shelters, and correctional facilities.

Nonetheless, most observers believe that deinstitutionalization was a sound policy decision, and research has demonstrated that with a comprehensive range of community support services including day treatment and residential settings for people in crisis, job training, employment opportunities, and housing, people with serious mental illness can live in the community. Managed care has supported the deinstitutionalization movement and has further reduced the numbers and lengths of inpatient hospitalizations. Further, a rising consumer movement and coalitions to advocate for people with mental illness, such as the National Alliance for the Mentally Ill (https://www.nami.org/) confirm that the majority of affected individuals prefer and benefit from community life.

TYPES OF DISORDERS

Psychiatrists have identified a range of mental disorders, from phobias (intense, irrational, and persistent fears) to depression to schizophrenia. Psychiatric diagnoses are made based on criteria that are described in the fifth edition of the *Diagnostic and Statistical Manual of Mental Disorders* (*DSM-V*) issued by the American Psychiatric Association in 2013. (See Chapter 3 for a discussion of the new diagnostic manual.) Some disorders are relatively mild and affect an individual's life in only a minor way. Others can be overwhelming, completely debilitating, and life threatening.

Anxiety disorders, which include phobias, and depression are the two most common mental disorders. In "Any Anxiety Disorder among Adults" (2015, http://www.nimh.nih.gov/health/statistics/prevalence/any-anxiety-disorder-among-adults.shtml), the National Institutes of Health indicates that in a given year 18.1% of the adults in the United States have an anxiety disorder, and 4.1% of these are considered "severe." On average, anxiety disorders begin at age 11, and women are more likely to be affected than men. The types of anxiety disorders and the lifetime prevalence in adults aged 18 years and older in the United States include post-traumatic stress disorder (PTSD; 3.5%), generalized anxiety disorder (3.1%), panic disorder (2.7%), obsessive-compulsive disorder (OCD; 1%), and phobias—specific phobia (8.7%), social phobia (6.8%), and agoraphobia (0.8%). Many people suffer from more than one mental disorder at a time (comorbidity). For example, millions of Americans suffer from substance (drug or alcohol) abuse combined with one or more other mental disorders.

Children suffer from many of the same mental disorders that afflict adults. The lifetime prevalence of anxiety disorder in adolescents aged 13 to 18 years is 25.1%. The types of anxiety disorders and the lifetime prevalence in adolescents aged 13 to 18 years in the United States include PTSD (4%), panic disorder (2.3%), generalized anxiety disorder (1%), and phobias—specific phobia (15.1%), social phobia (5.5%), and agoraphobia (2.4%). Children may also be affected by developmental disorders such as autism spectrum disorders. Children with disorganized thinking and difficulty communicating verbally, and those who have trouble understanding and navigating the world around them, may be diagnosed with autism or another pervasive developmental disorder.

These disorders may be among the most disabling because they are associated with serious learning difficulties and impaired intelligence.

AUTISM SPECTRUM DISORDERS

Autism is a spectrum of disorders affecting a person's ability to communicate and interact with others. Autism spectrum disorders (ASDs) are conditions that result from a neurological disorder that typically appears during the first three years of childhood and continues throughout life. These disorders were first described in 1943 by Leo Kanner (1894–1981), who reported on 11 children who displayed an unusual lack of interest in other people but were extremely interested in unusual aspects of the inanimate environment. Autistic children appear unattached to parents or caregivers, assume rigid or limp body postures when held, suffer impaired language, and exhibit behavior such as head banging, violent tantrums, and screaming. They are often self-destructive and uncooperative and experience delayed mental and social skills.

Autism is associated with a variety of neurological symptoms such as seizures and persistence of reflexes—involuntary muscle reactions and responses (e.g., the sucking reflex when the area around the mouth is stimulated) that are normal in infancy but usually disappear during normal child development. The NIMH reports in "Autism Spectrum Disorder" (2015, http://www.nimh.nih.gov/health/topics/autism-spectrum-disorders-asd/index.shtml) that one out of every 68 children may be diagnosed with an ASD and the prevalence of autism is four to five times more frequent in boys than in girls. The CDC also observes that the prevalence of ASD appears to have increased from 2000 to 2010 but this may be the result of a broader definition of ASD and improved diagnoses. (See Table 8.2.)

TABLE 8.2

Prevalence of autism spectrum disorders, 2000–10

Surveillance year	Birth year	Number of ADDM sites reporting	Prevalence per 1,000 children (range)	This is about 1 in X children...
2000	1992	6	6.7 (4.5–9.9)	1 in 150
2002	1994	14	6.6 (3.3–10.6)	1 in 150
2004	1996	8	8.0 (4.6–9.8)	1 in 125
2006	1998	11	9.0 (4.2–12.1)	1 in 110
2008	2000	14	11.3 (4.8–21.2)	1 in 88
2010	2002	11	14.7 (5.7–21.9)	1 in 68

SOURCE: "Identified Prevalence of Autism Spectrum Disorders," in *Autism Spectrum Disorders (ASDs): Data & Statistics*, Centers for Disease Control and Prevention, Division of Birth Defects, National Center on Birth Defects and Developmental Disabilities, August 12, 2015, http://www.cdc.gov/ncbddd/autism/data.html (accessed January 4, 2016)

ASDs were once thought to have psychological origins or occur as the result of bad parenting, but these hypotheses have been discarded in favor of biological and genetic explanations of causality. The cause of autism remains unknown, but the disorder has been associated with older parents, prematurity and low birth weight, maternal rubella infection, phenylketonuria (an inherited disorder of metabolism), tuberous sclerosis (an inherited disease of the nervous system and skin), lack of oxygen at birth, and encephalitis (inflammation of the brain). There is considerable evidence of the heritability of autism and gene variants and mutations associated with autism have been identified.

In "Developing a Predictive Gene Classifier for Autism Spectrum Disorders Based upon Differential Gene Expression Profiles of Phenotypic Subgroups" (*North American Journal of Medicine & Science*, vol. 6, no. 10, 2013), Valerie W. Hu and Yinglei Lai of George Washington University explain that up to 20% of ASD cases can be associated with a genetic abnormality but that no single gene or genetic variant causes more than 2% of ASD. Autism is not a single-gene disorder; rather, it is a complex disorder that results from simultaneous genetic variations in multiple genes as well as interactions between genetic, epigenetic (heritable changes in gene function that do not involve a change in deoxyribonucleic acid sequence), and environmental factors. Hu and Lai suggest that rather than single genes, panels of genes may be more useful biomarkers for the diagnosis of different types of ASD.

ASD varies from mild to severe, and the prognosis depends on the extent of the individual's disabilities and whether he or she receives the early, intensive interventions that are associated with improved outcomes. Treatment of autism spectrum disorders is individualized and may include applied behavior analysis, medications, dietary management and supplements, music therapy, occupational therapy, physical therapy, speech and language therapy, and vision therapy.

DEPRESSION

According to William C. Reeves et al., in "Mental Illness Surveillance among Adults in the United States" (*Morbidity and Mortality Weekly Report*, vol. 60, no. 3, September 2, 2011), depression affects about 8.7% of the U.S. population. Women are affected more often than men. The prevalence of depression is higher among women and non-Hispanic African Americans, compared with other populations. The NIMH reports in "Major Depression among Adults" (2015, http://www.nimh.nih.gov/health/statistics/prevalence/major-depression-among-adults.shtml) that 6.7% of the U.S. adult population suffers from depression in a given year and that 4.3% of cases cause severe impairment.

TABLE 8.3

Symptoms of depression

Persistent sad, anxious, or "empty" mood
Feelings of hopelessness, pessimism
Feelings of guilt, worthlessness, helplessness
Loss of interest or pleasure in hobbies and activities
Decreased energy, fatigue, being "slowed down"
Difficulty concentrating, remembering, making decisions
Difficulty sleeping, early-morning awakening, or oversleeping
Appetite and/or weight changes
Thoughts of death or suicide; suicide attempts
Restlessness, irritability
Persistent physical symptoms

SOURCE: "Signs & Symptoms," in *Depression*, National Institute of Mental Health, 2015, http://www.nimh.nih.gov/health/topics/depression/index.shtml#part_145397 (accessed January 4, 2016)

Defining Depression

Depression is a "whole body" illness, involving physical, mental, and emotional problems. A depressive disorder is not a temporary sad mood, and it is not a sign of personal weakness or a condition that can be willed away. People with depressive illness cannot just "pull themselves together" and hope that they will become well. Without treatment, the symptoms can persist for months or even years. Table 8.3 lists the symptoms that characterize depression. Not everyone who is depressed experiences all the symptoms. Some people have few symptoms, and some have many. Like other mental illnesses, the severity and duration of the symptoms of depression vary.

There are several types of depressive disorders. The most common form is dysthymic disorder (dysthymia), a less severe but chronic form of depression that by definition lasts at least two years in adults or at least one year in children. Dysthymic disorders commonly appear for the first time in children, teens, and young adults, and although they may not disable people as severely as other forms of depression, these disorders can ruin lives by robbing them of joy, energy, and productivity. According to the NIMH, in "Dysthymic Disorder among Adults" (2015, http://www.nimh.nih.gov/health/statistics/prevalence/dysthymic-disorder-among-adults.shtml), 1.5% of American adults suffer from dysthymic disorder.

Major depression is a more severe and disabling form. It is a leading cause of disability among Americans aged 15 to 44 years.

Causes of Depression

Combinations of genetic, psychological, and environmental factors are involved in the development of depressive disorders. Some types of depression run in families, and twin studies demonstrate that genetic factors determine susceptibility to depression. Major depression seems to recur in generation after generation of some families, but it also occurs in people with no family history of depression.

Studies of the brain support the premise that depression may have a biological and chemical basis. Although brain imaging studies clearly indicate that there are differences in the brain between those who suffer from depression and those who do not, it is not yet known if these differences cause the depression or result from it. Researchers speculate that the problem may be caused by the complex neurotransmission (chemical messaging) system of the brain and that people suffering from depression have either too much or too little of certain neurochemicals in the brain. Researchers also believe that depressed patients with normal levels of neurotransmitters may suffer from an inability to regulate them. Most antidepressant drugs that are currently used to treat the disorder attempt to correct these chemical imbalances.

A person's psychological makeup is another factor in depressive disorders. People who are easily overwhelmed by stress or who suffer from low self-esteem or a pessimistic view of themselves, of life, and of the world tend to be prone to depression. Events outside the person's control can also trigger a depressive episode. A major change in the patterns of daily living, such as a serious loss, a chronic illness, a difficult relationship, or financial problems, can trigger the onset of depression.

Treatment of Depression

Antidepressant medications that alter brain chemistry have been used to treat depressive disorders. Antidepressant medications—including selective serotonin reuptake inhibitors (SSRIs) such as fluoxetine hydrochloride, tricyclic antidepressants such as amitriptyline, and monoamine oxidase inhibitors—work by influencing the function of neurotransmitters such as dopamine or norepinephrine. SSRIs have fewer reported side effects (such as sedation, headache, weight gain or loss, and nausea) than tricyclic antidepressants.

Antidepressants do not offer immediate relief from symptoms; most take full effect in about four weeks, and some take up to eight weeks to achieve optimal therapeutic effect. Patients must be closely monitored by health professionals for side effects, dosage, and effectiveness. The most common side effects of antidepressants include headache, nausea, sleeplessness or drowsiness, agitation, sexual problems, dry mouth, constipation, bladder problems, and blurred vision.

Psychotherapy has also been demonstrated as effective therapy for mild to moderate depression. Talking about problems with mental health professionals can help patients better understand their feelings. Two types of short-term therapy lasting 10 to 20 weeks appear to improve symptoms of depression. Interpersonal psychotherapy (IPT) concentrates on helping patients improve personal relationships with family and friends. Cognitive behavioral therapy (CBT) attempts to help patients replace negative thoughts and feelings with more positive, optimistic approaches and actions.

CBT is based on the premise that thinking influences emotions and behavior, that feelings and actions originate with thoughts. CBT posits that it is possible to change the way people feel and act, even if their circumstances do not change. It teaches the advantages of feeling calm when faced with undesirable situations. CBT clients learn that they will confront undesirable events and circumstances whether they become troubled about them or not. When they are troubled about events or circumstances, they have two problems: the troubling event or circumstance, and the troubling feelings about the event or circumstance. Clients learn that when they do not become troubled about trying events and circumstances, they can reduce the number of problems that they face by half.

IPT helps people to look at their relationships with friends and family and make changes to resolve problems. IPT is short-term therapy that has demonstrated effectiveness for the treatment of depression. According to the International Society for Interpersonal Psychotherapy, IPT does not assume that mental illness arises exclusively from problematical interpersonal relationships. It does emphasize, however, that mental health and emotional problems occur within an interpersonal context. For this reason, the therapy aims to intervene specifically in social functioning to relieve symptoms.

In "Antidepressant Drug Effects and Depression Severity" (*Journal of the American Medical Association*, vol. 303, no. 1, January 6, 2010), a meta-analysis that reviews the results of six studies spanning 30 years of antidepressant drug treatment, Jay C. Fournier et al. suggest that people with severe depression benefit most from antidepressant medications, whereas there is little or no benefit for people with the less-severe symptoms of mild depression. The researchers assert that the benefit of antidepressant medication is comparable to placebo for people with mild to moderate symptoms.

Light therapy, which has been used to treat seasonal affective disorder (SAD, depression that occurs during the short, dark days of winter and resolves spontaneously as the days lengthen and grow brighter) also may be effective treatment for depression. Raymond W. Lam et al. report in "Efficacy of Bright Light Treatment, Fluoxetine, and the Combination in Patients with Nonseasonal Major Depressive Disorder: A Randomized Clinical Trial" (*JAMA Psychiatry*, vol. 73, no. 1, January 2016) that bright light treatment, both alone and in combination with fluoxetine, an SSRI, was effective treatment for adults with nonseasonal major depressive disorder. Lam et al. conclude, "the combination treatment had the most consistent effects."

Electrical stimulation of the brain, known as electroconvulsive therapy (ECT; formerly called shock therapy), may also be used to treat people with severe depression that has not responded to medication. Electric shocks that are administered to one side of the patient's head while he or she is under general anesthesia cause brain seizures that somehow relieve depression. The mechanism by which ECT works is as yet unknown. The treatment requires multiple sessions to achieve results. Because ECT has the potential for serious side effects (e.g., reactions to anesthesia and memory loss) and because of the history of abuses of the treatment, ECT is a controversial treatment and is reserved for people with the most treatment-resistant depression.

Children Also Suffer from Depression

The most frequently diagnosed mood disorders in children and adolescents are major depressive disorder, dysthymic disorder, and bipolar disorder. Children who are depressed are not unlike their adult counterparts. They may be teary and sad, lose interest in friends and activities, and become listless, self-critical, and hypersensitive to criticism. They feel unloved, helpless, and hopeless about the future, and they may think about suicide. Depressed children and adolescents may also be irritable, aggressive, and indecisive. They may have problems concentrating and sleeping and often become careless about their appearance and hygiene. Depressed children often display anxiety symptoms, such as clinging to parents or not wanting to go to school. They also experience more somatic symptoms, such as general aches and pains, stomachaches, and headaches, than adults with depression.

Dysthymic disorder usually begins in childhood or early adolescence and is a chronic but milder depressive disorder with fewer symptoms. The child or adolescent is depressed every day for at least one year. Because the average duration of the disorder is about four years, some children become so accustomed to feeling depressed that they may not identify themselves as being depressed or complain about symptoms. In "Dysthymic Disorder among Children" (2015, http://www.nimh.nih.gov/health/statistics/prevalence/dysthymic-disorder-among-children.shtml), the NIMH estimates a lifetime prevalence of 11.2% of adolescents aged 13 to 18 years. Of these, 3.3% suffer a "severe" depressive disorder.

Reactive depression is the most common mental health problem in children and adolescents. It is not considered a mental disorder, and many health professionals consider occasional bouts of reactive depression as entirely consistent with normal adolescent development. It is characterized by transient depressed feelings in response to some negative experience, such as a rejection from a boyfriend or girlfriend or a failing grade. Sadness or listlessness spontaneously resolves in a few hours or may last as long as two weeks. Distraction, in the form of a change of activity or setting, helps improve the mood of affected individuals.

BIPOLAR DISORDER

Bipolar disorder, also known as manic depression, is characterized by alternating periods of persistently elevated, expansive, or irritable mood—called mania—and periods of depression. During a manic episode, a person may feel inflated self-esteem and decreased need for sleep and be unusually talkative and easily distracted. He or she may also have flights of ideas, racing thoughts, increased goal-directed activity such as shopping, and excessive involvement in high-risk activities. According to the NIMH, in "Bipolar Disorder among Adults" (2015, http://www.nimh.nih.gov/health/statistics/prevalence/bipolar-disorder-among-adults.shtml), bipolar disorder affects about 2.6% of the U.S. adult population, and the median age (the middle value; half of all people are younger and half are older) of onset is 25.

During the early stages of the illness patients may experience few symptoms or even symptom-free periods between relatively mild episodes of mania and depression. Table 8.4 describes the symptoms of bipolar disorder. As the illness progresses, however, manic and depressive episodes become more serious and more frequent. Patients are less likely to experience intermissions, manic euphoria is increasingly replaced by irritability, and depressions deepen. Some individuals suffer psychotic episodes during periods of mania or depression. Bipolar disorder is one of the most lethal illnesses. According to Frederick K. Goodwin and Kay Redfield Jamison, in *Manic-Depressive Illness* (2007), "Patients with depressive and manic-depressive illnesses are far more likely to commit suicide than individuals in any other psychiatric or medical risk group. The mortality rate for untreated manic-depressive patients is higher than it is for most types of heart disease and many types of cancer."

The onset of bipolar illness is usually a depressive episode during adolescence. Manic episodes may not appear for months or even years. During manic episodes adolescents are tireless, overly confident, and tend to have rapid-fire or pressured speech. They may perform tasks and schoolwork quickly and energetically but in a wildly disorganized manner. Manic adolescents may seriously overestimate their capabilities, and the combination of bravado and loosened inhibitions may prompt them to participate in high-risk behaviors, such as vandalism, drug abuse, or unsafe sex. The NIMH reports in "Bipolar Disorder among Children" (2016, http://www.nimh.nih.gov/health/statistics/prevalence/bipolar-disorder-among-children.shtml) that the lifetime prevalence of bipolar disorder may be as high as 3% of adolescents aged 13 to 18 years. The disorder can run in families, and treatment for children and adolescents is similar to the treatment that is given to adults.

Treatments for Bipolar Disorder

Lithium has been widely used to treat bipolar disorder since the 1960s, and it is still the mood-stabilizing drug of choice for bipolar disorder. During the 1970s psychiatrists also began using anticonvulsant drugs, including carbamazepine, clonazepam, and valproic acid or divalproex sodium, to treat patients who could not tolerate lithium or for whom the drug did not work. Other anticonvulsants, such as gabapentin, lamotrigine, and oxcarbazepine, have also been used to treat the mania that is associated with bipolar disorder. Antimanic and other antipsychotic agents, such as olanzapine, risperidone, and zipraisidone, are often combined with antidepressants to relieve depressive symptoms and to promote better sleep patterns, an important factor in maintaining patients' mood stability These

TABLE 8.4

Symptoms of bipolar disorder

Symptoms of mania or a manic episode include:	Symptoms of depression or a depressive episode include:
Mood changes	**Mood changes**
• An overly long period of feeling "high," or an overly happy or outgoing mood • Extreme irritability.	• An overly long period of feeling sad or hopeless • Loss of interest in activities once enjoyed, including sex.
Behavioral changes	**Behavioral changes**
• Talking very fast, jumping from one idea to another, having racing thoughts • Being unusually distracted • Increasing activities, such as taking on multiple new projects • Being overly restless • Sleeping little or not being tired • Having an unrealistic belief in your abilities • Behaving impulsively and engaging in pleasurable, high-risk behaviors.	• Feeling overly tired or "slowed down" • Having problems concentrating, remembering, and making decisions • Being restless or irritable • Changing eating, sleeping, or other habits • Thinking of death or suicide, or attempting suicide.

SOURCE: "Symptoms of Bipolar Disorder Are Described Below," in *Bipolar Disorder*, National Institute of Mental Health, 2015, http://www.nimh.nih.gov/health/publications/bipolar-disorder-in-adults/index.shtml (accessed January 4, 2016)

medication strategies have proven effective in treating bipolar disorder; however, many patients still experience a residual pattern of ups and downs.

Medications may become less effective over time and have to be changed. Another major concern among practitioners and patients are medication side effects, especially of lithium. Because therapeutic blood levels of the drug are close to fatal levels, patients taking lithium must consume adequate amounts of water and salt to prevent dehydration, which would cause lithium blood levels to rise to toxic levels. People who take lithium must have their blood level of the drug checked frequently, and they must also be aware of the signs of lithium poisoning. Long-term use of the drug has been shown to cause kidney damage; however, adequate consumption of water and careful dosage monitoring are believed to reduce the risk of kidney disease.

The NIMH also explains that a combination of psychotherapy and medication may help people with bipolar disorder to live symptom-free for longer periods and to recover from episodes more quickly. Research is under way to find out whether psychotherapy may delay the start of bipolar disorder in children who are at high risk for the illness.

When medication and psychotherapy are not effective, ECT may prove beneficial. Although ECT may cause short-term side effects such as confusion, disorientation, and memory loss, these side effects generally subside after treatment.

SCHIZOPHRENIA

A person who hears voices, becomes violent, and sometimes ends up being homeless, muttering, and shouting incomprehensibly, frequently suffers from schizophrenia. This disease generally presents in adolescence, causing hallucinations, paranoia, delusions, and social isolation. The effects begin slowly and, initially, are often considered to be the normal behavioral changes of adolescence. Gradually, voices take over in the schizophrenic's mind, obliterating reality and directing the person to all kinds of erratic behaviors. Suicide attempts and violent attacks are not uncommon to schizophrenics. In an attempt to escape the torment that is inflicted by their brains, many schizophrenics turn to drugs. The NIMH observes in "Schizophrenia" (2015, http://www.nimh.nih.gov/health/publications/schizophrenia-booklet-12-2015/index.shtml) that people who have schizophrenia abuse alcohol and/or drugs more often than the general population.

The NIMH reports that about 1% of the U.S. population suffers from schizophrenia and similar disorders. Although the precise causes of schizophrenia are unknown, for years researchers have hypothesized that genetic susceptibility is a risk factor for schizophrenia and bipolar disorder. According to Jenny van Dongen and Dorret I. Boomsma, in "The Evolutionary Paradox and the Missing Heritability of Schizophrenia" (*American Journal of Medical Genetics*, pt. 162B, no. 2, March 2013), "Schizophrenia is among the most heritable psychiatric disorders."

Imaging studies of the brain reveal abnormal brain development in children who have schizophrenia, and imaging studies of adults with the disease find enlargement of the ventricles of the brain. Some studies suggest that the brain of a person with schizophrenia manufactures too much dopamine, a chemical that is vital to normal nerve activity. Conventional drug treatment focuses on blocking dopamine receptors in the brain, but not all people with schizophrenia respond to treatment. This type of treatment can produce serious side effects. Newer antipsychotic medications that are used to treat the disorder, such as risperidone, have fewer side effects than previously used medications. Regardless, patients who take these medications must be monitored closely for serious side effects such as the loss of the white blood cells that fight infection.

ANXIETY DISORDERS

Everyone experiences some degree of anxiety almost every day. In the 21st century a certain amount of anxiety is unavoidable and, in some cases, may even be beneficial. For example, mild anxiety before an exam or a job interview may actually improve performance. Anxiety before surgery, giving a speech, or driving in bad weather is normal.

Nevertheless, when anxiety becomes extreme or when an attack of anxiety strikes suddenly, without an apparent external cause, it can be debilitating and destructive. Its symptoms may include nervousness, fear, a "knot" in the stomach, rapid heartbeat, or increased blood pressure. If the anxiety is severe and long lasting, more serious problems may develop. People suffering from anxiety for extended periods may have headaches, ulcers, irritable bowel syndrome, insomnia, and depression. Because anxiety tends to create various other emotional and physical symptoms, a "snowball" effect can occur in which these problems produce even more anxiety.

Chronic anxiety can interfere with an individual's ability to lead a normal life. Mental health professionals consider a person who has prolonged anxiety as having an anxiety disorder. In "Any Anxiety Disorder among Adults" (2015, http://www.nimh.nih.gov/health/statistics/prevalence/any-anxiety-disorder-among-adults.shtml), the NIMH estimates that in any given year, approximately 18.1% of Americans aged 18 years and older suffer from anxiety disorders, and 22% of these cases (4.1% of the U.S. population) are severe.

Panic Disorder

Extremely high levels of anxiety may produce panic attacks that are both unanticipated and seemingly without cause. In one type of panic attack, called unexpected, the sufferer is unable to predict when an attack will occur. Other types of panic attacks are linked to a particular location, circumstance, or event and are called situationally bound or situationally predisposed panic attacks. These panic episodes can last as long as 30 minutes and are marked by an overwhelming sense of impending doom while the person's heart races and breathing quickens to the point of gasping for air. Sweating, weakness, dizziness, terror, and feelings of unreality are also typical. Individuals undergoing a panic attack fear they are going to lose control, "lose their mind," or even die.

Repeated panic attacks may be called a panic disorder. The NIMH estimates in "Panic Disorder among Adults" (2015, http://www.nimh.nih.gov/health/statistics/prevalence/panic-disorder-among-adults.shtml) that 2.7% of Americans suffer from panic disorders and 44.8% of these cases (1.2% of the U.S. population) are severe. Panic disorders are twice as common in women as in men and usually begin in early adulthood.

Research reveals that people who experience panic attacks tend to suppress their emotions. Researchers hypothesize that this tendency leads to an emotional buildup for which a panic attack is a form of release. Interestingly, most people who suffer from panic attacks do not experience anxiety between attacks.

The usual treatment for panic disorder is CBT combined with antianxiety drugs to treat the fear of the attacks. Sometimes antidepressant medications are used, even though people suffering from anxiety disorders are usually not clinically depressed. Relaxation therapy has also proved beneficial.

Phobias

Phobias are defined as unreasonable fears that are associated with a particular situation or object. The most common of the many varieties of phobias are specific phobias. Fear of bees, snakes, rodents, heights, odors, blood, needles, and storms are examples of common specific phobias. Specific phobias, especially animal phobias, are common in children, but they can occur at any age. According to the NIMH, in "Specific Phobia among Adults" (2015, http://www.nimh.nih.gov/health/statistics/prevalence/specific-phobia-among-adults.shtml), 8.7% of American adults suffer from specific phobias, and 21.9% of these cases (1.9% of the U.S. population) are severe. Most people with a phobia understand that their fears are unreasonable, but this awareness does not make them feel any less anxious.

Some specific phobias, such as a fear of heights, usually do not interfere with daily life or cause as much distress as more severe forms, such as agoraphobia. People suffering from severe phobias may rearrange their lives drastically to avoid the situations they fear will trigger panic attacks.

SOCIAL PHOBIAS. Social phobias (also called social anxiety disorders) can be more serious than specific phobias. A person with social phobia is intensely afraid of being judged by others. At social gatherings the person with social phobia expects to be singled out, scrutinized, judged, and found lacking. People with social phobias are usually very anxious about feeling humiliated or embarrassed. They are often so crippled by their own fears that they may have a hard time thinking clearly, remembering facts, or carrying on normal conversations. The individual with social phobia may tremble, sweat, or blush and often fears fainting or losing bladder or bowel control in social settings. In response to these overwhelming fears, the person with social phobia tries to avoid public situations and gatherings of people. The NIMH estimates in "Social Phobia among Adults" (2015, http://www.nimh.nih.gov/health/statistics/prevalence/social-phobia-among-adults.shtml) that 6.8% of adults in the United States suffer from social phobias, and 29.9% of these cases (2% of the U.S. population) are severe. Social phobias tend to start about age 13 and, if not treated, can continue throughout life.

Because social phobics fear being the center of attention or the subject of criticism, public speaking, asking questions, eating in front of others, or even attending social events creates anxiety. Social phobias should not be confused with shyness, which is a normal variation in personality. Social phobias can be disabling, preventing sufferers from attending school, working, and having friends.

AGORAPHOBIA. Many people who experience panic attacks go on to develop agoraphobia, the fear of crowds and open spaces. The term comes from the Greek word *agora*, which means "marketplace." This type of phobia is a severely disabling disorder that often traps its victims, rendering them virtual prisoners in their own home, unable to work, shop, or attend social activities.

Agoraphobia normally develops slowly, following an initial unexpected panic attack. For example, on an ordinary day, while shopping, driving to work, or doing errands, the individual is suddenly struck by a wave of terror that is characterized by symptoms such as trembling, a pounding heart, profuse sweating, and difficulty in breathing normally. The person desperately seeks safety and reassurance from friends or family. The panic subsides and all is well until another panic attack occurs.

The person with agoraphobia begins to avoid all places and situations where an attack occurred and then begins to avoid places where an attack could possibly occur or where it might be difficult to escape and get help. Gradually, the victim becomes more and more limited in the choice of places that are "safe." Eventually, the person with agoraphobia cannot venture outside the immediate neighborhood or leave the house. The fear ultimately expands to touch every aspect of the victim's life.

In "Agoraphobia among Adults" (2015, http://www.nimh.nih.gov/health/statistics/prevalence/agoraphobia-among-adults.shtml), the NIMH explains that 0.8% of American adults suffer from agoraphobia, and 40.6% of these cases (0.3% of the U.S. population) are classified as severe. Agoraphobia usually begins during the late teens or 20s and the average age of onset is 20.

PHOBIA TREATMENT PROGRAMS. Phobia treatment programs use a wide variety of CBT techniques to help patients overcome their fears. In addition, drugs may be used to ease the symptoms of anxiety, fear, and depression and to help the person return to a normal life more quickly. Antidepressants have been shown to help people who suffer from panic attacks and agoraphobia, and antianxiety drugs are useful in treating the generalized anxiety that frequently accompanies phobias.

Obsessive-Compulsive Disorder

Obsessive-compulsive disorder (OCD) is an anxiety disorder that is marked by unwanted, often unpleasant recurring thoughts (obsessions) and repetitive, often mechanical behaviors (compulsions). The repetitive behaviors, such as continually checking to be certain windows and doors are locked or repeated hand washing, are intended to dispel the obsessive thoughts that trigger them—that an intruder will enter the house through an unlocked door or window or that disease will be prevented by hand washing. The vicious cycle of obsessions and compulsions only serves to heighten anxiety; OCD can debilitate those who have the disorder.

The symptoms of OCD generally appear during childhood or adolescence. Imaging studies using positron emission tomography (PET) reveal that people with OCD have different patterns of brain activity than those without the disorder. Furthermore, the PET scans show that the part of the brain that is most affected by OCD (the striatum) changes and responds to both medication and behavioral therapy.

In "Obsessive Compulsive Disorder among Adults" (2015, http://www.nimh.nih.gov/health/statistics/prevalence/obsessive-compulsive-disorder-among-adults.shtml), the NIMH estimates that 1% of the U.S adult population suffers from OCD, and more than half of these cases (50.6% or 0.5% of the U.S. population) are severe.

Many of the medications that are used to treat other anxiety disorders appear effective for patients with OCD, as has a behavioral type of therapy called "exposure and response prevention," during which patients with OCD learn new ways to manage their obsessive thoughts without resorting to compulsive behaviors.

Anxiety among Children and Adolescents

Children and adolescents suffer from many of the same anxiety disorders as do adults. Taken together, the different types of anxiety disorders constitute the mental disorders that are most prevalent among children and adolescents. In "Any Anxiety Disorder among Children" (2015, http://www.nimh.nih.gov/health/statistics/prevalence/any-anxiety-disorder-among-children.shtml), the NIMH reports that about one-quarter (25.1%) of 13- to 18-year-olds will have an anxiety disorder at some point, and 5.9% will have "severe" anxiety disorders.

Separation anxiety disorder is a type of anxiety disorder that is found specifically in children. It is normal for infants, toddlers, and very young children to experience anxiety when separated from their parents or caregivers. For example, nearly every child experiences at least a momentary pang of separation anxiety on the first day of preschool or kindergarten. When this condition occurs in older children or adolescents and it is severe enough to impair social, academic, or job functioning for at least one month, it is considered separation anxiety disorder. The risk factors that are associated with separation anxiety disorder include stress, the illness or death of a family member, geographic relocation, and physical or sexual assault.

Children with separation anxiety may be clingy, and often they harbor fears that accidents or natural disasters will forever separate them from their parents. Because they fear being apart from their parents, they may resist attending school or going anywhere without a parent. Separation anxiety can produce physical symptoms such as dizziness, nausea, or palpitations. It is often associated with symptoms of depression. Young children with separation anxiety may have difficulty falling asleep alone in their room and may have recurrent nightmares.

According to the U.S. Department of Health and Human Services (HHS), research suggests that some children develop OCD following an infection with a specific type of streptococcus. These conditions are known as pediatric autoimmune neuropsychiatric disorders associated with streptococcal infections. It is believed that antibodies intended to combat the strep infection mistakenly attack a region of the brain and trigger an inflammatory reaction, which in turn leads to the development of OCD.

ATTENTION-DEFICIT/HYPERACTIVITY DISORDER

Attention-deficit disorder (ADD) and attention-deficit/hyperactivity disorder (ADHD) are psychiatric disorders that usually begin or become apparent in children in preschool and elementary school. Children with ADHD cannot sit still, have difficulty controlling their impulsive actions, and are unable to focus on projects long enough to complete them. Those who are diagnosed with ADD have the same symptoms but do not display hyperactivity. Although teachers originally dubbed ADHD a "learning problem," the disorder affects more than just schoolwork. Children with ADHD have trouble socializing, are often unable to make friends, and suffer from low self-esteem. If left untreated, ADHD can leave children unable to cope academically or socially, possibly leading to depression.

According to the NIMH, in "Attention Deficit/ Hyperactivity Disorder among Children" (2015, http://www.nimh.nih.gov/health/statistics/prevalence/attention-deficit-hyperactivity-disorder-among-children.shtml), 9% of 13- to 18-year-olds will have ADHD, and 1.8% of cases will be severe. ADHD frequently coexists with other mental health problems, such as a learning disability, anxiety and depression, bipolar disorder, or antisocial behavior. Children diagnosed with ADHD are usually affected into their teen years, but for most, symptoms subside in adulthood, and adults become more adept at controlling their behavior. Regardless, vigilance is warranted because research reveals an increased incidence in juvenile delinquency and subsequent encounters with the criminal justice system among adults who were diagnosed with ADHD during their youth.

In "Attention-Deficit/Hyperactivity Disorder among Adults" (2015, http://www.nimh.nih.gov/health/statistics/prevalence/attention-deficit-hyperactivity-disorder-among-adults.shtml), the NIMH reports that 4.1% of adults will have ADHD at some point during their lives, and 42.3% of these cases (1.7% of the U.S. adult population) will be severe.

The reported incidence of ADHD has increased in the 21st century, possibly because of better diagnosis, changing expectations, or insufficient supportive social structures. In the absence of clear criteria for ADHD or guidelines by which to diagnose it, researchers fear that the disorder may be under- or overdiagnosed. The cause of ADHD is as yet unknown. According to the NIMH, many studies suggest that genes play a large role. The NIMH also notes that ADHD is likely caused by a combination of environmental factors, and brain injuries as well as social environment may contribute. A biological explanation of ADHD arose because its symptoms respond to treatment with stimulants such as methylphenidate, which increase the availability of dopamine—the neurotransmitter that is vital for purposeful movement, motivation, and alertness. As a result, researchers theorize that ADHD may be caused by the unavailability of dopamine in the central nervous system.

Recent research supports the heritability of ADHD. Twin studies, such as Ingo Langner et al.'s "Twin and Sibling Studies Using Health Insurance Data: The Example of Attention Deficit/Hyperactivity Disorder" (*PLoS One*, vol. 8, no. 4, April 24, 2013), find that when ADHD is present in one twin, it is significantly more likely to be present in an identical twin than in non-twin siblings. These findings support inheritance as an important risk in a proportion of children with ADHD.

Although imaging studies reveal differences in the brains of children with ADHD, and scientists have found a link between the inability to pay attention and the diminished utilization of glucose in parts of the brain, some researchers question whether these changes cause the disorder. They argue that the observed changes may result from the disorder or simply coexist with it. As a result, some mental health professionals and educators concede that some children are legitimately diagnosed with ADHD and that others are mislabeled. They speculate that the latter group may be simply high-spirited, undisciplined, or misbehaving.

Treatment for ADHD

Much controversy about ADHD has focused on its treatment. NIMH research indicates that there are two effective treatment methods for elementary-school children with ADHD: a closely monitored medication regimen and a combination of medication and behavioral interventions. Behavioral interventions include psychotherapy, CBT, social skills training, support groups, and parent-educator skills training.

Although some researchers still question the wisdom of treatment with potentially addicting, powerful stimulants, prescription stimulants (such as methylphenidate, dextromethamphetamine, and amphetamine) have proved to be safe and effective for short-term treatment of ADHD. Another prescription medication that is used to treat ADHD, atomoxetine, is a nonstimulant drug, but it carries the risk of serious side effects, including cardiovascular symptoms, psychotic symptoms, and increased suicidal tendencies.

In "ADHD throughout the Years" (March 15, 2016, http://www.cdc.gov/ncbddd/adhd/timeline.html), the CDC observes that over time, the criteria used to diagnose the condition have changed, which in turn has affected the estimate of the percentage of children affected. There has been a consistent increase in parent-reported ADHD diagnoses. The CDC notes that it is not clear whether this increase represents a change in the number of children with ADHD, or a change in the number of children who were diagnosed with ADHD.

DISRUPTIVE DISORDERS

Children and adolescents with disruptive disorders, which include oppositional defiant disorder (ODD) and conduct disorder, display antisocial behaviors. Like separation anxiety, the diagnosis of a disruptive disorder largely depends on assessing whether behavior is age appropriate. For example, just as clinging may be considered normal for a toddler but abnormal behavior in an older child, toddlers and very young children often behave aggressively (e.g., grabbing toys and even biting one another). When, however, a child older than age five displays such aggressive behavior, it may indicate an emerging oppositional defiant or conduct disorder.

It is important to distinguish isolated acts of aggression or the normal childhood and adolescent phases of testing limits from the pattern of ongoing, persistent defiance, hostility, and disobedience that is the hallmark of ODD. Children with ODD are argumentative, lose their tempers, refuse to adhere to rules, blame others for their own mistakes, and are spiteful and vindictive. Their behaviors often alienate them from family and peers and cause problems at school.

Family strife, volatile marital relationships, frequently changing caregivers, and inconsistent child-rearing practices may increase the risk for the disorder. Some practitioners consider ODD a gateway condition to conduct disorder. According to Roy H. Lubit, in "Oppositional Defiant Disorder" (Medscape.com, October 7, 2015), estimates of the prevalence of ODD range from 1% to 11%, depending on the population and the way the disorder is evaluated. Prepubescent boys are diagnosed more often with ODD than girls of the same age, but after puberty the rates in both sexes are equal. About half of children with ADHD also have ODD.

Children or adolescents with conduct disorder are aggressive. They may fight, sexually assault, or behave cruelly to people or animals. Because lying, stealing, vandalism, truancy, and substance abuse are common behaviors, adults, social service agencies, and the criminal justice system often view affected young people as "bad" rather than as mentally ill. In "Facts for Families, No. 33: Conduct Disorders" (August 2013, http://www.aacap.org/cs/root/facts_for_families/conduct_disorder), the American Academy of Child and Adolescent Psychiatry describes an array of generally antisocial behaviors that when exhibited by children or adolescents suggest a diagnosis of conduct disorder. These actions and behaviors include:

- Bullying, threatening, or intimidating others
- Initiating physical fights
- Using a weapon such as a bat, brick, knife, or gun that can cause serious physical harm
- Being physically cruel to people or animals
- Stealing from a victim while confronting him or her
- Engaging in coercive or forced sexual activity
- Deliberately setting fires with the intention of causing damage
- Deliberately destroying others' property
- Breaking into a building, house, or car
- Lying to obtain goods or favors or to avoid obligations
- Stealing items without confronting a victim
- Staying out at night despite parental objections
- Running away from home
- Being truant from school

Conduct disorder severely compromises the lives of affected children and adolescents. Their schoolwork suffers, as do their relationships with adults and peers. The HHS finds that youths with conduct disorders have higher rates of injury and sexually transmitted infections and are likely to be expelled from school and have problems with the law. Rates of depression, suicidal thoughts, suicide attempts, and suicide are all higher in children and teens who are diagnosed with conduct disorder. Children in whom the disorder presents before the age of 10 years are predominantly male. Early onset places them at a greater risk for adult antisocial personality disorder. More than a quarter of severely antisocial children become antisocial adults.

As of March 2016, there were no medications that had proven effective in treating conduct disorder. Although psychosocial interventions can reduce their antisocial behavior, children or adolescents with a conduct disorder still create high levels of stress for the entire family. Support programs train parents how to positively reinforce appropriate behaviors and how to strengthen the emotional bonds between parent and child. Identifying and intervening with high-risk children to enhance their social interaction and prevent academic failure can mitigate some of the potentially harmful long-term consequences of conduct disorder. In "The Evidence Base for the Assessment and Treatment of Attention-Deficit/Hyperactivity and Oppositional Defiant Disorder" (*Colorado Journal of Psychiatry and Psychology: Child and Adolescent Mental Health*, vol. 1, no. 1, May 2015), Mary N. Cook, Gautam Rajendran, and Jason Williams note that the combination of parent training, which educates parents about the strategies for managing their child's behavior, and parent-child interaction therapy (PCIT) is effective for young children with conduct disorders. (PCIT teaches parents how to strengthen their attachment and how to be effective authority figures by giving directions in age-appropriate, positive ways, while setting consistent limits and learning how to appropriately implement consequences.)

EATING DISORDERS

Much of American society is preoccupied with body image. Advertisers of many products suggest that to be thin and beautiful is to be happy. Many prominent weight-loss programs reinforce this suggestion. A well-balanced, low-fat food plan, combined with exercise, can help most overweight people achieve a healthier weight and lifestyle. Dieting to achieve a healthy weight is quite different from dieting obsessively to become "model" thin, which can have consequences ranging from mildly harmful to life threatening. In *Eating Disorders: About More than Food* (2014, http://www.nimh.nih.gov/health/publications/eating-disorders-new-trifold/eating-disorders-pdf_148810.pdf), the NIMH observes that eating disorders frequently coexist with other mental disorders, including depression, substance abuse, and anxiety disorders. Although eating disorders affect males and females, rates among females are 2.5 times greater than among males.

Research indicates that certain foods are addictive and that some people can become addicted to behaviors, such as fasting, bingeing, purging, and using laxatives, that are associated with disordered eating. People with bulimia may talk of being "hooked" on certain foods and needing to feed their "habits." This addictive behavior can carry over into other areas of a person's life, resulting, for example, in substance abuse. Many people with eating disorders suffer from comorbidities (having more than one disease or disorder at the same time), such as severe depression, which increases their risk for suicide. In "G2B Reviews: Stress at the Intersection of Anxiety, Addiction and Eating Disorders" (*Genes, Brain and Behavior*, vol. 14, no. 1, January 2015), Andrew Holmes notes that some researchers view eating disorders as addictions in which anxiety and stress lead to "functional disturbances in brain circuits mediating feeding behaviors that, in turn, may go on to cause abnormal patterns of eating."

Anorexia Nervosa

Anorexia nervosa (AN) involves severe weight loss, a minimum of 15% below normal body weight. People with anorexia literally starve themselves, although they may be very hungry. For reasons that researchers do not yet fully understand, people with anorexia are irrationally fearful about gaining weight. They are often obsessed with food and weight, develop strange eating habits, refuse to eat with other people, and exercise strenuously to burn calories and prevent weight gain. Individuals with anorexia continue to believe they are overweight even when they are dangerously thin.

The medical complications of anorexia are similar to starvation. When the body attempts to protect its most vital organs (the heart and the brain) it goes into "slow gear." Monthly menstrual periods stop, and breathing, pulse, blood pressure, and thyroid function slow down. The nails and hair become brittle, and the skin dries. Water imbalance causes constipation, and the lack of body fat causes an inability to withstand cold temperatures. Depression, weakness, personality changes, and a constant obsession with food are also symptoms of the disease. The person suffering from anorexia may have outbursts of anger and hostility or may withdraw socially. In the most serious cases, anorexia is fatal.

In "Eating Disorders among Adults—Anorexia Nervosa" (2015, http://www.nimh.nih.gov/health/statistics/prevalence/eating-disorders-among-adults-anorexia-nervosa.shtml), the NIMH estimates that 0.9% of females and 0.3% of males will suffer from AN at some point during their lives.

Bulimia Nervosa

People who have bulimia nervosa (BN) eat compulsively and then purge (get rid of the food) through self-induced vomiting, use of laxatives, diuretics, strict diets, fasts, or exercise, or a combination of several of these compensatory behaviors. The NIMH reports in "Eating Disorders among Adults—Bulimia Nervosa" (2015, http://www.nimh.nih.gov/health/statistics/prevalence/eating-disorders-among-adults-bulimia-nervosa.shtml) that an estimated 1% of people will suffer from bulimia in their lifetime.

Many people with bulimia are at a healthy body weight or higher because of their frequent binge-purge behavior, which can occur from once or twice per week to several times per day. People with BN who maintain normal weight may manage to keep their eating disorder secret for years. Like AN, BN usually begins during adolescence, but many sufferers do not seek help until they are in their 30s or 40s.

Binge eating disorder (BED) and purging are dangerous. Although it occurs rarely, bingeing can cause esophageal ruptures, and purging can result in life-threatening heart conditions because the body loses vital minerals. The acid in vomit erodes tooth enamel and the lining of the esophagus, throat, and mouth and can cause scarring on the hands when fingers are pushed down the throat to induce vomiting. The esophagus may become inflamed, and glands in the neck may become swollen.

Causes of Eating Disorders

Mounting evidence suggests that there is a genetic component to susceptibility to eating disorders. For example, in "The Epidemiology of Eating Disorders: Genetic, Environmental, and Societal Factors" (*Clinical Epidemiology*, vol. 17, no. 6, February 2014), Deborah Mitchison and Phillipa J. Hay reviewed 149 published studies about the heritability of anorexia nervosa and bulimia nervosa and the overlap of genetic and environmental factors that influence the development of eating disorders. Six studies calculated heritability or genetic contribution estimates of AN, BN, and BED. Estimates ranged from 22% to 76% for AN, 52% to 62% for BN, and 57% for BED. Mitchison and Hay also find associations between eating disorder prevalence and a history of sexual or physical abuse.

People with bulimia and anorexia seem to have different personalities. Those with bulimia are likely to be impulsive (acting without considering the consequences) and are more likely to abuse alcohol and drugs. People with anorexia tend to be perfectionists, good students, and competitive athletes. They usually keep their feelings to themselves and rarely disobey their parents. However, people with these disorders share certain traits: they lack self-esteem, they have feelings of helplessness, and they fear gaining weight. In both disorders the eating problems appear to develop as a way of handling stress and anxiety.

The person with bulimia consumes huge amounts of food in a search for comfort and stress relief. The bingeing, however, brings only guilt and depression. By contrast, people with anorexia restrict food intake to gain a sense of control and mastery over some aspect of their lives. Controlling their body weight offers them two advantages: they can take control of their body and can gain approval from others.

Treatment of Eating Disorders

Generally, a physician treats the medical complications of the disorder, while a nutritionist counsels the patient about specific diet and eating plans. To help the person with an eating disorder face his or her underlying problems and emotional issues, psychotherapy is usually necessary. People with eating disorders, whether they are normal weight, overweight, or obese, should seek help from a mental health professional such as a psychiatrist, psychologist, or clinical social worker for their eating behavior. Sometimes the challenge is to convince people with eating disorders to seek and obtain treatment; other times it is difficult to gain their adherence to treatment. Many anorexics deny their illness, and getting and keeping anorexic patients in treatment can be difficult. Treating bulimia is similarly difficult. Many bulimics are easily frustrated and want to leave treatment if their symptoms are not quickly relieved.

Several approaches are used to treat eating disorders. CBT teaches people how to monitor their eating and change unhealthy eating habits. It also teaches them how to change the way they respond to stressful situations.

Like other forms of psychotherapy, CBT and IPT may be used in conjunction with medications. Because eating disorders frequently recur, it is recommended that successful short-term treatment be combined with ongoing maintenance therapy, such as monthly sessions following completion of the short-term phase.

Group therapy can be helpful for bulimics, who are relieved to find that they are not alone in their binge-eating behaviors. A combination of behavioral therapy and family systems therapy is often the most effective with anorexics. Family systems therapy considers the family as the unit of treatment and focuses on relationships and communication within the family rather than on the personality traits or symptoms that are displayed by individual family members. Family systems therapy considers the family as an entity that is more than the sum of its individual members and uses systems theory to identify family members' roles within the system as a whole. Problems are dealt with by modifying the system rather than by trying to change an individual family member. People with eating disorders who also suffer from depression may benefit from antidepressant and antianxiety medications to help relieve coexisting mental health problems.

Recovery from eating disorders is uneven. The Eating Disorders Coalition for Research, Policy, and Action characterizes recovery as a process that frequently entails multiple rehospitalizations, limited ability to work or attend school, and limited capacity for interpersonal relationships.

In "The Myths of Motivation: Time for a Fresh Look at Some Received Wisdom in the Eating Disorders?" (*International Journal of Eating Disorders*, vol. 45, no. 1, January 2012), Glenn Waller of the Vincent Square Eating Disorders Clinic in London observes that the lack of motivation to change, arising from feelings of helplessness or hopelessness, may impede recovery from eating disorders. He opines that behavioral strategies to enhance motivation should be explored to improve the effectiveness of eating disorders treatment.

PRESCRIBING PSYCHOACTIVE MEDICATION TO CHILDREN

In "Treatment of Children with Mental Illness" (2009, http://www.nimh.nih.gov/health/publications/treatment-of-children-with-mental-illness-fact-sheet/nimh-treatment-children-mental-illness-faq_34669.pdf), a publication aimed at the parents of children with a range of mental disorders, the NIMH acknowledges public concern that psychotropic medication is being prescribed to very young children and that the safety and efficacy (the ability of an intervention to produce the intended diagnostic or therapeutic effect in optimal circumstances) of most psychotropic medications, especially for children under the age of six years, have not yet been established. Several widely used drugs have not received approval from the U.S. Food and Drug Administration (FDA) for use in young children simply because there are not enough data to support their use.

Data are lacking because historically there were ethical concerns about involving children in clinical trials to determine not only the most effective treatments but also the proper dosage, the potential side effects, and the long-term effects of drug use on learning and development. Policies about research involving children affect the FDA approval process and recommendations for use. For example, methylphenidate is approved for use in children aged six years and older, but its use was not evaluated in children younger than age six. In contrast, dextromethamphetamine received approval for use in children as young as three years old because by the time approval was sought, study guidelines permitted participation of younger children. Highlighting the discrepancies in the approved starting ages of patients for certain drugs, Table 8.5 lists the brand and generic names of prescription medications that are used to treat ADHD in children and adolescents and indicates FDA approval of their use in children aged six years and older and aged three years and older. By contrast, none of the drugs that is prescribed to treat anxiety is FDA approved for use in people under the age of 18 years.

Because the FDA approval process often requires years of research to demonstrate safety and efficacy, and practitioners are eager to provide symptom relief for severely troubled children, many recommend off-label use of medications. Off-label treatment may involve the use of a medication that has not yet received official FDA approval for use in children or the use of a drug the FDA has approved for use in children for a different condition. As such, they are prescribed off label when used in pediatric and adolescent medicine. The NIMH observes that some off-label use is supported by data from well-controlled studies but cautions that other off-label prescribing, particularly to very young children whose responses to these drugs have not been scrutinized, should be performed prudently.

TABLE 8.5

Prescription drugs used to treat attention deficit hyperactivity disorder

Trade name	Generic name	Approved age
Adderall	amphetamine	3 and older
Adderall XR	amphetamine (extended release)	6 and older
Concerta	methylphenidate (long acting)	6 and older
Daytrana	methylphenidate patch	6 and older
Desoxyn	methamphetamine hydrochloride	6 and older
Dexedrine	dextroamphetamine	3 and older
Dextrostat	dextroamphetamine	3 and older
Focalin	dexmethylphenidate	6 and older
Focalin XR	dexmethylphenidate (extended release)	6 and older
Metadate ER	methylphenidate (extended release)	6 and older
Metadate CD	methylphenidate (extended release)	6 and older
Methylin	methylphenidate (oral solution and chewable tablets)	6 and older
Ritalin	methylphenidate	6 and older
Ritalin SR	methylphenidate (extended release)	6 and older
Ritalin LA	methylphenidate (long acting)	6 and older
Strattera	atomoxetine	6 and older
Vyvanse	lisdexamfetamine dimesylate	6 and older

Notes: "Extended release" means the medication is released gradually so that a controlled amount enters the body over a period of time. "Long acting" means the medication stays in the body for a long time. Not all Attention deficit hyperactivity disorder (ADHD) medications are approved for use in adults.

SOURCE: "Treatments," in *Attention Deficit Hyperactivity Disorder: What Is Attention Deficit Hyperactivity Disorder (ADHD, ADD)?* National Institutes of Mental Health, 2015

In "Treatment of Children with Mental Illness," the NIMH notes that there is strong support for the safety and efficacy of several medications for a variety of conditions, specifically psychostimulants for ADHD. The NIMH also observes that in addition to medications, other treatments for young people with mental disorders should be considered. Psychotherapy, family therapy, educational courses, and behavior management techniques can help everyone involved cope with the disorder.

POST-TRAUMATIC STRESS DISORDER

In "Post-traumatic Stress Disorder among Adults" (2015, http://www.nimh.nih.gov/health/statistics/prevalence/post-traumatic-stress-disorder-among-adults.shtml), the NIMH defines post-traumatic stress disorder (PTSD) as "an anxiety disorder that can develop after exposure to a terrifying event or ordeal in which there was the potential for or actual occurrence of grave physical harm. People with PTSD have persistent frightening thoughts and memories of their ordeal, may experience sleep problems, feel detached or numb, or be easily startled." The NIMH reports that an estimated 3.5% of U.S. adults suffer from PTSD, and 36.6% of these cases are considered severe (1.3% of the U.S. population).

PTSD can result from a range of distressing incidents, such as war, personal or sexual attack, being held captive, child abuse, car accidents, train wrecks, plane crashes, bombings, shootings, or natural disasters such as floods or earthquakes. Symptoms of PTSD include reliving the event and experiencing severe emotional and physical reactions to memories of the event, avoiding activities and places associated with the trauma, feeling detached from others, difficulty sleeping or concentrating and feeling unusually irritable or angry. Table 8.6 lists common responses to a traumatic event.

Although about half of people diagnosed with PTSD recover within three months without treatment, many sufferers require professional treatment. Treatment usually involves psychotherapy, medication, or both. Besides CBT, PTSD may be treated with exposure therapy, which helps people to face and manage their fear; cognitive restructuring, which helps people better understand their memories; or stress inoculation training, which helps people to reduce anxiety by viewing their memories differently. There are two FDA-approved medications for treating adults with PTSD—Zoloft (sertraline) and Paxil (paroxetine).

PTSD increases risk for suicide. In "Suicide Risk among 1.3 Million Veterans Who Were on Active Duty

TABLE 8.6

Common responses to a traumatic event

Cognitive	Emotional	Physical	Behavioral
• poor concentration • confusion • disorientation • indecisiveness • shortened attention span • memory loss • unwanted memories • difficulty making decisions	• shock • numbness • feeling overwhelmed • depression • feeling lost • fear of harm to self and/or loved ones • feeling nothing • feeling abandoned • uncertainty of feelings • volatile emotions	• nausea • lightheadedness • dizziness • gastro-intestinal problems • rapid heart rate • tremors • headaches • grinding of teeth • fatigue • poor sleep • pain • hyperarousal • jumpiness	• suspicion • irritability • arguments with friends and loved ones • withdrawal • excessive silence • inappropriate humor • increased/decreased eating • change in sexual desire or functioning • increased smoking • increased substance use or abuse

SOURCE: "Common Responses to a Traumatic Event," in *Helping Patients Cope with a Traumatic Event*, Centers for Disease Control and Prevention, undated, http://www.cdc.gov/masstrauma/factsheets/professionals/coping_professional.pdf (accessed January 5, 2016)

during the Iraq and Afghanistan Wars" (*Annals of Epidemiology*, vol. 25, no. 2, February 2015), Han K. Kang et al. note that PTSD is a significant risk factor for suicide. Kang et al. report that when comparing war veterans with PTSD to those without PTSD, veterans with PTSD had significantly higher rates of suicide.

SUICIDE

Suicide may be the ultimate expression or consequence of depression or another serious mental disorder. Not all people who suffer from depression contemplate suicide, nor do all those who attempt suicide suffer from depressive or other mental illnesses. Regardless, except for certain desperate medical situations, suicide in the United States is generally considered to be an unacceptable act. It is often referred to as a "long-term solution to a short-term problem."

In *Health, United States, 2014* (2015, http://www.cdc.gov/nchs/data/hus/hus14.pdf), the National Center for Health Statistics (NCHS) observes that in 2013 suicide ranked as the 10th-leading cause of death in the United States. It was the seventh-leading cause of death in males. In 2013 more than 40,000 deaths were attributed to suicide. Suicide rates were highest for males aged 65 years and older (30.9 per 100,000) and aged 45 to 64 (29 per 100,000 population). The rates were much lower for females at all ages, including those aged 45 to 64 years (9.4 per 100,000) and those aged 25 to 44 (6.8 per 100,000). (See Figure 8.5.)

Who Commits Suicide?

Suicide occurs among men and women of all racial, occupational, religious, and social groups, as well as all age groups, with the exception of the very young. The NCHS reports in *Health, United States, 2014* that between 2003 and 2013, suicide rates increased 50% among females aged 15 to 24 years, 19% among females ages 25 to 44, 36% among females ages 45 to 64, and 21% among females age 65 and older. Among males, rates increased 23% for those aged 45 to 64 years and 9% or less for the other male age groups.

The number of completed suicides does not give an accurate picture of the problem because for every completed suicide there are many unsuccessful suicide attempts. Furthermore, research reveals that more than half of the people who engage in suicidal behavior are not counted because they do not seek medical care or treatment.

Why Do People Commit Suicide?

People commit suicide for various reasons. Notes left by people who have killed themselves usually tell of life crises that they believed were unbearable. Many describe enduring chronic pain, losing loved ones, being unable to pay bills, or finding themselves incapable of living independently, and depression, substance abuse, physical abuse, and sexual abuse are all considered risk factors for suicide attempts by adolescents

Some suicides are committed on an irrational, impulsive whim. Researchers observe that even among those who are most determined to commit suicide, the desire is not as much to die as it is to escape the life they are leading and to end the pain they are suffering. Whatever the cause of their despair, they are desperately crying out for help.

Follow-up studies on suicide survivors reveal their intense ambivalence about actually dying. Not all survivors are glad to be alive, but for most, the attempted suicide marked a definite turning point. It was an urgent and dramatic signal that their problems demanded serious and immediate attention. Most survivors said that what they really wanted was to change their lives.

FIGURE 8.5

Suicide death rates, by age and sex, 2003–13

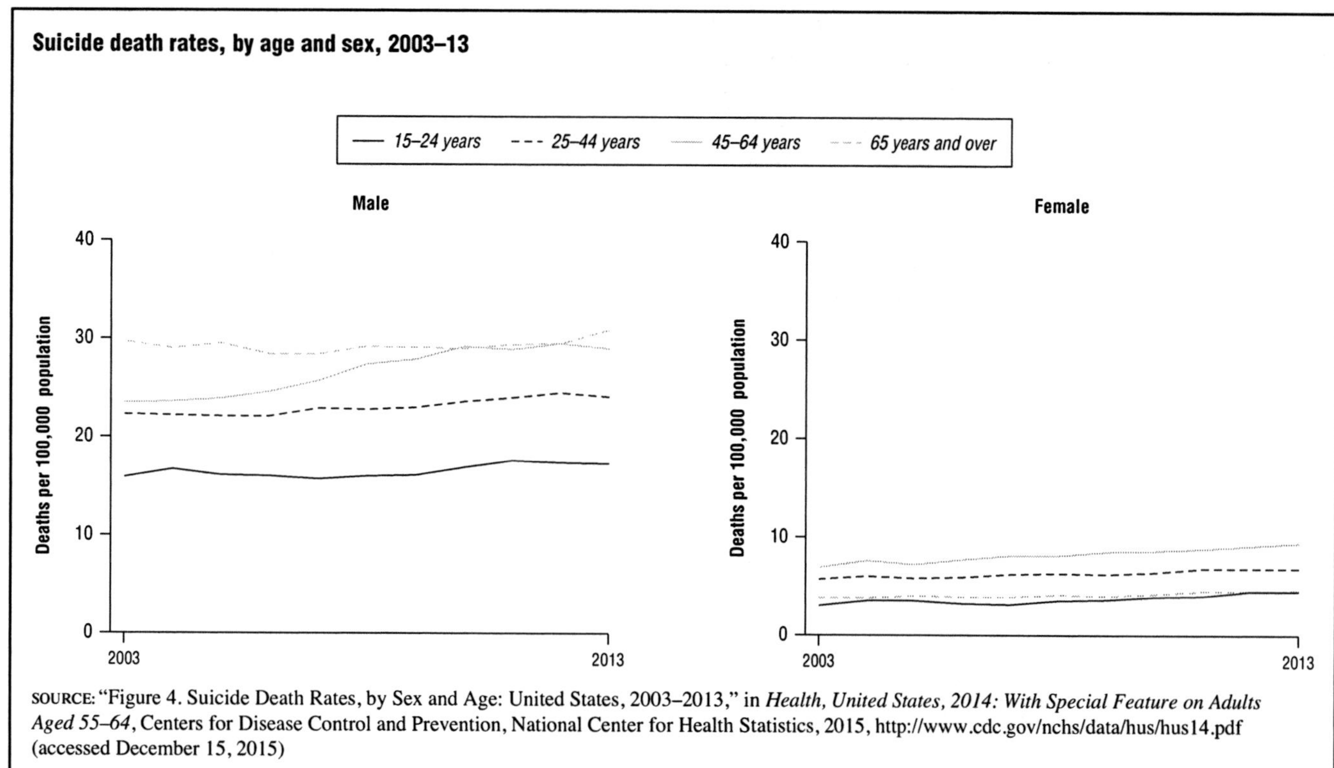

SOURCE: "Figure 4. Suicide Death Rates, by Sex and Age: United States, 2003–2013," in *Health, United States, 2014: With Special Feature on Adults Aged 55–64*, Centers for Disease Control and Prevention, National Center for Health Statistics, 2015, http://www.cdc.gov/nchs/data/hus/hus14.pdf (accessed December 15, 2015)

Suicide Is Increasing among White Non-Hispanic Americans

Anne Case and Angus Deaton looked at Gallup data from the Gallup Healthways Well-Being Index for the United States, the Gallup World Poll (which covers nearly all of the countries in Europe, the Organisation for Economic Co-operation and Development, and Latin America), and suicide data from the CDC and World Health Organization. In *Suicide, Age, and Wellbeing: An Empirical Investigation* (June 2015, http://scholar.princeton.edu/sites/default/files/deaton/files/suicide_aging_and_wellbeing_boulders_revised_june_8_2015.pdf), Case and Deaton find no correlation between life satisfaction, well-being, and suicide. They observe that in the United States, suicide rates have risen in recent years but there has been no decrease in self-reported well-being. Case and Deaton point out that for white non-Hispanics, the suicide rate is rising, driven by increasing suicide rates in middle age and offset by decreasing rates among older adults.

In a related article, "Rising Morbidity and Mortality in Midlife among White Non-Hispanic Americans in the 21st Century," published in the *Proceedings of the National Academy of Sciences* (vol. 112, no. 49, November 2015), Case and Deaton observe that midlife suicide is driving increased mortality among white non-Hispanic Americans. They cite several possible reasons for psychological distress that may be driving the growing number of suicides. They assert that people with only a high school education may not have as many opportunities for gainful, stable employment as they did in generations past and many middle-aged Americans have been unable to save enough money for a comfortable retirement. Case and Denton also note that there has been a deterioration of family support systems; for example, the divorce rate of people aged 50 years and older has doubled to 25% between 1990 and 2012.

Suicide among the Terminally Ill

Not all suicides are categorized as the acts of people who are mentally ill. Some people consider suicides committed by people who are terminally ill as rational choices. They argue that people who are terminally ill have the right to die—that is, the right to control the manner of their death. Patients with terminal diseases often worry that they will suffer long and painful deaths and that they stand a good chance of losing everything: health, independence, jobs, insurance, homes, and contact with loved ones and friends.

Researchers find that factors with significant impact on the quality of life include security, family, love, pleasurable activity, and freedom from pain and suffering. Sufferers of debilitating disease may lose all of these. For some, suicide is a last recourse to relieve pain, suffering, insecurity, dependence, or hopelessness.

The right to die and to choose the time and manner of death remains a hotly debated topic throughout the world. In the United States just five states (California, Montana,

Oregon, Vermont, and Washington) have legalized physician-assisted suicide. Since 1994 Oregon's Death with Dignity Act has allowed a terminally ill adult to request a prescription for a lethal dose of drugs. The legislation contains many restrictions that are intended to protect both patients and the physicians who prescribe the drugs. In an analysis of the law's application, Ronald A. Lindsay of the Center for Inquiry in Amherst, New York, observes in "Oregon's Experience: Evaluating the Record" (*American Journal of Bioethics*, vol. 9, no. 3, March 2009) that none of the untoward consequences feared by the law's staunchest opponents (specifically that it would affect "vulnerable groups disproportionately, that legal assisted dying could not be confined to the competent terminally ill who voluntarily request assistance, and that the practice would result in frequent abuses") had materialized. Lindsay asserts that Oregon's experience "argues in favor of legalization of assistance in dying."

In March 2008 Washington became the second state to permit physician-assisted suicide. Like the Oregon legislation, Washington's law aims to restrict the practice to minimize the potential for abuse. Patients must make two requests, more than two weeks apart, and one must be in writing. The patient must be of sound mind and not suffering from depression, and two physicians must approve the request for a lethal dose of drugs. In 2009 Montana became the third state to legalize physician-assisted suicide, and in 2013 Vermont became the fourth state to make physician-assisted suicide legal. California became the fifth state to legalize physician-assisted suicide in October 2015, when after much debate it passed guidelines similar to those in effect in Oregon.

Suicide's Warning Signs

Researchers believe that most suicidal people convey their intentions to someone among their friends and family, either openly or indirectly. The people they signal are those who know them well and are in the best position to recognize the signs and provide help. Comments such as "You'd be better off without me," "No one will have to worry about me much longer," or even a casual "I've had it" may be signals of upcoming attempts. Some people who are suicidal put their affairs in order. They draw up wills, give away prized possessions, or act as if they are preparing for a long trip. They may even talk about going away.

Often, the indicator is a distinct change in personality or behavior. A normally happy person may become increasingly depressed, a regular churchgoer may stop attending services, or an avid runner may quit exercising. These types of changes, if added to expressions of worthlessness or hopelessness, can indicate not only that the person is seriously depressed but also that he or she may have decided to commit suicide. Although the vast majority of people who are depressed are not suicidal, most of the suicide-prone are depressed. Researchers and health care practitioners caution that suicide threats and attempts should not be discounted as harmless bids for attention. Anyone thinking, talking about, or planning suicide should receive immediate professional evaluation and treatment.

CHAPTER 9
COMPLEMENTARY AND ALTERNATIVE MEDICINE

The National Center for Complementary and Integrative Health (NCCIH; formerly the National Center for Complementary and Alternative Medicine), was established in 1998 and is one of the 27 institutes and centers of the National Institutes of Health (NIH). In "NCCIH Facts-at-a-Glance and Mission" (January 9, 2015, https://nccih.nih.gov/about/ataglance), the NCCIH states that its mission is to "define, through rigorous scientific investigation, the usefulness and safety of complementary and alternative medicine [CAM] interventions and their roles in improving health and health care." To determine a method's or product's effectiveness and safety, the organization uses a hierarchy of evidence. (See Figure 9.1.) Studies indicate that data on the efficacy (the ability of an intervention to produce the intended diagnostic or therapeutic effect in optimal circumstances) and safety of complementary therapies span a continuum ranging from expert opinions, anecdotes, and case studies to encouraging information that has been obtained from large, well-developed clinical trials.

In "Complementary, Alternative, or Integrative Health: What's in a Name?" (March 2016, https://nccih.nih.gov/health/integrative-health), the NCCIH distinguishes between complementary, alternative, and integrative medicine in the following manner:

- Alternative medicine is therapy or treatment that is used instead of conventional medical treatment. One example of alternative medicine is using herbal preparations containing valerian, chamomile, and hops rather than over-the-counter or prescription relaxants or sleep aids. The NCCIH observes that exclusive use of alternative medicine is rare; most people use unconventional approaches along with conventional therapies.
- Complementary medicine is alternative therapy or treatment that is used along with conventional medicine, not in place of it. An example of complementary medicine is the addition of relaxation techniques or movement awareness therapies (such as the Alexander technique, Pilates, and the Feldenkrais method) to the traditional approaches of physical and occupational therapy that are used to rehabilitate people who have had a stroke. Complementary medicine appears to offer health benefits, but often there is little scientific evidence to support its utility.
- Integrative medicine is the coordinated combination of conventional medical treatment and CAM therapies that have been scientifically researched and have demonstrated that they are both safe and effective. An example of integrative medicine is teaching stress management and relaxation techniques to people with high blood pressure and heart disease along with the use of traditional approaches such as weight management, exercise, and prescription drugs to reduce the risks and complications of heart disease.

Despite the classification system that is outlined by the NCCIH, complementary and integrative health care continues to be known by a variety of names (nontraditional medicine, unorthodox medical practices, and holistic health care) and reflects a wide range of philosophies, including the need for or reliance on scientific evidence of effectiveness. Generally, alternative therapies tend to be untested and unproven, whereas complementary and integrative practices that are used in conjunction with mainstream medicine are often those with a substantial scientific basis of demonstrated safety and efficacy.

It is, however, important to bear in mind that many complementary and alternative practices for which there is no current research demonstrating safety and efficacy are not alternative medicine at all but are the longstanding, traditional practices in the cultures from which they arose. These time-honored practices are only deemed "alternative" in countries and cultures where allopathic Western medicine prevails. For example, homeopathy, which is described in detail in this chapter, is a demonstrably safe

FIGURE 9.1

Hierarchy of evidence

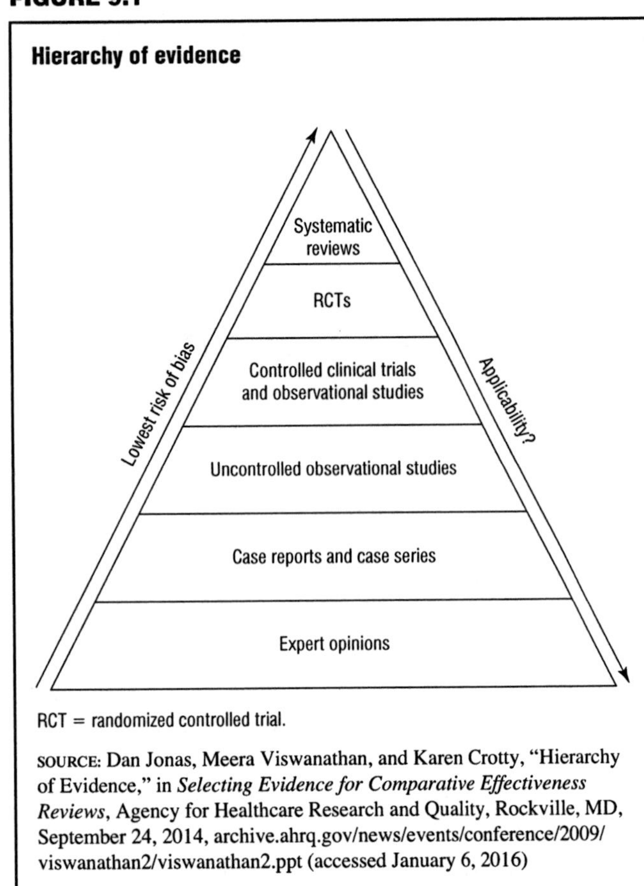

RCT = randomized controlled trial.

SOURCE: Dan Jonas, Meera Viswanathan, and Karen Crotty, "Hierarchy of Evidence," in *Selecting Evidence for Comparative Effectiveness Reviews*, Agency for Healthcare Research and Quality, Rockville, MD, September 24, 2014, archive.ahrq.gov/news/events/conference/2009/viswanathan2/viswanathan2.ppt (accessed January 6, 2016)

and effective 200-year-old system of complementary and alternative medicine used throughout the world.

THE GROWING POPULARITY OF CAM

Many people have turned to CAM approaches out of frustration with mainstream medicine. Some CAM users are interested in natural, as opposed to pharmaceutical, solutions to health problems, whereas others want to take charge of their health and are seeking self-care approaches to maintaining health and wellness. Helping this movement along is information technology, which is enabling easy access to sources of CAM information on the Internet and in print and electronic media, and advertising and marketing of new CAM products and methods. Combined data from the 2002, 2007, and 2012 National Health Interview Surveys were reported by Tainya C. Clarke et al. in "Trends in the Use of Complementary Health Approaches among Adults: United States, 2002–2012" (*National Health Statistics Reports*, no. 79, February 10, 2015) and showed that 36% of American adults ages 18 to 44 used CAM approaches in 2002, 40% of this group used CAM in 2007, and 37% in 2012. Table 9.1 shows trends in the use of complementary health approaches in 2002, 2007, and 2012.

In 2012 the most frequently used complementary health approach was the use of natural products which includes dietary supplements; nearly 18% of adults said they used vitamins, minerals, herbs, and probiotics (live bacteria that replace or add to the beneficial bacteria normally present in the gastrointestinal tract). (See Figure 9.2.) Mind-body practices such as deep breathing, yoga, and tai chi were used by more than 10% of American adults.

From 2002 to 2012 the percentage of adults practicing yoga nearly doubled. (See Figure 9.3, which shows age-adjusted percentages for each of the three years.) Although use of yoga increased among people of all ages, the increase was smaller among older age groups. (See Figure 9.4.) Use of yoga grew among adults of all races and ethnicities. It nearly doubled among Hispanics and non-Hispanic African Americans from 2007 to 2012. (See Figure 9.5.)

Clarke et al. report that in 2012 the most commonly used natural products were fish oil/omega-3 fatty acids. Found in certain plants and nuts as well as in fatty fish, omega-3 fatty acids lower triglycerides and may reduce the risk of death, heart attack, dangerous abnormal heart rhythms, and strokes. The second most used natural product was glucosamine (an amino sugar that the body produces and distributes in cartilage and other connective tissue that has been used to help prevent and treat arthritis and joint pain), followed by probiotics and prebiotics (carbohydrates that cannot be digested by the body but serve as food for probiotics) and melatonin (a hormone involved in sleep-wake cycles that is often used to promote sleep). (See Table 9.2.)

Children's Use of CAM

According to Lindsey I. Black et al., in "Use of Complementary and Alternative Medicine among Children Aged 4–17 Years in the United States: National Health Interview Survey, 2007–2012" (*National Health Statistics Report*, no. 78, February 10, 2015), the use of complementary health approaches among children did not change from 2007 to 2012, remaining at about 12%. Black et al. report that as with adults, use of complementary health approaches was more frequent among children with chronic health conditions such as anxiety, musculoskeletal conditions, and recurrent headaches and among those with higher family income and parental educational attainment. (See Table 9.3.) Not surprisingly, parents' use of complementary health approaches strongly influences the use of such approaches by their children.

Black et al. note that as with adults, CAM use among children most often relied on natural products, followed by chiropractic and osteopathic care, and yoga, tai chi, or qigong. Children's use of yoga increased from 2.3% in 2007 to 3.1% in 2012.

The natural products children used most frequently in 2012 were fish oil, melatonin, pro- and prebiotics, and Echinacea (traditionally used to treat or prevent colds,

TABLE 9.1

Trends in the use of selected complementary health approaches, 2002, 2007, and 2012

Complementary health approach	2002 Number (in thousands)	2002 Age-adjusted percent[a]	2007 Number (in thousands)	2007 Age-adjusted percent[a]	2012 Number (in thousands)	2012 Age-adjusted percent[a]
Nonvitamin, nonmineral dietary supplements	38,183	18.9	38,797	17.7	40,579	17.7
Deep-breathing exercises[b]	23,457	11.6	27,794	12.7	24,218	10.9
Yoga, tai chi, and qi gong	11,766	5.8	14,436	6.7	22,281	10.1
Chiropractic or osteopathic manipulation[c]	15,226	7.5	18,740	8.6	19,369	8.4
Meditation[d]	15,336	7.6	20,541	9.4	17,948	8.0
Massage therapy	10,052	5.0	18,068	8.3	15,411	6.9
Special diets[e]	6,765	3.3	6,040	2.8	6,853	3.0
Homeopathic treatment[f]	3,433	1.7	3,909	1.8	5,046	2.2
Progressive relaxation	6,185	3.0	6,454	2.9	4,766	2.1
Guided imagery	4,194	2.1	4,866	2.2	3,846	1.7
Acupuncture	2,136	1.1	3,141	1.4	3,484	1.5
Energy healing therapy	1,080	0.5	1,216	0.5	1,077	0.5
Naturopathy	498	0.2	729	0.3	957	0.4
Hypnosis	505	0.2	561	0.2	347	0.1
Biofeedback	278	0.1	362	0.2	281	0.1
Ayurveda	154	0.1†	214	0.1†	241	0.1

[a]The denominator used in the calculation of percentages was all sample adults.
[b]In 2012, deep-breathing exercises included deep-breathing exercises as part of hypnosis; biofeedback; Mantra meditation (including Transcendental Meditation, Relaxation Response, and Clinically Standardized Meditation); mindfulness meditation (including Vipassana, Zen Buddhist meditation, mindfulness-based stress reduction, and mindfulness-based cognitive therapy); spiritual meditation (including centering prayer and contemplative meditation); guided imagery; progressive relaxation; yoga; tai chi; or qi gong. In 2002 and 2007, the use of deep-breathing exercises was asked broadly and not if used as part of other complementary health approaches. No trend analyses were conducted on the use of deep-breathing exercises.
[c]In 2002, the use of chiropractic care was asked broadly, and osteopathic approach was not specified on the survey. No trend analyses were conducted on the use of chiropractic or osteopathic manipulation.
[d]In 2012, meditation included Mantra meditation (including Transcendental Meditation, Relaxation Response, and Clinically Standardized Meditation); mindfulness meditation (including Vipassana, Zen Buddhist meditation, mindfulness-based stress reduction, and mindfulness-based cognitive therapy); spiritual meditation (including centering prayer and contemplative meditation); and meditation used as a part of other practices (including yoga, tai chi, and qi gong). In 2002 and 2007, the use of meditation was asked broadly and not if practiced as part of other complementary health approaches.
[e]Respondents used one or more named special diets for 2 weeks or more in the past 12 months. Special diets included vegetarian (including vegan), macrobiotic, Atkins, Pritikin, and Ornish diets.
[f]No distinction was made between persons who sought treatment from a homeopathic practitioner and those who self-medicated.
Notes: Estimates were age-adjusted using the projected 2000 U.S. population as the standard population and using four age groups: 18–24, 25–44, 45–64, and 65 and over. The denominators for statistics shown exclude persons with unknown complementary and alternative medicine information. Estimates are based on household interviews of a sample of the civilian noninstitutionalized population.

SOURCE: Adapted from Tainya C. Clarke et al., "Table 1. Trends in the Use of Complementary Health Approaches during the Past 12 Months, by Type of Approach: United States, 2002, 2007, and 2012," in "Trends in the Use of Complementary Health Approaches among Adults: United States, 2002–2012," *National Health Statistics Reports*, no. 79, February 10, 2015, http://www.cdc.gov/nchs/data/nhsr/nhsr079.pdf (accessed January 7, 2016)

flu, and other infections). (See Table 9.4.) The conditions for which children most frequently used complementary approaches were back/neck pain, head or chest colds, other musculoskeletal complaints and anxiety/stress. (See Table 9.5.)

In "Complementary and Alternative Medicine Use by Pediatric Specialty Outpatients" (*Pediatrics*, vol. 131, no. 2, February 1, 2014), Denise Adams et al. report that CAM use is high among children with chronic illnesses. Vitamins and minerals and herbal and homeopathic remedies were the most popular products used by children, and the most popular practices were massage, chiropractic manipulation, faith healing, aromatherapy, and relaxation techniques.

USE OF CAM FOR CHILDREN WITH AUTISM SPECTRUM DISORDERS. Roger S. Aikins et al. compare in "Utilization Patterns of Conventional and Complementary/Alternative Treatments in Children with Autism Spectrum Disorders and Developmental Disabilities in a Population-Based Study" (*Journal of Behavioral and Developmental Pediatrics*, vol. 35, no. 1, January 2014) the use of conventional treatments and CAM in preschoolers with autism spectrum disorders and other developmental disabilities. The researchers find use of CAM is common in families of young children with autism spectrum disorders, and it is not due to the lack of availability of conventional treatment, which has been suggested by other research. Aikins et al. find that CAM is predicted by higher parental educational attainment.

Aikins et al. find that most families using CAM chose low risk treatment such as probiotics and gluten-free or other alternative diets. About 9% of those surveyed used therapies the researchers considered potentially unsafe or unproven, such as antifungal medications, chelation therapy (use of an agent to bind to iron or lead in the blood to eliminate the metal's toxic effect), and vitamin B_{12} injections.

Why Do People Seek CAM?

People turn to complementary health approaches for many different reasons. One of the attractions is its emphasis on the "whole person," rather than on simply the diseased organ or body part. Complementary therapies

FIGURE 9.2

10 most common complementary health approaches among adults, 2012

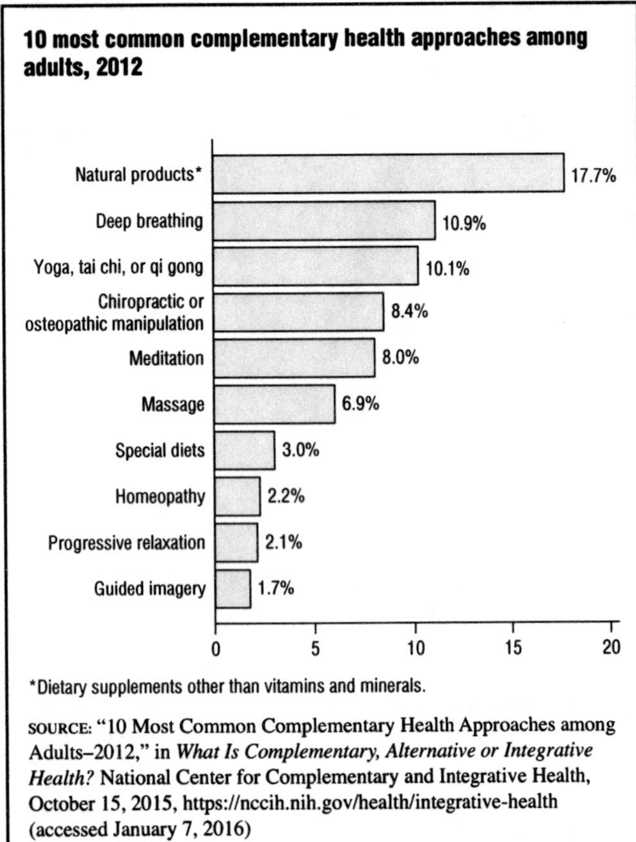

*Dietary supplements other than vitamins and minerals.

SOURCE: "10 Most Common Complementary Health Approaches among Adults–2012," in *What Is Complementary, Alternative or Integrative Health?* National Center for Complementary and Integrative Health, October 15, 2015, https://nccih.nih.gov/health/integrative-health (accessed January 7, 2016)

FIGURE 9.3

Use of yoga, tai chi, and qigong among adults, 2002, 2007, and 2012

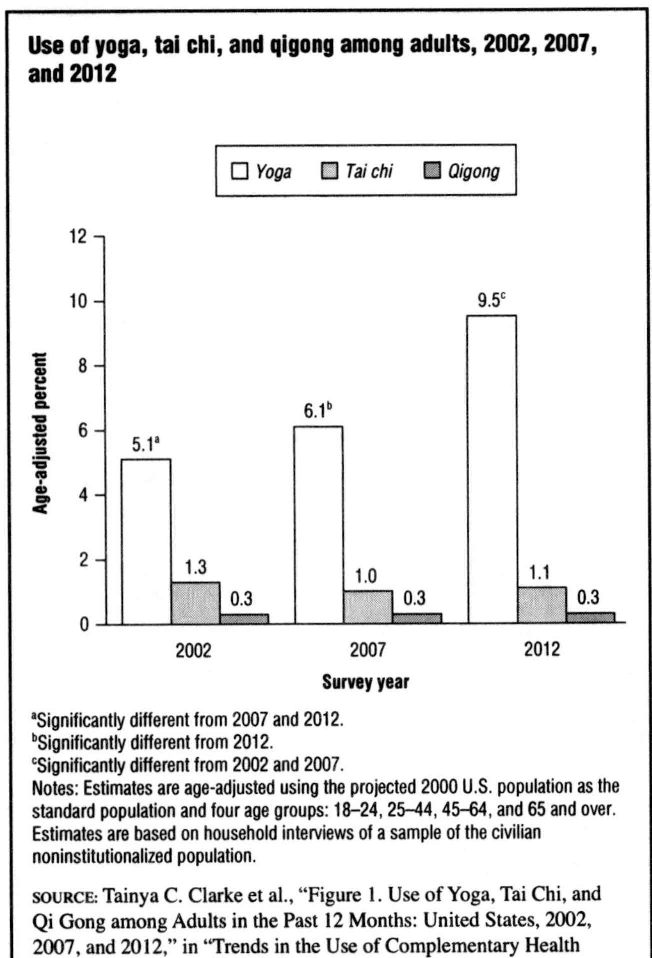

[a]Significantly different from 2007 and 2012.
[b]Significantly different from 2012.
[c]Significantly different from 2002 and 2007.
Notes: Estimates are age-adjusted using the projected 2000 U.S. population as the standard population and four age groups: 18–24, 25–44, 45–64, and 65 and over. Estimates are based on household interviews of a sample of the civilian noninstitutionalized population.

SOURCE: Tainya C. Clarke et al., "Figure 1. Use of Yoga, Tai Chi, and Qi Gong among Adults in the Past 12 Months: United States, 2002, 2007, and 2012," in "Trends in the Use of Complementary Health Approaches among Adults: United States, 2002–2012," *National Health Statistics Reports*, no. 79, February 10, 2015, http://www.cdc.gov/nchs/data/nhsr/nhsr079.pdf (accessed January 7, 2016)

and practitioners tend to consider patients as human beings rather than as simply physical bodies, and nearly all emphasize the mind-body connection and pay attention to emotional wellness and spirituality.

In "Wellness-Related Use of Common Complementary Health Approaches among Adults: United States, 2012" (*National Health Statistics*, no. 85, November 4, 2015), Barbara J. Stussman et al. report selected reasons for the use of natural product supplements, yoga, and spinal manipulation identified by the 2012 Adult Alternative Medicine supplement to the National Health Interview Survey. Stussman et al. find that dietary supplements and yoga were more frequently used for wellness than to treat a specific health condition while spinal manipulation was used more often as treatment for a specific health problem. Wellness or disease prevention was the most frequently cited reason for using dietary supplements (83.3%) followed by improving immune function (42%), improving energy (31%), focusing on the whole person—mind, body and spirit (26.5%), and improving memory or concentration (22.2%).

Figure 9.6 shows five wellness-related benefits survey respondents attributed to their use of complementary health approaches. For example, more than three-quarters (80%) of those who do yoga feel they are less stressed, about two-thirds (67.2%) feel better emotionally, and more than half (59.3%) credit yoga with improved sleep. Other reported benefits of yoga include prompting users to exercise more regularly (63.2%), eat healthier (42.6%), cut back or stop smoking cigarettes (25.2%), and cut back or stop drinking alcohol (12.4%).

Some patients seek alternative therapies when conventional medicine fails to relieve their symptoms or when traditional treatment produces unpleasant side effects. In "Reasons Why Older Americans Use Complementary and Alternative Medicine: Costly or Ineffective Conventional Medicine and Recommendations from Health Care Providers, Family, and Friends" (*Educational Gerontology*, vol. 39, no. 9, 2013), Elizabeth M. Tait et al. looked at why older adults use CAM. The researchers report that most older adults said they used complementary health because a health care provider recommended it or it was recommended by family, friends, or coworkers. Others said it was because conventional medicine was ineffective or too costly.

FIGURE 9.4

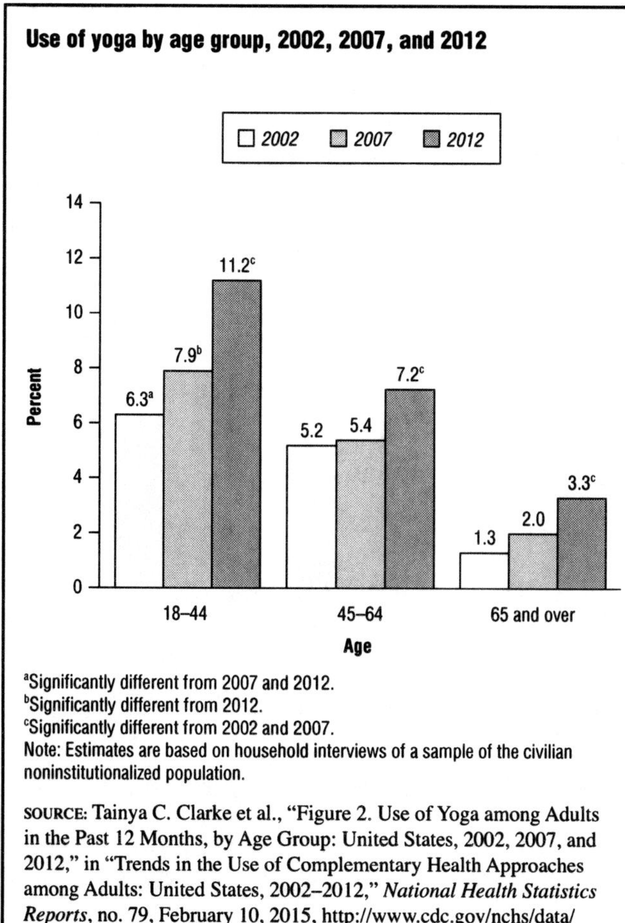

[a]Significantly different from 2007 and 2012.
[b]Significantly different from 2012.
[c]Significantly different from 2002 and 2007.
Note: Estimates are based on household interviews of a sample of the civilian noninstitutionalized population.

SOURCE: Tainya C. Clarke et al., "Figure 2. Use of Yoga among Adults in the Past 12 Months, by Age Group: United States, 2002, 2007, and 2012," in "Trends in the Use of Complementary Health Approaches among Adults: United States, 2002–2012," *National Health Statistics Reports*, no. 79, February 10, 2015, http://www.cdc.gov/nchs/data/nhsr/nhsr079.pdf (accessed January 7, 2016)

All Kinds of People Use Complementary Health Approaches

Besides people who distrust or question conventional medical treatment, there are other groups that make frequent use of complementary health approaches. Gwen Wyatt et al. observe in "Complementary and Alternative Medicine Use, Spending, and Quality of Life in Early Stage Breast Cancer" (*Nursing Research*, vol. 59, no. 1, January–February 2010) that as many as 80% of women with breast cancer use complementary therapies to improve their quality of life during cancer treatment. The researchers find that biologically based therapies (primarily nutritional supplements) and mind-body therapies were used most often by a majority of the sample.

Cancer patients are not, however, the only ones to seek complementary approaches. In "Any Difference? Use of a CAM Provider among Cancer Patients, Coronary Heart Disease (CHD) Patients and Individuals with No Cancer/CHD" (*BMC Complementary and Alternative Medicine*, vol. 12, no. 1, January 12, 2012), Agnete E. Kristoffersen, Arne J. Norheim, and Vinjar M. Fønnebø report that a survey of people in Norway found that the proportion of cancer patients seeing a complementary health practitioner was not statistically different from patients with coronary heart disease or individuals without cancer or coronary heart disease. The researchers do not find widespread use of complementary health approaches among cancer patients (only 8% reported visiting a complementary health practitioner during the 12 months prior to the survey), and they observe that their findings are only slightly lower than the rates that are reported by other surveys, such as a study in the United Kingdom that reported just 9.2%.

Lauren M. Denneson, Kathryn Corson, and Steven K. Dobscha examined complementary health use among U.S. military veterans with chronic pain and published their findings in "Complementary and Alternative Medicine Use among Veterans with Chronic Noncancer Pain" (*Journal of Rehabilitation Research and Development*, vol. 48, no. 9, 2011). The researchers find that 82% of subjects reported using at least one complementary health therapy during the past year, and nearly all (99%) expressed a willingness to try complementary health treatment for pain. The most preferred complementary health approach was massage therapy, and the least preferred was chiropractic care.

Complementary Health Use in Hospitals

In the 21st century many complementary health practices have been incorporated into mainstream medicine. The Institute of Medicine finds in *Complementary and Alternative Medicine in the United States* (2005) that the integration of complementary and conventional medicine is occurring in many settings including hospitals, physicians' offices, and health maintenance organizations.

In "CE: Integrative Care: The Evolving Landscape in American Hospitals" (*American Journal of Nursing*, vol. 115, no. 10, October 2015), Margo A. Halm and Julie Katseres reports the results of a 2010 hospital survey about CAM use, including the finding that 42% of hospitals said they offer CAM services. Hospitals with known integrative care programs offer a range of services including massage therapy, acupuncture, guided imagery, biofeedback, music therapy, pet therapy, therapeutic touch, yoga, tai chi/qigong, and nutritional supplements.

The 2010 survey reported that hospitals are motivated to offer CAM services in response to patient demand (85%), clinical effectiveness (70%), and by its consistency with their organizational mission (58%). To choose which therapies to offer, hospitals rely largely on patient demand (78%), followed by evidence of effectiveness (74%) and practitioner availability (58%).

TYPES OF COMPLEMENTARY HEALTH APPROACHES

Complementary health approaches may be categorized into four broad domains. There is some overlap between these CAM domains:

- Mind-body interventions—mind-body medicine is a range of practices that aims to use the power of the

FIGURE 9.5

Use of yoga by race and Hispanic origin, 2002, 2007, and 2012

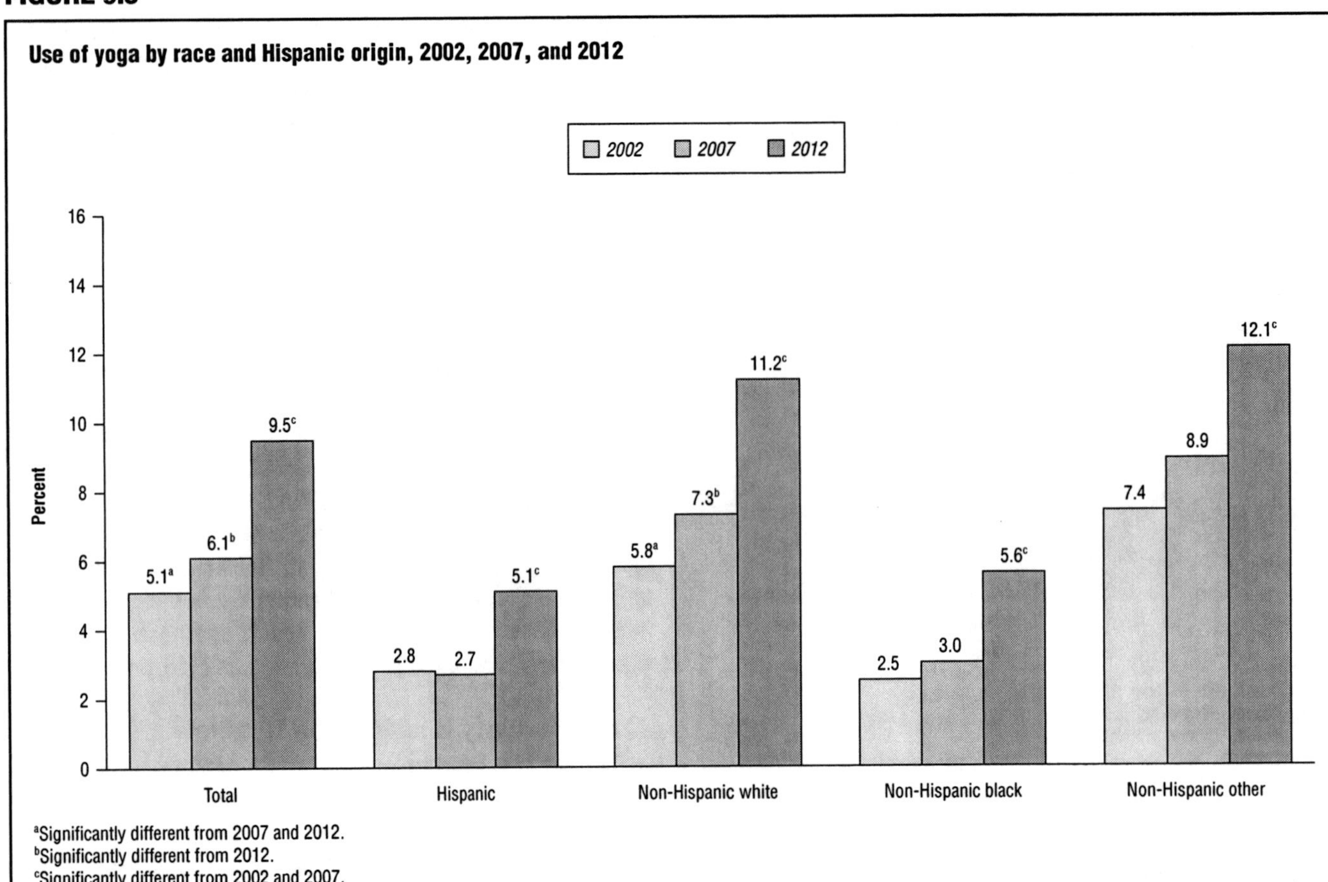

[a]Significantly different from 2007 and 2012.
[b]Significantly different from 2012.
[c]Significantly different from 2002 and 2007.
Notes: Estimates are age-adjusted using the projected 2000 U.S. population as the standard population and four age groups: 18–24, 25–44, 45–64, and 65 and over. Estimates are based on household interviews of a sample of the civilian noninstitutionalized population.

SOURCE: Tainya C. Clarke et al., "Figure 3. Use of Yoga among Adults in the Past 12 Months, by Hispanic Origin and Race: United States, 2002, 2007, and 2012," in "Trends in the Use of Complementary Health Approaches among Adults: United States, 2002–2012," *National Health Statistics Reports*, no. 79, February 10, 2015, http://www.cdc.gov/nchs/data/nhsr/nhsr079.pdf (accessed January 7, 2016)

mind to influence the symptoms of disease and healing. Increasingly, this type of alternative medicine has gained acceptance among medical professionals. Mind-body therapies (such as relaxation techniques, patient support groups, and art, dance, and music therapies) are now widely used by practitioners of conventional medicine. Less widely accepted mind-body techniques include meditation, breathing, hypnosis, and prayer.

- Biologically based therapies—this type of treatment uses organic (naturally occurring) substances such as herbs, food, and vitamins to treat symptoms of disease and improve health and wellness. Examples of biologically based therapies include dietary supplements, herbal remedies, and the hotly debated use of hormones such as human growth hormone and dehydroepiandrosterone (the most plentiful steroid hormone in the body) to combat disease and to slow aging.
- Manipulative and body-based practices—movement therapies, manipulative methods, and bodywork are another type of CAM. Examples of these methods are massage therapy, chiropractic, and osteopathic manipulation (also referred to as craniosacral manipulative therapy).
- Energy medicine—these techniques aim to influence energy fields that practitioners of this form of CAM believe exist in and around the body. Also called biofield therapies, some are "touch" therapies, and others do not involve direct contact with any part of the body. Reiki and qigong are examples of biofield therapies. Other forms of energy therapies known as bioelectromagnetic-based therapies use magnetic energy, electromagnetic fields, pulsed fields, alternating current, or direct current fields to influence "energy flow."

There also are whole medical systems. Many of these alternative medicine systems developed before conventional Western medicine or independent of it. Alternative medicine systems are based on different beliefs and philosophies and, as a result, approach diagnosis and treatment of disease quite differently from traditional Western medicine. Examples of alternative medicine systems that

TABLE 9.2

Percentage of adults who used selected dietary supplements, 2007 and 2012

Dietary supplements[a]	2007 Number (in thousands)	2007 Age-adjusted percent[b]	2012 Number (in thousands)	2012 Age-adjusted percent[b]
Fish oil[c]	10,923	4.8	18,848	7.8
Glucosamine or chondroitin	7,236	3.2	6,450	2.6
Probiotics or prebiotics	865	0.4	3,857	1.6
Melatonin	1,296	0.6	3,065	1.3
Coenzyme Q–10 (CoQ10)	2,691	1.2	3,265	1.3
Echinacea	4,848	2.2	2,261	0.9
Cranberry (pills or capsules)	1,560	0.7	1,934	0.8
Garlic supplements	3,278	1.4	1,927	0.8
Ginseng	3,345	1.5	1,752	0.7
Ginkgo biloba	2,977	1.3	1,619	0.7
Green tea pills (not brewed tea) or EGCG (pills)[d]	1,528	0.7	1,503	0.6
Combination herb pill	3,446	1.5	1,463	0.6
MSM (methylsulfonylmethane)	1,312	0.6	1,051	0.4
Milk thistle (silymarin)	1,001	0.4	988	0.4
Saw palmetto	1,682	0.7	988	0.4
Valerian	877	0.4	801	0.3

[a]Respondents may have used more than one nonvitamin, nonmineral dietary supplement.
[b]The denominator used in the calculation of percentages was all sample adults.
[c]In 2007, fish oil was described as fish oil or omega 3 or DHA fatty acid. In 2012, fish oil was described as fish oil or omega 3 or DHA or EPA fatty acid.
[d]EGCG is epigallocatechin gallate.
Notes: Estimates were age-adjusted using the projected 2000 U.S. population as the standard population and using four age groups: 18–24, 25–44, 45–64, and 65 and over. Estimates are based on household interviews of a sample of the civilian noninstitutionalized population.

SOURCE: Tainya C. Clarke et al., "Table 3. Adults Aged 18 and over Who used Selected Types of Nonvitamin, Nonmineral Dietary Supplements during the Past 30 Days: United States, 2007 and 2012," in "Trends in the Use of Complementary Health Approaches among Adults: United States, 2002–2012," *National Health Statistics Reports*, no. 79, February 10, 2015, http://www.cdc.gov/nchs/data/nhsr/nhsr079.pdf (accessed January 7, 2016)

began in Western cultures are homeopathy and naturopathic medicine. Alternative medicine systems that developed in other cultures include acupuncture, Ayurvedic medicine, and traditional Chinese medicine.

ALTERNATIVE MEDICINE SYSTEMS

Practically every culture has a medicine system; some societies developed more than one system, tradition, or philosophy to explain the causes of disease and suggest therapies to relieve symptoms. This section considers two alternative medicine systems that had their origins in Western culture (homeopathy and naturopathic medicine) and three that developed in non-Western cultures (acupuncture, Ayurvedic medicine, and traditional Chinese medicine).

Homeopathic Medicine

Homeopathic medicine (also called homeopathy) is based on the belief that "like cures like" and uses very diluted amounts of natural substances to encourage the body's own self-healing mechanisms. If taken in higher doses or in stronger concentrations, the natural substances that are used by homeopathy to stimulate self-healing would likely produce the symptoms the diluted substances aim to relieve.

Homeopathy was developed by the German physician Samuel Hahnemann (1755–1843) during the 1790s. First experimenting on healthy subjects and himself, Hahnemann discovered that he could produce symptoms of particular diseases by injecting small doses of various herbal substances. This discovery inspired him to try another experiment: giving sick people extremely diluted formulations of substances that would produce the same symptoms they suffered from in an effort to evoke natural recovery and regeneration.

Hahnemann believed that homeopathic remedies (substances that caused symptoms similar to those caused by the disease but not diluted forms of the disease-causing agents) worked by activating the "vital force," the organizing energy system that governs health in a human being. There is no comparable belief in Western medicine, but the idea of vital force bears some resemblance to the Ayurvedic concept of *prana* and to qi (also called chi) in Chinese medicine.

Homeopathy gained a foothold in the United States during the 1830s, when it appeared able to stem some epidemics, such as cholera (a devastating infectious disease that produces severe diarrhea), but by the 1900s it fell out of favor as traditional medical practice experienced greater success treating the diseases of the day. During the 1970s there was renewed interest in homeopathy in the United States, and by 2016 believers credited homeopathy with gentle, effective, and nontoxic treatment of many infections, emotional problems, and learning disorders. Although proponents assert that homeopathic medicine speeds healing, it cannot treat traumatic injuries, such as broken bones, or genetic diseases.

TABLE 9.3

Percentages of children aged 4–17 who used complementary health approaches, 2007 and 2012

Selected characteristic	Any complementary health approach use[a] 2007 Age-adjusted percent[b]	Any complementary health approach use[a] 2012 Age-adjusted percent[b]
Total	**12.0**	**11.6**
Sex		
Boys	10.5	9.7
Girls	13.5	13.5
Age (years)[c]		
4–11	9.8	9.3
12–17	15.0	14.7
Hispanic origin and race		
Hispanic	8.2	6.1
Non-Hispanic white, single race	14.7	14.9
Non-Hispanic black or African American, single race	5.5	5.5
Non-Hispanic all other races	13.6	14.2
Parent's education[d]		
Less than high school diploma	4.1	2.1
High school diploma or GED[e]	8.1	6.9
More than high school	15.2	15.0
Poverty status[f]		
Poor	7.0	5.7
Near poor	8.5	9.1
Not poor	14.9	14.8
Health insurance[g]		
Private	14.1	14.6
Public	8.1	7.6
Uninsured	10.4	8.4

[a]Complementary health approach definition was a "yes" response to chelation therapy; nonvitamin, nonmineral dietary supplements; vegetarian or vegan diet; macrobiotic diet; Atkins diet; Pritikin diet; Ornish diet; acupuncture; Ayurveda; homeopathic treatment; naturopathy; Native American or Medicine Man; Shaman; Curandero, Machi, or Parchero; Yerbero or Hierbista; Sobador; Huesero; chiropractic or osteopathic manipulation; massage; Feldenkrais; Alexander technique; Pilates; Trager psychophysical integration; biofeedback; mantra meditation; Transcendental Meditation; relaxation; clinically standard meditation; spiritual meditation; guided imagery; progressive relaxation; yoga, tai chi, or qi gong (with deep breathing); hypnosis; and energy healing.
[b]The denominator used in the calculation of percentages was all sample children.
[c]Estimates for age groups are not age-adjusted.
[d]Refers to the education level of the parent with the higher level of education, regardless of that parent's age.
[e]GED is General Educational Development high school equivalency diploma.
[f]Based on family income and family size using the U.S. Census Bureau's poverty thresholds for the previous calendar year. "Poor" persons are defined as below the poverty threshold. "Near poor" persons have incomes of 100% to less than 200% of the poverty threshold. "Not poor" persons have incomes that are 200% of the poverty threshold or greater.
[g]Based on a hierarchy of mutually exclusive categories. Children with more than one type of health insurance were assigned to the first appropriate category in the hierarchy. "Uninsured" includes children who had no coverage as well as those who had only Indian Health Service coverage or had only a private plan that paid for one type of service such as accidents or dental care.
Notes: Estimates are based on household interviews of a sample of the civilian noninstitutionalized population. Estimates are age-adjusted using the projected 2000 U.S. population as the standard population and using two age groups: 4–11 and 12–17.

SOURCE: Lindsey I. Black et al., "Adapted from Table. 2. Age-Adjusted Percentages of Children Aged 4–17 Years Who Used Any Complementary Health Approaches during the Past 12 Months, by Selected Characteristics: United States, 2007 and 2012," in "Use of Complementary Health Approaches among Children Aged 4–17 Years in the United States: National Health Interview Survey, 2007–2012," *National Health Statistics Reports*, no. 78, February 10, 2015, http://www.cdc.gov/nchs/data/nhsr/nhsr078.pdf (accessed January 7, 2016)

Iris Bell and Nancy N. Boyer considered homeopathic treatment for middle ear infections and respiratory infections in children and published their findings in "Homeopathic Medications as Clinical Alternatives for Symptomatic Care of Acute Otitis Media and Upper Respiratory Infections in Children" (*Global Advances in Health and Medicine*, vol. 2, no. 1, January 2013). The researchers conclude that homeopathy speeds symptom relief in these conditions as well as and with lower risk than conventional drug approaches and that it reduces antibiotic treatment for otitis media.

Bell and Boyer assert that scientific evidence counters detractors' claims that homeopathic remedies are biologically inactive placebos and observe that homeopathy has gained U.S. consumer acceptance as evidenced by annual expenditures of $2.9 billion on homeopathic remedies. They conclude, "Homeopathy appears equivalent to and safer than conventional standard care in comparative effectiveness trials, but additional well-designed efficacy trials are indicated."

Naturopathic Medicine

As its name suggests, naturopathic medicine, or naturopathy, uses naturally occurring substances to prevent, diagnose, and treat disease. This alternative medicine system, one of the oldest, has its origins in Native American culture and as well as in Greek, Chinese, and Indian philosophies of health and illness.

Naturopathy was introduced in the United States by the German physician Benedict Lust (1872–1945), and its popularity rose, declined, and was rekindled during the same period as homeopathy. Lust opened a school of naturopathic medicine in New York City. He and James Foster, a physician in Idaho who used natural healing techniques, christened their blend of herbal medicine, manipulative therapies, homeopathy, nutrition, and psychology naturopathy.

The overarching principles of modern naturopathic medicine are "first, do no harm" and "nature has the power to heal." Naturopathy seeks to treat the whole person because disease is seen as arising from many causes rather than from a single cause. Naturopathic physicians are taught that "prevention is as important as cure" and to view creating and maintaining health as equally important as curing disease. They are instructed to identify and treat the causes of diseases rather than acting only to relieve symptoms. Naturopathy also requires practitioners to serve as teachers to encourage patients to assume personal responsibility for their health and actively participate in self-care.

Naturopathic physicians' treatment methods include nutritional counseling and the addition of dietary

TABLE 9.4

Percentages of children who used selected dietary supplements, 2007 and 2012

Nonvitamin, nonmineral dietary supplements	Used selected nonvitamin, nonmineral dietary supplements[a]			
	2007		2012	
	Number (in thousands)	Age-adjusted percent[b]	Number (in thousands)	Age-adjusted percent[b]
Fish oil[c]	394	0.7	664	1.1
Melatonin	87[e]	0.1[e]	419	0.7
Probiotics or prebiotics	[d]	0.3[e]	294	0.5
Echinacea	434	0.8	205	0.4
Garlic supplements	78[e]	0.1[e]	80[e]	0.1[e]
Combination herb pill	290[e]	0.5[e]	68[e]	0.1[e]
Ginseng	[e]		63[e]	0.1[e]
Cranberry (pills, capsules)	33[e]	0.1[e]	31[e]	0.1[e]
Glucosamine or chondroitin	[e]		42[e]	0.1[e]

[a]Respondents may have used more than one nonvitamin, nonmineral dietary supplement.
[b]The denominator used in the calculation of percentages was all sample children.
[c]In 2007, fish oil was described as fish oil or omega-3 or DHA fatty acid. In 2012, fish oil was described as fish oil or omega-3 or DHA or EPA fatty acid.
[d]Difference is not statistically significant.
[e]Estimates are considered unreliable. Data have a relative standard error (RSE) greater than 30% and less than or equal to 50% and should be used with caution. Data not shown have an RSE greater than 50%.
Notes: Estimates are based on household interviews of a sample of the civilian noninstitutionalized population. Estimates were age-adjusted using the projected 2000 U.S. population as the standard population and using two age groups: 4–11 and 12–17.

SOURCE: Lindsey I. Black et al., "Adapted from Table. 3. Frequencies and Age-Adjusted Percentages of Children Aged 4–17 Years Who Used Selected Types of Nonvitamin, Nonmineral Dietary Supplements for Health Reasons in the Past 30 Days, by Type of Product Used: United States, 2007 and 2012," in "Use of Complementary Health Approaches among Children Aged 4–17 Years in the United States: National Health Interview Survey, 2007–2012," *National Health Statistics Reports*, no. 78, February 10, 2015, http://www.cdc.gov/nchs/data/nhsr/nhsr078.pdf (accessed January 7, 2016)

TABLE 9.5

Numbers and percentages of children aged 4–17 who used complementary health approaches, by the condition for which it was used, 2007 and 2012

Disease or condition[a]	2007		2012	
	Number (in thousands)	Age-adjusted percentage[b]	Number (in thousands)	Age-adjusted percentage[b]
Back or neck pain	686	8.8	602	8.9
Head or chest cold	409	6.5	294	5.1
Other musculoskeletal conditions	345	5.0	416	6.0
Anxiety or stress	293	4.4	221	3.4
ADHD or ADD[c]	150	2.3	131	2.2
Insomnia or trouble sleeping	134	2.0	110	1.7
Constipation	[d]		70[d]	1.2[d]
Respiratory allergy	68[d]	1.2[d]	69[d]	1.0[d]
Sore throat other than strep or tonsillitis	94[d]	1.4[d]	50[d]	0.9[d]
Sinusitis	117[d]	2.0[d]	45[d]	0.7[d]
Abdominal pain	66[d]	1.0[d]	44[d]	0.6[d]
Depression	178[d]	0.9[d]	41[d]	0.6[d]
Asthma	112	1.8[d]	34[d]	0.5[d]

[a]Respondents may have used more than one modality to treat a disease or condition, but were counted only once under each disease or condition treated. The questions about using a modality to treat a disease or condition were only asked of respondents who had used the modality within the past 12 months. The exception to this is the questions about using nonvitamin, nonmineral dietary supplements to treat a disease or condition, which were only asked of respondents who had used nonvitamin, nonmineral dietary supplements within the past 30 days.
[b]The denominator used in the calculation of percentages was the number of children who used complementary health approaches within the past 12 months, excluding persons with unknown information about whether a complementary health approach was used to treat the specified condition.
[c]ADHD is attention deficit hyperactivity disorder and ADD is attention deficit disorder.
[d]Estimates are considered unreliable. Data have a relative standard error (RSE) greater than 30% and less than or equal to 50% and should be used with caution. Data not shown have an RSE greater than 50%.
Notes: Estimates are based on household interviews of a sample of the civilian noninstitutionalized population. Estimates are age-adjusted using the 2000 U.S. population as the standard population and using two age groups: 4–11 and 12–17.

SOURCE: Lindsey I. Black et al., Adapted from "Table 5. Frequencies and Age-Adjusted Percentages of Children Aged 4–17 Years Who Used Complementary Health Approaches in the Past 12 Months for Specific Conditions, among Those Who Used Complementary Health Approaches, by the Condition for Which It Was Used: United States, 2007 and 2012," in "Use of Complementary Health Approaches among Children Aged 4–17 Years in the United States: National Health Interview Survey, 2007–2012," *National Health Statistics Reports*, no. 78, February 10, 2015, http://www.cdc.gov/nchs/data/nhsr/nhsr078.pdf (accessed January 7, 2016)

supplements, herbs, or vitamins to a patient's diet; hydrotherapy (water-based therapies, usually involving whirlpool or other baths); exercise; manipulation; massage; heat therapy; and electrical stimulation. They are trained to

FIGURE 9.6

Perceived wellness benefits from using selected complementary health approaches, 2012

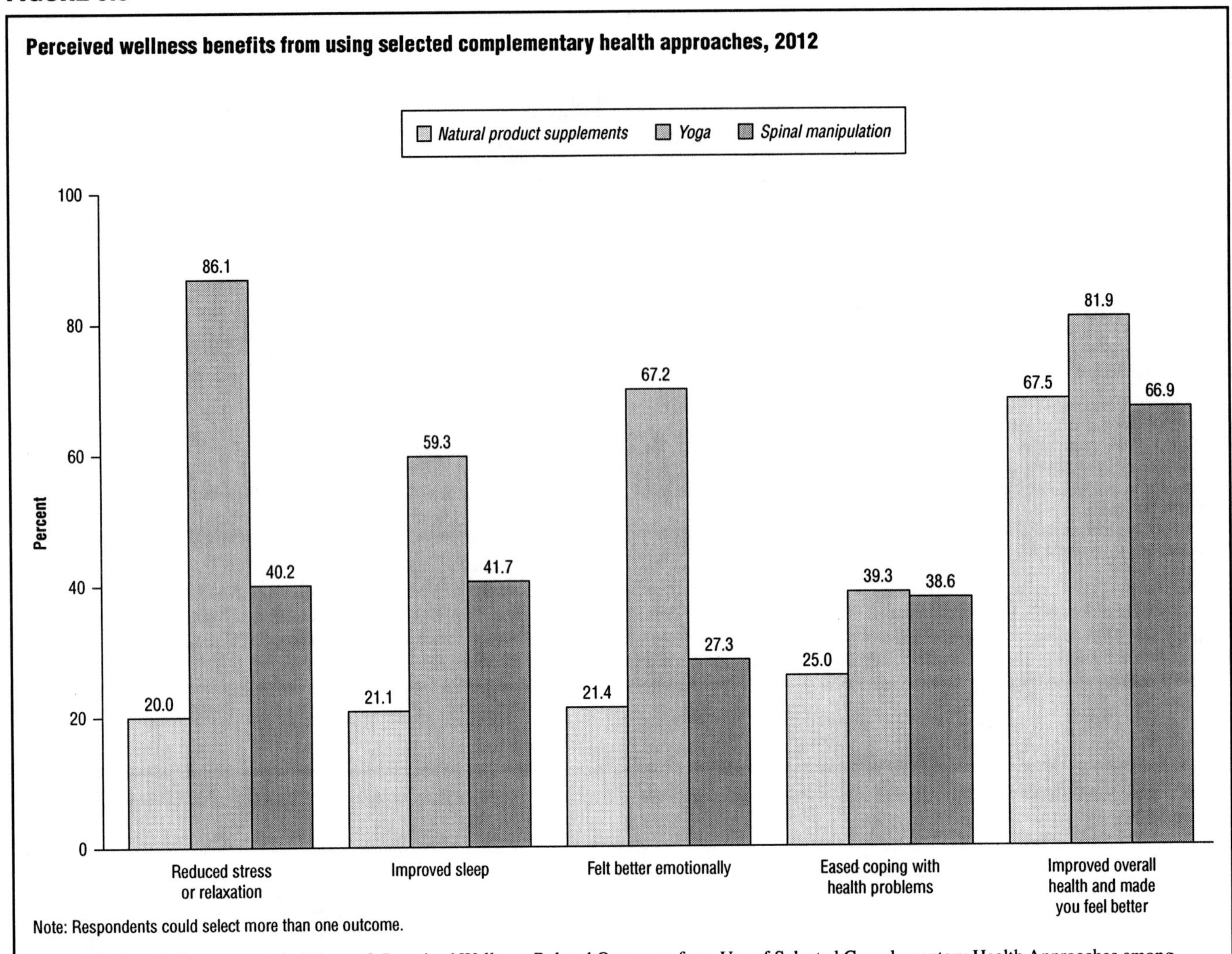

Note: Respondents could select more than one outcome.

SOURCE: Barbara J. Stussman et al., "Figure 6. Perceived Wellness-Related Outcomes from Use of Selected Complementary Health Approaches among Users Aged 18 and over: United States, 2012," in "Wellness-Related Use of Common Complementary Health Approaches among Adults: United States, 2012," *National Health Statistics Reports*, no. 85, November 4, 2015, http://www.cdc.gov/nchs/data/nhsr/nhsr085.pdf (accessed January 7, 2016)

prescribe herbal medicines and homeopathic remedies, perform minor surgical procedures such as setting broken bones, and offer counseling services to help patients resolve emotional problems and modify their lifestyles to improve their health and wellness. Because naturopathy draws on Chinese and Indian medical techniques, naturopathic physicians often use Chinese herbs, acupuncture, and Ayurvedic medicine to treat disease.

There is little published research examining the efficacy of naturopathy as a system of treatment, some studies have been conducted to evaluate the individual therapies that are frequently recommended by naturopathic physicians. For example, diet and lifestyle changes have proved extremely valuable in treating heart disease and diabetes, and the use of acupuncture to treat pain has gained widespread acceptance. In "Acupuncture for PTSD, Naturopathy for Cardiovascular Risk; Yoga for Osteoarthritis; Chasteberry for PMS; and Antioxidants for Cardiovascular Events" (*Explore*, vol. 9, no. 6, November–December 2013), Richard Glickman-Simon and Brian S. Alper find that naturopathic care consisting of dietary and lifestyle counseling, during an initial one-hour session followed by six 30-minute sessions at work-site clinics, plus nutritional medicine and/or dietary supplementation may reduce the rate of metabolic syndrome (factors such as abdominal obesity, high triglycerides and low high-density lipoprotein cholesterol, high blood pressure and high fasting blood sugar), thereby reducing cardiovascular risk.

Acupuncture

Acupuncture is a Chinese practice that dates back more than 5,000 years. Although Sir William Osler (1849–1919) called acupuncture the best available treatment for low back pain during the late 1800s, it was not widely used to treat pain in the United States until the 1970s. Chinese medicine describes acupuncture (the insertion of extremely thin, sterile needles into any of 360 specific points on the body) as a way to balance qi, the body's vital life force that flows over the surface of the body and through internal organs. Traditional Western medicine explains the acknowledged effectiveness of acupuncture as the result of triggering the release of pain-relieving substances called endorphins, which occur naturally in the body, and neurotransmitters and neuropeptides, which influence brain chemistry.

There have been many studies on acupuncture's potential usefulness, but historically the results have been mixed due to complexities with study design and size. For example, a 2009 systematic review, "Evidence from the Cochrane Collaboration for Traditional Chinese Medicine Therapies" (*Journal of Alternative and Complementary Medicine*, vol. 15, no. 9, September 2009) by Eric Manheimer et al., considered 26 studies of acupuncture and concluded that, although they suggested benefit, most of the studies were of poor quality. Nonetheless, there are many reports of acupuncture's effectiveness in reducing postoperative and chemotherapy nausea and vomiting as well as in the treatment of addiction, stroke rehabilitation, headache, menstrual cramps, tennis elbow, fibromyalgia, osteoarthritis, low back pain, carpal tunnel syndrome, and asthma.

Glickman-Simon and Alper reviewed several trials of acupuncture as treatment for post-traumatic stress disorder (PTSD; a serious mental disorder that occurs in response to a life-threatening or catastrophic event). They find that acupuncture may improve symptoms of PTSD, and may be as effective as cognitive behavioral therapy and selective serotonin reuptake inhibitors.

There is growing evidence that acupuncture may be helpful for other conditions such as depression and weight loss. For example, in "Effect of Combined Manual Acupuncture and Massage on Body Weight and Body Mass Index Reduction in Obese and Overweight Women: A Randomized, Short-Term Clinical Trial" (*Journal of Acupuncture and Meridian Studies*, vol. 8, no. 2, April 2015), Junfeng He et al. report that although the precise mechanism of action is not yet known, acupuncture appears to suppress appetite, regulate obesity-related peptides, and improve fat metabolism.

Ayurvedic Medicine

Ayurvedic medicine (also called Ayurveda, which means "science of life") is believed to be the oldest medical tradition and has been practiced in India and Asia for more than 5,000 years. With an emphasis on preventing disease and promoting wellness, its practitioners view emotional health and spiritual balance as vital for physical health and disease prevention. Ayurveda is a medical system that considers diet, hygiene, sleep, lifestyle, and healthy relationships as powerful influences on health.

Practitioners aim to balance the three *doshas*—fundamental human qualities that they believe reside in varying concentrations in different parts of the human body. The *doshas* are thought to be disturbed by improper diet, sleep deprivation, travel, coffee, alcohol, or excessive exposure to the sun and are balanced with diet, exercise, detoxification (ritual cleansing of toxins), yoga, spiritual counseling, herbal medicine, breathing exercises, and chanting.

In "Ayurveda: Between Religion, Spirituality, and Medicine" (*Evidence-Based Complementary and Alternative Medicine*, November 28, 2013), Christian S. Kessler et al. explain that Ayurveda is recognized by the World Health Organization as a medical science and that it is used by more than 1.4 billion people worldwide. In India and other neighboring countries, Ayurvedic medicine is legally viewed as comparable to conventional medicine.

Traditional Chinese Medicine

Traditional Chinese medicine (TCM) combines nutrition, acupuncture, massage, herbal medicine, and qigong (exercises to improve the flow of vital energy through the body) to help people achieve balance and unity of their mind, body, and spirit. TCM has been used for more than 3,000 years by about one-fourth of the world's population, and in the United States it has been embraced by naturopathic physicians, chiropractors, and other CAM practitioners.

One diagnostic technique that is noticeably different from Western medicine is the TCM approach to taking pulses. TCM practitioners take pulses at six different locations, including three points on each wrist, and pulses are described using 28 distinct qualities. Reading the pulses enables practitioners to evaluate qi.

TCM views balancing qi as central to health, wellness, and disease prevention and treatment. TCM also seeks to balance the feminine and masculine qualities of yin and yang using other techniques such as moxibustion (stimulating acupuncture points with heat) and cupping (increasing circulation by putting a heated jar on the skin of a body part).

Herbal medicine is the most commonly prescribed treatment; herbal preparations may be consumed as teas made from boiled fresh herbs or dried powders or in combined formulations known as patent medicines. More than 200 herbal preparations are used in TCM, and several, such as ginseng, ma huang, and ginger, have become popular in the United States. Ginseng is supposed to improve immunity and prevent illness; ma huang is a stimulant used to promote weight loss and relieve lung congestion; and ginger is prescribed to aid digestion, relieve nausea, reduce osteoarthritic knee pain, and improve circulation.

Many modern pharmaceutical drugs are derived from TCM herbal medicines. For example, ma huang components are used to make ephedrine and pseudoephedrine. Ginkgo biloba extract is used to treat cerebral insufficiency (lack of blood flow to the brain).

Research to determine the effectiveness of TCM has focused on the efficacy of specific herbs and combinations of herbs. For example, in "Chinese Herbal Medicine for Postinfectious Cough: A Systematic Review of Randomized Controlled Trials" (*Evidence-Based Complementary and Alternative Medicine*, November 20, 2013), Wei Liu, Hong-Li Jiang, and Bing Mao review 12 studies to assess the safety and efficacy of Chinese herbal medicine formulas containing ephedra, *Platycodon grandiflorus*, *Folium perilla*, almond, and *Schizonepeta tenuifolia* for persistent cough. The researchers conclude that Chinese herbal medicine effectively improves symptoms and is safe and well tolerated.

MIND-BODY INTERVENTIONS

Mind-body interventions (such as meditation, progressive relaxation, hypnosis, deep breathing exercises, and yoga) are practices based on the belief that the mind, body, and spirit are connected to one another and to environmental influences. Mind-body medicine recognizes the relationship between stress, altered mental states, and illness and aims to improve physical, mental, and emotional well-being. According to Kenneth R. Pelletier (1946–), a clinical professor at the University of Arizona School of Medicine and author of *The Best Alternative Medicine: What Works? What Does Not?* (2000), the guiding principles of mind-body medicine are:

- Stress and depression contribute to the development of, and hinder recovery from, chronic diseases because they create measurable hormonal imbalances.
- Psychoneuroimmunology explains how mental functioning provokes physical and biochemical changes that weaken immunity, lowering resistance to disease.
- Overall health improves when people are optimistic and have a positive outlook on life. Health and wellness are harmed by anger, depression, and chronic stress.
- The placebo effect (improved health and favorable physical changes in response to inactive medication such as a sugar pill) confirms the importance of mind-body medicine and is a valuable intervention.
- Social support from family, friends, coworkers, classmates, or organized self-help groups boosts the effectiveness of traditional and CAM therapies.

This section looks at two types of mind-body interventions: meditation and biofeedback. Other commonly used mind-body interventions include music and dance therapies, cognitive behavioral therapy, hypnosis, guided imagery and visualization, and a Chinese exercise discipline called tai chi chuan.

Meditation

Historically, meditation has been used in religious training and practices and to enhance spiritual growth, but it is also a powerful self-care measure that may be used to relieve stress and promote healing. Transcendental meditation, an Indian practice that involves sitting and silently chanting a mantra (a word repeated to quiet the mind), aims to produce a healthy state of relaxation.

During the 1960s the cardiologist Herbert Benson (1935–) studied meditation, and he and his colleagues at Harvard University Medical School showed that people who meditate can reduce heart and respiration rates, lower blood levels of the hormone cortisol, and increase alpha waves (smooth, regular electrical oscillations in the human brain that occur when a person is awake and relaxed). Benson developed a relaxation technique loosely based on transcendental meditation that he dubbed the "relaxation response," and this technique quickly gained recognition in the United States and Europe.

There have been many studies performed to evaluate physical and psychological responses to meditation, and its benefits are universally accepted in the CAM and conventional medical communities. Research has focused on understanding how meditation works and the conditions it may help relieve.

In "Meditation and Health: The Search for Mechanisms of Action" (*Social and Personality Compass*, vol. 7, no. 1, January 2013), Bethany E. Kok, Christian E. Waugh, and Barbara L. Fredrickson review the effects of meditation on health, which include:

- Improving immune function and resistance to diseases such as the common cold
- Reducing inflammation as measured by changes in interleukin-6 (IL-6), a marker of inflammation
- Reducing and boosting responses to vaccines, as measured by a rise in antibody titers
- Reducing blood pressure
- Reducing stress and pain perception

Madhav Goyal et al. report the results of a review of 47 studies performed to determine whether meditation improves stress-related outcomes such as anxiety, depression, and positive mood, as well as attention, substance use, eating habits, sleep, and pain in "Meditation Programs for Psychological Stress and Well-Being: A Systematic Review and Meta-analysis" (*JAMA Internal Medicine*, vol. 144, no. 3, March 2014). The researchers conclude that meditation may provide moderate improvement in negative aspects of psychological stress, including anxiety, depression, and pain but find no evidence that it was more effective than other treatment such as drugs or behavioral therapies.

In "Meditation: What You Need to Know" (November 2014, https://nccih.nih.gov/health/meditation/overview.htm), the NCCIH states that meditation may "reduce blood pressure, symptoms of irritable bowel syndrome, anxiety and depression, insomnia, and the incidence, duration, and severity of acute respiratory illnesses (such as influenza)."

Biofeedback

Biofeedback training aims to help people learn to regulate body functions such as heart rate and blood pressure. Sensitive monitoring devices are attached to the individual to measure and record a variety of physical responses such as skin temperature and electrical resistance, brain-wave activity, and respiration rate. There are also devices to monitor other functions such as bladder activity and acid in the stomach. By observing their own responses and following instructions given by highly trained technicians, most people are able to exert some degree of conscious control over these body functions. Biofeedback is especially effective for helping people learn to manage stress, and it has become a mainstream medical treatment for conditions such as high blood pressure, asthma, migraine headaches, and some types of urinary and fecal incontinence (inability to control bladder or bowel functions).

Frances J. Reyes reports in "Implementing Heart Rate Variability Biofeedback Groups for Veterans with Posttraumatic Stress Disorder" (*Biofeedback*, vol. 42, no. 4, Winter 2014) that biofeedback monitoring of heart rate variability (HRV) can help people suffering from post-traumatic stress disorder (PTSD is described in Chapter 8) because low HRV is associated with the heightened reactions characteristic of PTSD, and high HRV is associated with more flexible and balanced responses. Using biofeedback to help increase HRV can help to reduce the severity of and relieve PTSD symptoms.

BIOLOGICALLY BASED THERAPIES

Biologically based therapies include herbal medicines and remedies, dietary supplements, and the use of hormones to combat disease and improve health. Because herbal medicines are used in a variety of other complementary health practices, such as homeopathy, naturopathy, Ayurveda, and TCM, this section describes a hotly contested biologically based therapy: the use of dietary supplements.

Dietary Supplements

Most complementary, alternative, and integrative health practitioners as well as conventional medical practitioners agree that food sources are the best way to obtain nutrients. They also agree that it is difficult for many people to get sufficient quantities of specific vitamins or minerals from their daily diet. For example, many nutritionists feel that the diets of most Americans do not contain enough chromium and that most women do not consume adequate amounts of iron.

Advocates of dietary supplements believe the recommended dietary allowances (RDAs) are too low for some vitamins and minerals, and they observe that it is difficult to obtain higher than the RDA of certain vitamins without also consuming an excess of fat and calories. An example of this dilemma is vitamin E, an antioxidant that is found in high-fat vegetable and seed oils.

Another current controversy is whether to prescribe diets supplemented with specific vitamins for people without established vitamin deficiencies. Critics of dietary supplements believe that people should attempt to obtain as many needed nutrients from food sources as possible, without relying on dietary supplements. Furthermore, there is no consensus about dosages higher than the RDAs, although it is known that some vitamins and minerals, such as vitamins A and E and chromium, are toxic in high doses. For example, more than 400 International Units (IU) of vitamin E taken daily may increase the risk of stroke, and high doses of vitamin E are generally not advised for people taking medications to reduce blood clotting.

Unlike drugs, dietary supplements are considered to be foods; as a result, they go to market with far less testing and scrutiny and without U.S. Food and Drug Administration (FDA) approval. In *Healing Ways: An Integrative Health Sourcebook* (2016), Matilde Parente explains that "it can be difficult or impossible for consumers to know whether or not their botanical product of choice contains the part of the plant that is believed to contain the active ingredients—and in what proportion, potency, or purity."

The legislation governing supplements, the Dietary Supplement Health and Education Act of 1994, also established the Office of Dietary Supplements at the NIH. The mission of the office (2016, http://ods.od.nih.gov/About/MissionOriginMandate.aspx) is "to strengthen knowledge and understanding of dietary supplements by evaluating scientific information, stimulating and supporting research, disseminating research results, and educating the public to foster an enhanced quality of life and health."

ARE DIETARY SUPPLEMENTS EFFECTIVE? Many dietary supplements have undergone rigorous testing to determine whether they are effective for the conditions they claim to address. However, there are questions about the efficacy of several popular dietary supplements, and research continued in 2016 in an effort to resolve these questions. For example, the effectiveness of glucosamine (thought to play a role in cartilage formation) and chondroitin (which helps give cartilage elasticity, taken as a supplement to relieve arthritis pain) remains the subject of controversy. In "The Effect of Glucosamine and/or Chondroitin Sulfate on the Progression of Knee Osteoarthritis: A Report from the Glucosamine/Chondroitin Arthritis Intervention Trial" (*Arthritis and Rheumatism*, vol. 58, no. 10, October 2008), Allen D. Sawitzke et al. report the results of the NIH-sponsored Glucosamine/Chondroitin Arthritis Intervention Trial, which found that the combination was no more effective than placebo in slowing the joint space loss and the loss of cartilage in the knees of people with osteoarthritis.

Roger Chou et al. report in "Analgesics for Osteoarthritis: An Update of the 2006 Comparative Effectiveness Review" (*Comparative Effectiveness Review*, no. 38, October 2011) that in 2011 the Agency for Healthcare Research and Quality issued an updated report that compared the benefits and harms of oral nonsteroidal anti-inflammatory drugs (NSAIDs), such as acetaminophen, to chondroitin and glucosamine, and topical agents, such as cream containing capsaicin for osteoarthritis. According to Chou et al., the agency reviewed the results of 273 studies and concluded that "there were no clear differences between glucosamine or chondroitin and oral NSAIDs for pain or function" and that several rigorous trials suggest that glucosamine has some "small benefits over placebo for pain."

Marlene Fransen et al. confirm the effectiveness of glucosamine and chondroitin in "Glucosamine and Chondroitin for Knee Osteoarthritis: A Double-Blind Randomised Placebo-Controlled Clinical Trial Evaluating Single and Combination Regimens" (*Annals of the Rheumatics Diseases*, January 6, 2014). The researchers find the dietary supplements reduce joint space narrowing and pain in people with knee osteoarthritis.

ARE DIETARY SUPPLEMENTS NECESSARY? In "Should You Take Dietary Supplements?" (*NIH News in Health*, August 2013), the NIH reports that more than half of all Americans take at least one dietary supplement daily or periodically. Craig Hopp, an expert in botanicals research at the NIH observes, "There's little evidence that any supplement can reverse the course of any chronic disease." The NIH, however, states that there is evidence that some supplements can benefit health. Calcium supports bone health, and vitamin D helps the body absorb calcium. Antioxidant vitamins C and E help to prevent cell damage, and some research suggests that fish oil may promote heart health.

Some populations may need dietary supplements. For example, vegans who do not eat meat, fish, eggs, or dairy may need to supplement their diets with vitamin B_{12}, which helps to maintain the health of nerves and blood cells. Folic acid is important for women of childbearing age to prevent neural tube defects in their children.

SOME DIETARY SUPPLEMENTS MAY BE HARMFUL. Because many dietary supplements are naturally occurring and available without a prescription, some consumers mistakenly believe that using them could not possibly be harmful. This is not the case because dietary supplements have the potential to interact unfavorably with specific foods and medicines or even cause harm when taken on their own. For example, vitamin K reduces the effectiveness of blood thinners, and ginkgo can increase blood thinning. St. John's wort, an herb used to relieve depression, can increase the breakdown of drugs, making them less effective.

Eric A. Klein et al. confirm in "Vitamin E and the Risk of Prostate Cancer" (*Journal of the American Medical Association*, vol. 306, no. 14, October 2011) the risks associated with vitamin E consumption. Based on the results of a population study, the researchers find that rather than reducing the risk of developing prostate cancer, vitamin E consumption increased the risk. A study of 35,000 healthy men aged 50 years and older found that those who took 400 IU of vitamin E per day had a 17% increase in prostate cancer.

In *Healing Ways*, Parente points out that the effects of dietary supplements can vary from one person to another. For example, DHEA, a hormone that is naturally made in the body, may pose some safety risks including acne, hair loss, stomach upset and high blood pressure, even when used short term. Parente notes that DHEA also may interact with other dietary supplements such as ginger, ginkgo, ginseng, licorice, and soy and cautions that it should not be used by children or breast-feeding mothers.

MANIPULATIVE AND BODY-BASED METHODS

Manipulative therapies, such as osteopathic manipulation and chiropractic, and body-based methods (also known as bodywork), such as therapeutic massage, are CAM practices that have been tremendously popular during the last two decades. Clarke et al. report that the use of manipulative therapies was the fourth most commonly used complementary health approach and grew from 7.5% in 2002 to 8.6% in 2007 and was essentially unchanged in 2012 (8.4%).

Enthusiasm for these complementary health approaches is at least in part attributed to their demonstrated ability to relieve aches and pains that are associated with musculoskeletal injuries and stress more effectively than treatment that is prescribed by conventional medical practitioners. As a result, these therapeutic modalities have made inroads into mainstream medicine.

In "Massage for Low Back Pain: An Updated Systematic Review within the Framework of the Cochrane Back Review Group" (*Spine*, vol. 34, no. 16, July 15, 2009), Andrea Furlan et al. review 13 trials of massage for back pain. In two of the studies, massage proved more effective than a sham therapy. In eight studies comparing massage with other back pain treatment, massage was comparable to exercise and was superior to treatments involving joint mobilization, relaxation therapy, physical therapy, acupuncture, and self-care education.

Amy T. Wang et al. recount in "Massage Therapy after Cardiac Surgery" (*Seminars in Thoracic and Cardiovascular Surgery*, vol. 22, no. 3, Autumn 2010) their experiences with massage therapy of cardiac surgery patients at the Mayo Clinic in Rochester, Minnesota. The researchers observe that following surgery, patients experience pain, anxiety, and tension that not only cause the patient to suffer but can also "impair immune function and slow wound healing." Wang et al. opine that massage therapy can effectively relieve these postoperative problems, thus enabling patients to realize the full benefits of surgery.

In "Durability of Effect of Massage Therapy on Blood Pressure" (*International Journal of Preventive Medicine*, vol. 4, no. 5, May 2013), Mahshid Givi of Isfahan (Iran) University of Medical Sciences reports that a study to determine whether massage has an enduring blood pressure–reducing effect finds that 72 hours after receiving massage therapy, subjects' blood pressure was lower when compared to subjects in a control group that did not receive massage therapy.

Parente observes that massage has shown to be effective for chronic neck and low back pain, muscle soreness related to sports, osteoarthritis of the knee, chronic tension headaches, and fibromyalgia. There also is evidence that massage can help to relieve pain and improve mood, anxiety, and fatigue among people with cancer and acquired immunodeficiency syndrome.

Chiropractic

In "What Is Chiropractic?" (2016, http://www.acatoday.org/Patients/Why-Choose-Chiropractic/What-is-Chiropractic), the American Chiropractic Association (ACA) defines chiropractic as "a health care profession that focuses on disorders of the musculoskeletal system and the nervous system, and the effects of these disorders on general health. Chiropractic care is used most often to treat neuromusculoskeletal complaints, including but not limited to back pain, neck pain, pain in the joints of the arms or legs, and headaches." Doctors of chiropractic (also known as chiropractors) do not use or prescribe drugs or perform surgery. Instead, they rely on adjustment and manipulation of the musculoskeletal system, particularly the spinal column.

Many chiropractors use nutritional therapy and prescribe dietary supplements, and some use a technique known as applied kinesiology to diagnose and treat disease. Applied kinesiology is based on the belief that every organ problem is associated with the weakness of a specific muscle.

Besides manipulation, chiropractors also use a variety of other therapies to support healing and relax muscles before they make manual adjustments. These treatments include the following:

- Heat and cold therapy to relieve pain, speed healing, and reduce swelling
- Hydrotherapy to relax muscles and stimulate blood circulation
- Immobilization such as casts, wraps, traction, and splints to protect injured areas
- Electrotherapy to deliver deep-tissue massage and boost circulation
- Ultrasound to relieve muscle spasms and reduce swelling

In "Frequently Asked Questions about Chiropractic" (2016, http://www.acatoday.org/Patients/Why-Choose-Chiropractic/Chiropractic-Frequently-Asked-Questions), the ACA explains that chiropractors use their hands or an instrument to manipulate the spine and joints to improve joint function, reduce inflammation and relieve pain. These manipulations are termed "adjustments," and while they rarely cause discomfort, there have been some reports of injuries associated with high-velocity upper neck manipulation, including a rare form of stroke. The ACA reports that the incidence of these injuries is just one to three in 100,000 patients treated.

Visits to chiropractors are most often for the treatment of low back pain, neck pain, and headaches. Critics of chiropractic are concerned about injuries that may result from powerful "high velocity" manual adjustments, and some physicians question chiropractors' abilities to establish medical diagnoses. Others worry that people seeking chiropractic care instead of conventional medical care may be forgoing lifesaving diagnoses and treatment.

EFFECTIVENESS OF CHIROPRACTIC. In "Chiropractic: In Depth" (January 4, 2016, https://nccih.nih.gov/health/chiropractic/introduction.htm), the NCCIH reports that a review of the relevant literature reveals that spinal manipulation, which may also be performed by physical therapists, osteopaths, and some conventional medical doctors, may provide relief from low back pain. Spinal manipulation appears to be safe and as effective as conventional treatments. A 2010 review of the evidence for manual therapy treatment concluded that "spinal manipulation/mobilization may be helpful for several conditions in addition to back pain, including migraine and cervicogenic (neck-related) headaches, neck pain, upper- and lower-extremity joint conditions, and whiplash-associated disorders."

ENERGY THERAPIES

Energy therapies that purport to influence energy fields in and around the body are among the CAM practices that arouse the most suspicion from the conventional medical community. Some skeptics attribute the health benefits reported by patients who have received energy therapies to the placebo effect (a perceived beneficial result that occurs from the therapy because of the patient's expectation that the therapy will help). Despite a widespread lack of understanding and acceptance from traditional health care practitioners, some hospitals and pioneering practitioners are incorporating energy therapies into their treatment programs.

Reiki

An ancient Japanese technique, Reiki is bioenergetic healing that is intended to restore physical, emotional, mental, and spiritual balance. The therapy takes its name from two Japanese words. *Rei* means higher power, wisdom, and all that exists, and *ki* is the life force, or the energy that runs through all living things.

Based on the teachings of Mikao Usui (1865–1926), Reiki is a universal healing vibration that flows through the practitioner to the client. Practitioners act as a channel for Reiki energy, and as it passes through practitioners, it acts to strengthen and harmonize them simultaneously as it heals their clients.

There are more than a dozen styles of Reiki, each with its own subtle variations. Students studying with Usui Reiki masters receive a series of "attunements" and may progress through three levels or degrees of training. Level I connects the practitioner to the Reiki channel and initiates the flow of healing energy. Level II teaches distance or remote healing. Level III initiates the practitioner to the role of master and teacher.

Some practitioners use a variety of other therapies, including meditation, prayer, chanting, breathing, and movement education. Most often performed as hands-on bodywork, Reiki is thought to convey energy to calm nerves, relax muscles, and ease pain. During the second level of training, practitioners learn to deliver Reiki energy remotely, over long distances.

There are many case studies describing the effectiveness of Reiki to reduce anxiety and relieve discomfort, but as of 2016 there were few published reports of rigorous research designed to determine its efficacy. In "A Systematic Review of the Therapeutic Effects of Reiki" (*Journal of Complementary Medicine*, vol. 15, no. 11, November 2009), Sondra vanderVaart et al. find all of the studies on Reiki lacking in rigor. Although nine of 12 trials reported a significant therapeutic effect, the reviewers conclude that "the serious methodological and reporting limitations of limited existing Reiki studies preclude a definitive conclusion on its effectiveness. High-quality randomized controlled trials are needed to address the effectiveness of Reiki over placebo."

In "Effects of Reiki on Autonomic Activity Early after Acute Coronary Syndrome" (*Journal of the American College of Cardiology*, vol. 56, no. 12, September 2010), Rachel S. C. Friedman et al. find that Reiki improved heart rate variability and the emotional state in patients who were hospitalized for acute coronary syndrome. The researchers hypothesize that the beneficial effects of Reiki may be due to "the presence of another person, the presence of a person with healing intention, the light touch technique, or a combination of factors" and call for additional research to gain an understanding of its mechanism of action.

The dearth of rigorous research was also noted by Janine Joyce and G. Peter Herbison in "Reiki for Depression and Anxiety" (*Cochrane Library*, April 3, 2015). Joyce and Herbison sought to determine whether Reiki is effective treatment for anxiety and depression and finding just three small studies to review, concluded that there is insufficient evidence to say whether Reiki is helpful for people suffering from anxiety or depression.

COMPLEMENTING TRADITIONAL MEDICINE. Clinics and hospitals across the United States offer Reiki to surgical patients, women in labor, and those suffering from pain, anxiety, sleep disorders, headaches, asthma, and eating disorders. According to the Center for Reiki Research (2014, http://www.centerforreikiresearch.org/), 76 hospitals and clinics in the United States offered patients Reiki treatments in 2014.

In conventional medical settings, Reiki is usually presented as a method to reduce stress and promote relaxation, thereby enhancing the body's natural ability to heal itself. To gain credibility with traditional physicians and other mainstream professionals, Reiki therapists often downplay the spiritual benefits of the practice and avoid mentioning other CAM practices.

Although its effectiveness has not been documented in scientific studies, Reiki has gained acceptance because it is viewed as a complement, rather than as an alternative, to traditional Western medicine. Considered to be safe by many health care practitioners, it is well received by patients who seem to respond favorably to the time and attention, as well as to the healing energy, offered by Reiki therapists.

IMPORTANT NAMES AND ADDRESSES

Alzheimer's Association
225 N. Michigan Ave., 17th Floor
Chicago, IL 60601-7633
(312) 335-8700
1-800-272-3900
FAX: 1-866-699-1246
E-mail: info@alz.org
URL: http://www.alz.org/

American Academy of Child and Adolescent Psychiatry
3615 Wisconsin Ave. NW
Washington, DC 20016
(202) 966-7300
FAX: (202) 966-2891
URL: http://www.aacap.org/

American Academy of Pediatrics
141 Northwest Point Blvd.
Elk Grove Village, IL 60007-1098
(847) 434-4000
1-800-433-9016
FAX: (847) 434-8000
URL: http://www.aap.org/

American Association of Suicidology
5221 Wisconsin Ave. NW
Washington, DC 20015
(202) 237-2280
FAX: (202) 237-2282
URL: http://www.suicidology.org/

American Cancer Society
250 Williams St. NW
Atlanta, GA 30303
1-800-227-2345
URL: http://www.cancer.org/

American Chiropractic Association
1701 Clarendon Blvd., Ste. 200
Arlington, VA 22209
(703) 276-8800
FAX: (703) 243-2593
E-mail: memberinfo@acatoday.org
URL: http://www.acatoday.org/

American Congress of Obstetricians and Gynecologists
409 12th St. SW
Washington, DC 20024-2188
(202) 638-5577
1-800-673-8444
URL: http://www.acog.org/

American Diabetes Association
1701 N. Beauregard St.
Alexandria, VA 22311
1-800-342-2383
URL: http://www.diabetes.org/

American Heart Association
7272 Greenville Ave.
Dallas, TX 75231
1-800-242-8721
URL: http://www.americanheart.org/

American Lung Association
55 W. Wacker Dr., Ste. 1150
Chicago, IL 60601
1-800-548-8252
URL: http://www.lungusa.org/

American Parkinson Disease Association
135 Parkinson Ave.
Staten Island, NY 10305
(718) 981-8001
1-800-223-2732
FAX: (718) 981-4399
E-mail: apda@apdaparkinson.org
URL: http://www.apdaparkinson.org/

American Psychiatric Association
1000 Wilson Blvd., Ste. 1825
Arlington, VA 22209-3901
(703) 907-7300
1-888-357-7924
E-mail: apa@psych.org
URL: http://www.psych.org/

American Psychological Association
750 First St. NE
Washington, DC 20002-4242
(202) 336-5500
1-800-374-2721
URL: http://www.apa.org/

Arthritis Foundation
1355 Peachtree St. NE, Sixth Floor
Atlanta, GA 30309
(404) 872-7100
1-800-283-7800
URL: http://www.arthritis.org/

Autism Society
4340 East-West Hwy., Ste. 350
Bethesda, MD 20814
(301) 657-0881
1-800-328-8476
URL: http://www.autism-society.org/

Centers for Disease Control and Prevention
1600 Clifton Rd.
Atlanta, GA 30329-4027
1-800-232-4636
URL: http://www.cdc.gov/

Cystic Fibrosis Foundation
6931 Arlington Rd., Second Floor
Bethesda, MD 20814
(301) 951-4422
1-800-344-4823
E-mail: info@cff.org
URL: http://www.cff.org/

Epilepsy Foundation
8301 Professional Pl. East, Ste. 200
Landover, MD 20785-2353
1-800-332-1000
E-mail: ContactUs@efa.org
URL: http://www.epilepsyfoundation.org/

Huntington's Disease Society of America
505 Eighth Ave., Ste. 902
New York, NY 10018
(212) 242-1968
1-800-345-4372
E-mail: hdsainfo@hdsa.org
URL: http://www.hdsa.org/

March of Dimes Foundation
1275 Mamaroneck Ave.
White Plains, NY 10605
(914) 997-4488
URL: http://www.modimes.org/

Mental Health America
2000 N. Beauregard St., Sixth Floor
Alexandria, VA 22311
(703) 684-7722
1-800-969-6642
FAX: (703) 684-5968
URL: http://www.nmha.org/

Muscular Dystrophy Association
222 S. Riverside Plaza, Ste. 1500
Chicago, IL 60606
1-800-572-1717
E-mail: mda@mdausa.org
URL: http://www.mdausa.org/

National Center for Complementary and Integrative Health
National Institutes of Health
9000 Rockville Pike
Bethesda, MD 20892
(301) 519-3153
1-888-644-6226
FAX: 1-866-464-3616
E-mail: info@nccih.nih.gov
URL: https://nccih.nih.gov/

National Center for Health Statistics
3311 Toledo Rd.
Hyattsville, MD 20782-2003
(301) 458-4000
1-866-441-6247
URL: http://www.cdc.gov/nchs/

National Fibromyalgia Association
1000 Bristol St. N., Ste. 17-247
Newport Beach, CA 92660
(714) 921-0150
FAX: (714) 921-6920
E-mail: nfa@fmaware.org
URL: http://www.fmaware.org/

National Multiple Sclerosis Society
733 Third Ave., Third Floor
New York, NY 10017
(212) 463-7787
FAX: (212) 986-7981
E-mail: info@msnyc.org
URL: http://www.nationalmssociety.org/

National Osteoporosis Foundation
251 18th St. S, Ste. 630
Arlington, VA 22202
(703) 647-3000
1-800-231-4222
FAX: (703) 414-3742
E-mail: info@nof.org
URL: http://www.nof.org/

National Tay-Sachs and Allied Diseases Association
2001 Beacon St., Ste. 204
Boston, MA 02135
1-800-906-8723
FAX: (617) 277-0134
E-mail: info@ntsad.org
URL: http://www.ntsad.org/

Sickle Cell Disease Association of America
3700 Koppers St., Ste. 570
Baltimore, MD 21227
(410) 528-1555
1-800-421-8453
FAX: (410) 528-1495
E-mail: scdaa@sicklecelldisease.org
URL: http://www.sicklecelldisease.org/

United Network for Organ Sharing
700 N. Fourth St.
Richmond, VA 23219
(804) 782-4800
URL: http://www.unos.org/

RESOURCES

The Centers for Disease Control and Prevention (CDC) tracks nationwide health trends and reports its findings in several periodicals, especially in the *Advance Data* series, the annual *HIV Surveillance Report*, and the *Morbidity and Mortality Weekly Report*. The CDC's National Center for Injury Prevention and Control provides data about deaths and disability that are caused by accidents and violence. The National Center for Health Statistics (NCHS) provides a complete statistical overview of the nation's health in its annual *Health, United States*. The NCHS periodicals *National Vital Statistics Reports* and *Vital and Health Statistics* detail U.S. birth and death data and trends.

The National Health Interview Surveys offer information about the lifestyles, health behaviors, and health risks of Americans. The CDC publishes results from the Behavioral Risk Factor Surveillance System, which conducts surveys in each state asking adults questions about a wide range of behaviors affecting their health. The National Health and Nutrition Examination Survey, which is conducted by the National Institute of Mental Health (NIMH) and the NCHS, also helps characterize the health and well-being of Americans. Working with other agencies and professional organizations, the CDC helped create Healthy People 2020 (http://www.healthypeople.gov/2020/default.aspx), which serves as a blueprint for improving the health of Americans during the second decade of the 21st century.

Mental health and illness in the United States were detailed in the landmark report *Mental Health: A Report of the Surgeon General* (1999) and in follow-up reports, including *Achieving the Promise: Transforming Mental Health Care in America* (July 2003). In "Mental Health Surveillance among Children—United States, 2005–2011" (Ruth Perou et al., May 2013), the CDC provides estimates of how many children experience a mental disorder each year. The NIMH provides detailed information about mental health research and treatment of mental illness. The Harvard School of Medicine's National Comorbidity Surveys provide estimates of the incidence and prevalence of mental disorders.

The National Institutes of Health provides definitions, epidemiological data, and research findings about a comprehensive range of medical and public health subjects. The National Center for Complementary and Integrative Health defines and describes a range of alternative, complementary, and integrative medical practices.

Medical, public health, and nursing journals offer a wealth of disease-specific information and research findings. The studies cited in this edition are drawn from a wide range of professional publications, including the *American Journal of Preventive Medicine*, *BMC Medical Genetics*, *Circulation*, *Diagnosis*, *Journal of the American Medical Association*, *Lancet*, *New England Journal of Medicine*, and *Stroke*.

The American Cancer Society's *Cancer Facts and Figures, 2015* (2015) provided valuable data, as did the Alzheimer's Association, the American Diabetes Association, the American Heart Association, the American Lung Association, and the National Osteoporosis Foundation, all of which are excellent resources for information about the epidemiology of diseases, treatments, and clinical trials. Many other professional associations, voluntary medical organizations, and foundations dedicated to research, education, and advocacy related to other specific medical conditions and disabling diseases proved to be useful sources for up-to-date information in this edition.

INDEX

Page references in italics refer to photographs. References with the letter t *following them indicate the presence of a table. The letter* f *indicates a figure. If more than one table or figure appears on a particular page, the exact item number for the table or figure being referenced is provided.*

A

H

I

J

T

U

V

W

X

Y

Z

CPSIA information can be obtained
at www.ICGtesting.com
Printed in the USA
FFOW05n1647230916

9 781573 027007